Best Wishes

Rith Kay

May 2015

_____

Statistical Thinking for Non-Statisticians in Drug Regulation

Statistical Thinking for Non-Statisticians in Drug Regulation

SECOND EDITION

Richard Kay, PhD

Statistical Consultant, RK Statistics Ltd
Honorary Visiting Professor, School of Pharmacy, Cardiff University, UK

WILEY Blackwell

Registered Office
John Wiley & Sons, Ltd, The Atrium, Southern Gate, Chichester, West Sussex, PO19 8SQ, UK

Editorial Offices
9600 Garsington Road, Oxford, OX4 2DQ, UK
The Atrium, Southern Gate, Chichester, West Sussex, PO19 8SQ, UK
111 River Street, Hoboken, NJ 07030-5774, USA

For details of our global editorial offices, for customer services and for information about how to apply for permission to reuse the copyright material in this book please see our website at www.wiley.com/wiley-blackwell

Library of Congress Cataloging-in-Publication Data

Kay, R. (Richard), 1949– author.
Statistical thinking for non-statisticians in drug regulation / Richard Kay. – Second edition.
     p. ; cm.
  Includes bibliographical references and index.
  ISBN 978-1-118-47094-7 (cloth)
  I. Title.
  [DNLM: 1. Clinical Trials as Topic–methods. 2. Drug Approval. 3. Drug Industry. 4. Statistics as Topic. QV 771.4]
  R853.C55
  615.5′80724–dc23

                                        2014020541

A catalogue record for this book is available from the British Library.

Wiley also publishes its books in a variety of electronic formats. Some content that appears in print may not be available in electronic books.

Set in 9.5/13pt Meridien by SPi Publisher Services, Pondicherry, India
Printed and bound in Malaysia by Vivar Printing Sdn Bhd

1   2015

Contents

Preface to the second edition

The first edition of this book was submitted for publication over seven years ago. As predicted, there have been numerous developments, both in the world of pharmaceutical statistics and within the regulatory environment, which need to be presented and explained. In the intervening years, the FDA has published guidelines on Adaptive Designs and on Non-Inferiority Trials. The CHMP have updated their guidance on Missing Data, produced a guideline on the Clinical Evaluation of Diagnostic Agents and have undertaken a major exercise on the evaluation of the benefit–risk balance. In recent years, we have seen greater application of the use of observational studies within regulatory applications, particularly when dealing with orphan drugs, and also a willingness to consider the use of Bayesian methods. Although there is still considerable concern expressed about various elements of adaptive designs, we are beginning to understand where the boundaries are and what can be done without compromising the scientific integrity of the study. All of these aspects and more have led to me write this new edition.

There are five new chapters and several other chapters have been restructured. Chapter 15 looks at Bayesian Statistics, contrasting the Bayesian methodology with classical methods, presenting the advantages and concerns and discussing the use of these methods in pharmaceutical applications. Adaptive designs are discussed in Chapter 16 with sections on minimising bias and covering various types of adaptations. Some practicalities and recommendations regarding the circumstances under which such designs can be considered are also presented. We all recognise that the randomised controlled trial is the gold standard in terms of evaluating the efficacy and also the safety of a new medicine, but in some settings running such trials is not possible. Observational studies offer an alternative, but their ability to provide valid conclusions is heavily dependent on good design and conduct and careful analysis. Such designs are discussed in Chapter 17. In recent years, we have become much more formal in the statistical evaluation of safety data. Chapter 19 covers various aspects of safety data analysis, including the use of graphical methods, and goes on to detail potential approaches to the quantification of the benefit–risk balance both inside and outside of the regulatory submission. This chapter concludes with a discussion on methods for post-approval safety monitoring. Statistical methods for the evaluation of diagnostic methods and method comparison are discussed in Chapter 20.

Chapter 5 in the first edition of the book was entitled 'Multi-Centre Trials'. This chapter has been restructured and is now entitled 'Adjusting the Analysis'. This restructuring is based on my recent teaching experiences in explaining the rationale around adjusting the statistical analysis for baseline factors in a general way. Several other chapters contain sections similarly restructured as a result of my teaching experience. I hope that these changes make things clearer than maybe they were before. Chapter 18 entitled 'Meta-Analysis' is a major restructuring of the initial chapter on this topic and reflects the current uses of this methodology within the pharmaceutical industry.

I have received many encouraging comments on the first edition of this book and I would like to thank everyone who has given feedback. I hope that this revision is also well-received. My aim is to make statistical thinking and methods used within the pharmaceutical industry accessible to non-statisticians so that they are better able to communicate using statistical language, better able to understand statistical methods used in reports and publications and what can and cannot be concluded from the resulting analyses, and are better equipped to contribute to statistical arguments used within regulatory submissions and beyond. I continue to teach courses on statistics for non-statisticians, and many of the changes and additions that I make to my teaching materials and have made to this book have come out of my experiences on those courses. I would like to thank my students for their challenging questions; they make me think about better ways to explain things. Finally I would like to thank all of those who got in touch to point out mistakes in the first edition. I have corrected those but some may remain and indeed the new material may contain some more. I encourage the reader to provide feedback for this second edition and please do not hesitate to point out any mistakes, for which I am solely responsible.

Richard Kay
Great Longstone
March 2014

Preface to the first edition

This book is primarily concerned with clinical trials planned and conducted within the pharmaceutical industry. Much of the methodology presented is in fact applicable on a broader basis and can be used in observational studies and in clinical trials outside of the pharmaceutical sector; nonetheless, the primary context is clinical trials and pharmaceuticals. The development is aimed at non-statisticians and will be suitable for physicians, investigators, clinical research scientists, medical writers, regulatory personnel, statistical programmers, senior data managers and those working in quality assurance. Statisticians moving from other areas of application outside of pharmaceuticals may also find the book useful in that it places the methods that they are familiar with, in context in their new environment. There is substantial coverage of regulatory aspects of drug registration that impact on statistical issues. Those of us working within the pharmaceutical industry recognise the importance of being familiar with the rules and regulations that govern our activities, and statistics is a key aspect of this.

The aim of the book is not to turn non-statisticians into statisticians. I do not want you to go away from this book and 'do' statistics. It is the job of the statistician to provide statistical input to the development plan, to individual protocols, to write the statistical analysis plan, to analyse the data and to work with medical writing in producing the clinical report, and also to support the company in its interactions with regulators on statistical issues.

The aims of the book are really threefold. Firstly, to aid communication between statisticians and non-statisticians; secondly, to help in the critical review of reports and publications; and finally, to enable the more effective use of statistical arguments within the regulatory process. We will take each of these points in turn.

In many situations, the interaction between a statistician and a non-statistician is not a particularly successful one. The statistician uses terms such as power, odds ratio, p-value, full analysis set, hazard ratio, non-inferiority, type II error, geometric mean, last observation carried forward and so on, of which the non-statistician has a vague understanding, but maybe not a good enough understanding to be able to get an awful lot out of such interactions. Of course, it is always the job of a statistician to educate and every opportunity should be taken for imparting knowledge about statistics, but in a specific context, there may not be time for that. Hopefully this book will explain, in ways that are understandable, just what these terms mean and provide some insight into their interpretation and the context in which they are used. There is also a lot of confusion between what on the surface appear to be the same or similar things: significance level and *p*-value, equivalence and non-inferiority, odds ratio and relative risk, relative risk and hazard ratio (by the way this is a minefield!) and meta-analysis and pooling to name just a few. This book will clarify these important distinctions.

It is unfortunately the case that many publications, including some in leading journals, contain mistakes with regard to statistics. Things have improved over the years with the standardisation of the ways in which publications are put together and reviewed. For example, the CONSORT statement (see Section 16.5 [this is Section 21.5 in the 2nd edition]) has led to a distinct improvement in the quality of reporting. Nonetheless mistakes do slip through, in terms of poor design, incorrect analysis, incomplete reporting and inappropriate interpretation – hopefully not all at once! It is important therefore when reading an article that the non-statistical reader is able to make a judgement regarding the quality of the statistics and to notice any obvious flaws that may undermine the conclusions that have been drawn. Ideally, the non-statistician should involve their statistical colleagues in evaluating their concerns, but keeping a keen eye on statistical arguments within the publication may help to alert the non-statistician to a potential problem. The same applies to presentations at conferences, posters, advertising materials and so on.

Finally, the basis of many concerns raised by regulators, when they are reviewing a proposed development plan or assessing an application for regulatory approval, is statistical. It is important that non-statisticians are able to work with their statistical colleagues in correcting mistakes, changing aspects of the design, responding to questions about the data to hopefully overcome those concerns.

In writing this book, I have made the assumption that the reader is familiar with the general aspects of the drug development process. I have assumed knowledge of the phase I to phase IV framework, of placebos, control groups, and double-dummy together with other fundamental elements of the nuts and bolts of clinical trials. I have assumed however no knowledge of statistics! This may or may not be the correct assumption in individual cases, but it is the common denominator that we must start from, and also it is actually not a bad thing to refresh on the basics. The book starts with some basic issues in trial design in Chapter 1, and I guess most people picking up this book will be familiar with many of the topics covered there. But don't be tempted to skip this chapter; there are still certain issues, raised in this first chapter, that will be new and important for understanding arguments put forward in subsequent chapters. Chapter 2 looks at sampling and inferential statistics. In this chapter, we look at the interplay between the population and the sample, basic thoughts on measuring average and variability and then explore the process of sampling leading to the concept of the standard error as a way of capturing precision/reliability of the sampling process. The construction and interpretation of confidence intervals are covered in Chapter 3 together with testing hypotheses and the (dreaded!) *p*-value. Common statistical tests for various data types are developed in Chapter 4 which also covers different ways of measuring treatment effect for binary data, such as the odds ratio and relative risk.

Many clinical trials that we conduct are multi-centre and Chapter 5 looks at how we extend our simple statistical comparisons to this more complex structure. These ideas lead naturally to the topics in Chapter 6 which include the concepts of adjusted analyses, and more generally, analysis of covariance which allows adjustment for many baseline factors, not just centre. Chapters 2–6 follow a logical development sequence in which the basic building blocks are initially put in place and then used to deal with more and more complex data structures. Chapter 7 moves a little away from this development path and covers the important topic of 'intention-to-treat' and aspects of conforming with that principle through the definition of different analysis sets and dealing with missing data. In Chapter 8, we cover the very important design topics of power and the sample size calculation which then leads naturally to a discussion about the distinction between statistical significance and clinical importance in Chapter 9.

The regulatory authorities, in my experience, tend to dig their heels in on certain issues and one such issue is multiplicity. This topic, which has many facets, is discussed in detail in Chapter 10. Non-parametric and related methods are covered in Chapter 11. In Chapter 12, we develop the concepts behind the establishment of equivalence and non-inferiority. This is an area where many mistakes are made in applications, and in many cases, these slip through into published articles. It is a source of great concern to many statisticians that there is widespread misunderstanding of how to deal with equivalence and non-inferiority. I hope that this chapter helps to develop a better understanding of the methods and the issues. If you have survived so far, then Chapter 13 covers the analysis of survival data. When an endpoint is time to some event, for example, death, the data are inevitably subject to what we call censoring and it is this aspect of so-called survival data that has led to the development of a completely separate set of statistical methods. Chapter 14 builds on the earlier discussion on multiplicity to cover one particular manifestation of that, the interim analysis. This chapter also looks at the management of these interim looks at the data through data monitoring committees. Meta-analysis and its role in clinical development is covered in Chapter 15, and the book finishes with a general Chapter 16 on the role of statistics and statisticians in terms of the various aspects of design and analysis and statistical thinking more generally.

It should be clear from the last few paragraphs that the book is organised in a logical way; it is a book for learning rather than a reference book for dipping into. The development in later chapters will build on the development in earlier chapters. I strongly recommend, therefore, that you start on page 1 and work through. I have tried to keep the discussion away from formal mathematics. There are formulas in the book but I have only included these where I think this will enhance understanding; there are no formulas for formulas sake! There are some sections that are more challenging than others and I have marked with an asterisk those sections that can be safely sidestepped on a first (or even a second) run through the book.

The world of statistics is ever changing. New methods are being developed by theoreticians within university departments, and ultimately some of these will find their way into mainstream methods for design and statistical analysis within our industry. The regulatory environment is ever changing as regulators respond to increasing demands for new and more effective medicines. This book in one sense represents a snapshot in time in terms of what statistical methods are employed within the pharmaceutical industry and also in relation to current regulatory requirements. Two statistical topics that are not included in this book are Bayesian Methods and Adaptive (Flexible) Designs (although some brief mention is made of this latter topic in Section 14.5.2). Both areas are receiving considerable attention at the moment, and I am sure that within a fairly short period of time, there will be much to say about them in terms of the methodological thinking, examples of their application and possibly with regard to their regulatory acceptance but for the moment they are excluded from our discussions.

The book has largely come out of courses that I have been running under the general heading of 'Statistical Thinking for Non-Statisticians' for a number of years. There have been several people who have contributed from time to time and I would like to thank them for their input and support: Werner Wierich, Mike Bradburn and in particular Ann Gibb who gave these courses with me over a period of several years and enhanced my understanding through lively discussion and asking many challenging questions. I would also like to thank Simon Gillis who contributed to Chapter 16 [this is Chapter 21 in the 2nd edition] with his much deeper knowledge of the processes that go on within a pharmaceutical company in relation to the analysis and reporting of a clinical trial.

Richard Kay
Great Longstone
January 2007

Abbreviations

ADR	adverse drug reaction
AEs	adverse events
AIDAC	Anti-Infective Drugs Advisory Committee
ALKPH	alkaline phosphatase
ALT	alanine transaminase
ANCOVA	analysis of covariance
ANOVA	analysis of variance
ARR	absolute relative risk
AST	asparate transaminase
AUC	area under the curve
BILTOT	total bilirubin
BMD	bone mineral density
CDER	Center for Drug Evaluation and Research
CFC	Chlorofluorocarbon
CHMP	Committee for Medical Products for Human Use
CI	confidence interval
CMAX	maximum concentration
CMH	Cochran-Mantel-Haenszel
CNS	central nervous system
CPMP	Committee for Proprietary Medicinal Products
CR	complete response
crd	clinically relevant difference
CRF	Case Report Form
CSR	Clinical Study Report
CTC	common terminology criteria
dBP	diastolic blood pressure
DILI	drug-induced liver injury
df	degrees of freedom
DMCs	Data Monitoring Committees
DSMB	Data and Safety Monitoring Board
DSMC	Data and Safety Monitoring Committee
ECG	Electrocardiogram
EMEA	European Medicines Evaluation Agency
FDA	Food and Drug Administration
FEV$_1$	forced expiratory volume in one second
FNR	false negative rate
FPR	false positive rate
GP	General Practitioner

HAMA	Hamilton Anxiety Scale
HAMD	Hamilton Depression Scale
HER2	human epidermal growth factor receptor-2
HIV	human immunodeficiency virus
HR	Hazard Ratio
ICH	International Committee on Harmonisation
ITT	intention-to-treat
IVRS	Interactive Voice Response System
IWRS	Interactive Web Response System
KM	Kaplan-Meier
LLN	lower limit of normal
LR	likelihood ratio
LOCF	last observation carried forward
MCDA	multi-criteria decision analysis
MedDRA	*Med*ical *D*ictionary for *R*egulatory *A*ctivities
MH	Mantel-Haenszel
MI	myocardial infarction
NNH	number needed to harm
NNT	number needed to treat
NPV	negative predictive value
NS	not statistically significant
OR	odds ratio
ORR	objective response rate
OS	overall survival
PA	predictive accuracy
PD	progressive disease
PEF	peak expiratory flow
PFS	progression-free survival
PHN	post-hepatic neuralgia
PPV	positive predictive value
PR	partial response
PRR	proportional reporting ratio
RECIST	Response Evaluation Criteria in Solid Tumours
RR	relative risk
RRR	relative risk reduction
PT	preferred term
SAE	serious adverse event
SAP	Statistical Analysis Plan
sBP	systolic blood pressure
SD	stable disease
sd	standard deviation
se	standard error
SOC	system organ class
ULN	upper limit of normal
VAS	visual analogue scale
WHO	World Health Organization

CHAPTER 1

Basic ideas in clinical trial design

1.1 Historical perspective

As many of us who are involved in clinical trials will know, the randomised controlled trial is a relatively new invention. As pointed out by Pocock (1983) and others, very few clinical trials of the kind we now regularly see were conducted prior to 1950. It took a number of high-profile successes plus the failure of alternative methodologies to convince researchers of their value.

Example 1.1 The Salk Polio Vaccine trial

One of the largest trials ever conducted took place in the USA in 1954 and concerned the evaluation of the Salk polio vaccine. The trial has been reported extensively by Meier (1978) and is used by Pocock (1983) in his discussion of the historical development of clinical trials.
　　Within the project, there were essentially two trials, and these clearly illustrated the effectiveness of the randomised controlled design.

Trial 1: Original design: Observed control
1.08 million children from selected schools were included in this first trial. The second graders in those schools were offered the vaccine, while the first and third graders would serve as the control group. Parents of the second graders were approached for their consent, and it was noted that the consenting parents tended to have higher incomes. Also, this design was not blinded so that both parents and investigators knew which children had received the vaccine and which had not.

Trial 2: Alternative design: Randomised control
A further 0.75 million children in other selected schools in grades one to three were to be included in this second trial. All parents were approached for their consent, and those children where consent was given were randomised to receive either the vaccine or a placebo injection. The trial was double blind with parents, children and investigators unaware of who had received the vaccine and who had not.

The results from the randomised controlled trial were conclusive. The incidence of paralytic polio, for example, was 0.057 per cent in the placebo group compared to 0.016 per cent in the active group, and there were four deaths in the placebo group compared to none in the active group. The results from the observed control trial, however, were less convincing with a smaller observed difference (0.046 per cent vs. 0.017 per cent). In addition, in the cases where

---

Statistical Thinking for Non-Statisticians in Drug Regulation, Second Edition. Richard Kay.
© 2015 John Wiley & Sons, Ltd. Published 2015 by John Wiley & Sons, Ltd.

consent could not be obtained, the incidence of paralytic polio was 0.036 per cent in the randomised trial and 0.037 per cent in the observed control trial, event rates considerably lower than those among placebo patients and in the untreated controls, respectively. This has no impact on the conclusions from the randomised trial, which is robust against this absence of consent; the randomised part is still comparing like with like. In the observed control part however, the fact that the *no consent* (grade 2) children have a lower incidence than those children (grades 1 and 3) who were never offered the vaccine potentially causes some confusion in a non-randomised comparison; does it mean that grade 2 children naturally have lower incidence than those in grades 1 and 3? Whatever the explanation, the presence of this uncertainty reduced confidence in the results from the observed control trial.

The randomised part of the Salk Polio Vaccine trial has all the hallmarks of modern-day trials – randomisation, control group and blinding – and it was experiences of these kinds that helped convince researchers that only under such conditions can clear, scientifically valid conclusions be drawn.

1.2 Control groups

We invariably evaluate our treatments by making comparisons – active compared to control. It is very difficult to make absolute statements about specific treatments, and conclusions regarding the efficacy and safety of a new treatment are made relative to an existing treatment or placebo.

ICH E10 (2001): 'Note for Guidance on Choice of Control Group in Clinical Trials'

'Control groups have one major purpose: to allow discrimination of patient outcomes (for example, changes in symptoms, signs, or other morbidity) caused by the test treatment from outcomes caused by other factors, such as the natural progression of the disease, observer or patient expectations, or other treatment'.

Control groups can take a variety of different forms; here are just a few examples of trials with alternative types of control group:
- Active versus placebo
- Active A versus active B (vs. active C)
- Placebo versus dose level 1 versus dose level 2 versus dose level 3 (dose finding)
- Active A + active B versus active A + placebo (add-on)

The choice will depend on the objectives of the trial.

Open trials with no control group can nonetheless be useful in an exploratory, maybe early phase setting, but it is unlikely that such trials will be able to provide confirmatory, robust evidence regarding the performance of the new treatment.

Similarly, external concurrent or historical controls (groups of subjects external to the study either in a different setting or previously treated) cannot provide definitive evidence in most settings. We will discuss such trials in Chapter 17. The focus in this book however is the randomised controlled trial.

1.3 Placebos and blinding

It is important to have blinding of both the subject and the investigator wherever possible to avoid unconscious bias creeping in, either in terms of the way a subject reacts psychologically to treatment or in relation to the way the investigator interacts with the subject or records subject outcome.

ICH E9 (1998): 'Note for Guidance on Statistical Principles for Clinical Trials'

'Blinding or masking is intended to limit the occurrence of conscious or unconscious bias in the conduct and interpretation of a clinical trial arising from the influence which the knowledge of treatment may have on the recruitment and allocation of subjects, their subsequent care, the attitudes of subjects to the treatments, the assessment of the endpoints, the handling of withdrawals, the exclusion of data from analysis, and so on'.

Ideally, the trial should be *double-blind* with both the subject and the investigator being blind to the specific treatment allocation. If this is not possible for the investigator, for example, then the next best thing is to have an independent evaluation of outcome, both for efficacy and for safety. A *single-blind* trial arises when either the subject or investigator, but not both, is blind to treatment.

An absence of blinding can seriously undermine the validity of an endpoint in the eyes of regulators and the scientific community more generally, especially when the evaluation of that endpoint has an element of subjectivity. In situations where blinding is not possible, it is important to use hard, unambiguous endpoints and to use independent recording of that endpoint.

The use of placebos and blinding goes hand in hand. The existence of placebos enables trials to be blinded and accounts for the placebo effect – the change in a patient's condition that is due to the act of being treated, but is not caused by the active component of that treatment.

Note that having a placebo group does not necessarily imply that one group is left untreated. In many situations, oncology is a good example, the experimental therapy/placebo is added to an established active drug regimen; this is the add-on study.

1.4 Randomisation

Randomisation is clearly a key element in the design of our clinical trials. There are two reasons why we randomise subjects to the treatment groups:
- To avoid any bias in the allocation of the patients to the treatment groups
- To ensure the validity of the statistical test comparisons

Randomisation lists are produced in a variety of ways, and we will discuss several methods later. Once the list is produced, the next patient entering the trial receives the next allocation within the randomisation scheme. In practice, this process is managed by *packaging* the treatments according to the predefined randomisation list.

There are a number of different possibilities when producing these lists:
- Unrestricted randomisation
- Block randomisation
- Unequal randomisation
- Stratified randomisation
- Central randomisation
- Dynamic allocation and minimisation
- Cluster randomisation

1.4.1 Unrestricted randomisation

Unrestricted (or simple) randomisation is simply a random list of, for example, As and Bs. In a moderately large trial, with, say, $n = 200$ subjects, such a process will likely produce approximately equal group sizes. There is no guarantee however that this will automatically happen and in small trials, in particular, this can cause problems.

1.4.2 Block randomisation

To ensure balance in terms of numbers of subjects, we usually undertake *block randomisation* where a randomisation list is constructed by randomly choosing from the list of potential blocks. For example, there are six ways of allocating two As and two Bs in a *block* of size four:

AABB, ABAB, ABBA, BAAB, BABA, BBAA

and we choose at random from this set of six blocks to construct our randomisation list, for example,

ABBA   BAAB   ABAB   ABBA, ...

Clearly, if we recruit a multiple of four patients into the trial, we will have perfect balance and approximate balance (which is usually good enough) for any sample size.

In large trials, it could be argued that block randomisation is unnecessary. In one sense, this is true; overall balance will be achieved by chance with an unrestricted randomisation list. However, it is usually the case that large trials will be multi-centre trials, and not only is it important to have balance overall, but it is also important to have balance within each centre. In practice, therefore, we would allocate several blocks to each centre, for example, five blocks of size four if we are planning to recruit 20 patients from each centre. This will ensure balance within each centre and also overall.

How do we choose block size? There is no magic formula, but more often than not, the block size is equal to two times the number of treatments.

What are the issues with block size?

ICH E9 (1998): 'Note for Guidance on Statistical Principles for Clinical Trials'

'Care must be taken to choose block lengths which are sufficiently short to limit possible imbalance, but which are long enough to avoid predictability towards the end of the sequence in a block. Investigators and other relevant staff should generally be blind to the block length...'.

Shorter block lengths are better at producing balance. With two treatments, a block length of four is better at producing balance than a block length of 12. The block length of four gives perfect balance if there is a multiple of four patients entering, whereas with a block length of 12, perfect balance is only going to be achieved if there are a multiple of 12 patients in the study. The problem, however, with the shorter block lengths is that this is an easy code to crack and inadvertent unblinding can occur. For example, suppose a block length of four was being used in a placebo-controlled trial and also assume that experience of the active drug suggests that many patients receiving that drug will suffer nausea. Suppose the trial begins and the first two patients suffer nausea. The investigator is likely to conclude that both these patients have been randomised to active and that therefore the next two allocations are to placebo. This knowledge could influence his/her willingness to enter certain patients into the next two positions in the randomisation list, causing bias in the mix of patients randomised into the two treatment groups. Note the comment in the ICH guideline regarding keeping the investigator (and others) blind to the block length. While in principle this comment is sound, the drug is often delivered to a site according to the chosen block length, making it difficult to conceal information on block size. If the issue of inadvertent unblinding is going to cause problems, then more sophisticated methodologies can be used, such as having the block length itself varying, perhaps randomly chosen from two, four or six.

1.4.3 Unequal randomisation

All other things being equal, having equal numbers of subjects in the two treatment groups provides the maximum amount of information (the greatest power) with regard to the relative efficacy of the treatments. There may, however, be issues that override statistical efficiency:

- It may be necessary to place more patients on active compared to placebo in order to obtain the required safety information.
- In a three-group trial with active A, active B and placebo (P), it may make sense to have a 2:2:1 randomisation to give more power for the A versus B comparison as that difference is likely to be smaller than the A versus P and B versus P differences.

Unequal randomisation is sometimes needed as a result of these considerations. To achieve this, the randomisation list will be designed for the second example with double the number of A and B allocations compared to placebo.

For unequal randomisation, we would choose the block size accordingly. For a 2:1 randomisation to A or P, we could randomly choose from the blocks:

AAP, APA, PAA

1.4.4 Stratified randomisation

Block randomisation therefore forces the required balance in terms of the numbers of patients in the treatment groups, but things can still go wrong. For example, let's suppose in an oncology study with time to death as the primary endpoint that we can measure baseline risk (say, in terms of the size of the primary tumour) and classify patients as either high risk (H) or low risk (L) and further suppose that the groups turn out as follows:

A : HHLHLHHHHLLHHHLHHLHHH $\quad (H = 15, L = 6)$
B : LLHHLHHLLHLHLHLHHLLHLL $\quad (H = 10, L = 12)$

Note that there are 15 (71 per cent) high-risk patients and six (29 per cent) low-risk patients in treatment group A compared to a split of 10 (45 per cent) high-risk and 12 (55 per cent) low-risk patients in treatment group B.

Now suppose that the mean survival times are observed to be 21.5 months in group A and 27.8 months in group B. What conclusions can we draw? It is very difficult; the difference we have seen could be due to real treatment differences or could be caused by the imbalance in terms of differential risk across the groups, or a mixture of the two. Statisticians talk in terms of *confounding* (just a fancy way of saying *mixed up*) between the treatment effect and the effect of baseline risk. This situation is very difficult to unravel, and we avoid it by *stratified randomisation* to ensure that the *case mix* in the treatment groups is comparable.

This simply means that we produce separate randomisation lists for the high-risk and the low-risk patients, the strata in this case. For example, the following lists (which are block size four in each case):

H : ABBAAABBABABABABBBAAABBAABABBBAA
L : BAABBABAAABBBAABABABBBAABBAABAAB

will ensure firstly that we end up with balance in terms of treatment group sizes but also secondly that both the high- and low-risk patients will be equally split across those groups, that is, balance in terms of the mix of patients.

Having separate randomisation lists for the different centres in a multi-centre trial to ensure *equal* numbers of patients in the treatment groups within each centre is using *centre* as a stratification factor; this will ensure that we do not end up with treatment being confounded with centre.

ICH E9 (1998): 'Note for Guidance on Statistical Principles for Clinical Trials'

'It is advisable to have a separate random scheme for each centre, i.e. to stratify by centre or to allocate several whole blocks to each centre. Stratification by important

prognostic factors measured at baseline (e.g. severity of disease, age, sex, etc.) may sometimes be valuable in order to promote balanced allocation within strata'.

Where the requirement is to have balance in terms of several factors, a stratified randomisation scheme using all combinations of these factors to define the strata would ensure balance. For example, if balance is required for sex and age, then a scheme with four strata – males, <50 years; females, <50 years; males, ≥50 years; and females, ≥50 years – will achieve the required balance.

1.4.5 Central randomisation

In *central randomisation*, the randomisation process is controlled and managed from a centralised point of contact. Each investigator makes a telephone call through an *Interactive Voice Response System* (IVRS) or an *Interactive Web Response System* (IWRS) to this centralised point when they have identified a patient to be entered into the study and is given the next allocation, taken from the appropriate randomisation list. Blind can be preserved by simply specifying the number of the (pre-numbered) pack to be used to treat the particular patient; the computerised system keeps a record of which packs have been used already and which packs contain which treatment. Central randomisation has a number of practical advantages:

- It can provide a check that the patient about to be entered satisfies certain inclusion/exclusion criteria, thus reducing the number of protocol violations.
- It provides up-to-date information on all aspects of recruitment.
- It allows more efficient distribution and stock control of medication.
- It provides some protection against biased allocation of patients to treatment groups in trials where the investigator is not blind; the investigator knowing the next allocation could (perhaps subconsciously) select patients to include or not include based on that knowledge; with central randomisation, the patient is identified and information given to the system before the next allocation is revealed to them.
- It gives an effective way of managing multi-centre trials.
- It allows the implementation of more complex allocation schemes such as minimisation and dynamic allocation (but see comments later on these techniques).

Earlier, we discussed the use of stratified randomisation in multi-centre trials, and where the centres are large, this is appropriate. With small centres however, for example, in GP trials, this does not make sense and a stratified randomisation with *region* defining the strata may be more appropriate. Central randomisation would be essential to manage such a scheme.

Stratified randomisation with more than a small number of strata would be difficult to manage at the site level, and the use of central randomisation is then almost mandatory.

1.4.6 Dynamic allocation and minimisation

ICH E9 (1998): 'Note for Guidance on Statistical Principles for Clinical Trials'

'Dynamic allocation is an alternative procedure in which the allocation of treatment to a subject is influenced by the current balance of allocated treatments and, in a stratified trial, by the stratum to which the subject belongs and the balance within that stratum. Deterministic dynamic allocation procedures should be avoided and an appropriate element of randomisation should be incorporated for each treatment allocation'.

Dynamic allocation moves away from having a pre-specified randomisation list, and the allocation of patients evolves as the trial proceeds. The method looks at the current balance, in terms of the mix of patients and a number of pre-specified factors, and allocates the next patient in an optimum way to help redress any imbalances that exist at that time.

For example, suppose we require balance in terms of sex and age (≥65 vs. <65) and part way through the trial we see a mix of patients as in Table 1.1.

Treatment group A contains proportionately more males (12 out of 25 vs. 10 out of 25) than treatment group B but fewer patients over 65 years (7 out of 25 vs. 8 out of 25). Further suppose that the next patient to enter is male and aged 68 years. In terms of sex, we would prefer that this patient be placed in treatment group B, while for age, we would prefer this patient to enter in group A. The greater imbalance however is in relation to sex, so our overall preference would be for treatment group B to help *correct* for the current imbalance. The method of *minimisation* would simply put this patient in group B. ICH E9 however recommends that we have a *random element* to that allocation, and so, for example, we would allocate this patient to treatment group A with, say, probability of 0.7. Minimisation is a special case of dynamic allocation where the random assignment probability (0.7 in the example) is equal to one. Of course with a small number of baseline factors, for example, centre and two others, stratified randomisation will give good enough balance, and there is no need to consider the more complex dynamic allocation. This technique, however, has been proposed when there are more factors involved.

Since the publication of ICH E9 however, there has been considerable debate about the validity of dynamic allocation, even with the random element. There

Table 1.1 Current mix of patients

	A	B
Total	25	25
Male	12/25	10/25
Age ≥65	7/25	8/25

is a school of thought that has some sympathy within regulatory circles that supports the view that the properties of standard statistical methodologies, notably *p*-values and confidence intervals, are not strictly valid when such allocation schemes are used. As a result, regulators are very cautious.

CPMP (2003): 'Points to Consider on Adjustment for Baseline Covariates'

'*...techniques of dynamic allocation such as minimisation are sometimes used to achieve balance across several factors simultaneously. Even if deterministic schemes are avoided, such methods remain highly controversial. Thus applicants are strongly advised to avoid such methods'.*

So if you are planning a trial, then stick with stratification and avoid dynamic allocation. If you do have an ongoing trial that is using dynamic allocation, then be prepared at the statistical analysis stage to supplement the standard methods of calculating *p*-values with more complex methods that take account of the dynamic allocation scheme. These methods go under the name of *randomisation tests*.

See Roes (2004) for a comprehensive discussion of dynamic allocation.

1.4.7 Cluster randomisation

In some cases, it can be more convenient or appropriate not to randomise individual patients, but to randomise groups of patients. The groups, for example, could correspond to GPs so that each GP enters, say, four patients, and it is the 100 GPs that are randomised, 50 giving treatment A and 50 giving treatment B. Such methods are used but are more suited to phase IV than the earlier phases of clinical development. Many health interventions in third world countries are frequently evaluated using cluster randomisation.

Bland (2004) provides a review and some examples of cluster randomised trials, while Campbell, Donner and Klar (2007) give a comprehensive review of the methodology.

1.5 Bias and precision

When we are evaluating and comparing our treatments, we are looking for two things:
- An unbiased, correct view of how effective (or safe) the treatment is
- An accurate estimate of how effective (or safe) the treatment is

As statisticians, we talk in terms of *bias* and *precision*; we want to eliminate bias and to have high precision. Imagine having 10 attempts at hitting the bull's-eye on a target board as shown in Figure 1.1. Bias is about hitting the bull's-eye on average; precision is about being consistent.

These aspects are clearly set out in ICH E9.

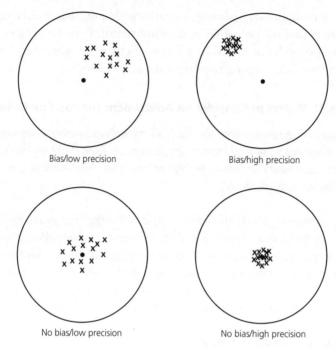

Figure 1.1 Bias and precision

ICH E9 (1998): 'Note for Guidance on Statistical Principles for Clinical Trials'

'Many of the principles delineated in this guidance deal with minimising bias and maximising precision. As used in this guidance, the term "bias" describes the systematic tendency of any factors associated with the design, conduct, analysis and interpretation of the results of clinical trials to make the estimate of a treatment effect deviate from its true value'.

What particular features in the design of a trial help to eliminate bias?
- Concurrent control group as the basis for a *treatment comparison*
- Randomisation to avoid bias in allocating subjects to treatments
- Blinding of both the subject and the investigator
- Pre-specification of the methods of statistical analysis

What particular features in the design of a trial help to increase precision?
- Large sample size
- Measuring the endpoints in a precise way
- Standardising aspects of the protocol that impact on patient-to-patient variation
- Collecting data on key prognostic factors and including those baseline factors as covariates in the statistical analysis
- Choosing a homogeneous group of patients

- Choosing the most appropriate design (e.g. using a crossover design rather than a parallel-group design where this is appropriate)   .

Several of the issues raised here may be unclear at this point; simply be aware that eliminating bias and increasing precision are the key issues that drive our statistical thinking from a design perspective. Also, be aware that if something should be sacrificed, then it is precision rather than bias. High precision in the presence of bias is of no value; you are simply then getting a more precise wrong answer! First and foremost, we require an unbiased view; increasing precision is then a bonus. Similar considerations are also needed when we choose the appropriate statistical methodology at the analysis stage.

One particular point to make clear, and this is a common misunderstanding, is that having a large sample size of itself does not remove bias. If there is a flaw in the trial design, or in the planned methods of statistical analysis, that causes bias, then beating the trial over the head with large patient numbers will not eliminate that bias and you will still be misled, regarding the true treatment difference perhaps even more so because the trial is large. As mentioned earlier, having a large sample size in a flawed clinical trial will just result in a more precise, incorrect answer!

1.6 Between- and within-patient designs

The simplest trial design of course is the *parallel-group design* assigning patients to receive either treatment A or treatment B. For example, suppose we have a randomised parallel-group design in hypertension with 50 patients per group and that the mean fall in diastolic blood pressure in each of the two groups is as follows:

A : $\bar{x}_1 = 4.6$ mmHg
B : $\bar{x}_2 = 7.1$ mmHg

One thing to note that will aid our discussion later is it would be easy (but incorrect) to conclude in light of the data that B is a more effective treatment than A because we have seen a greater fall on average with treatment B than with treatment A, but is that necessarily the case? One thing we have to remember is that the 50 patients in group A are a different group of patients from the 50 patients in group B and patients respond differently, so, the observed difference between the treatments could simply be caused by patient-to-patient variation. As we will see later, unravelling whether the observed difference is reflective of a real treatment difference or simply a chance difference caused by patient-to-patient variation with identical treatments is precisely the role of the *p*-value; but it is not easy.

This design is what we refer to as a *between-patient design*. The basis of the treatment comparison is the comparison between two independent groups of patients.

An alternative design is the *within-patient design*. Such designs are not universally applicable but can be very powerful under certain circumstances. One form of the within-patient design is the *paired design*:

- In ophthalmology – treatment A in the right eye and treatment B in the left eye.
- In a volunteer study in wound care – *create* a wound on each forearm and use dressing of type A on the right forearm and dressing of type B on the left forearm.

Here, the 50 subjects receiving A will be the same 50 subjects who receive B, and the comparison of A and B in terms of, say, mean healing time in the second example is a comparison based on identical *groups* of subjects. At least in principle, drawing conclusions regarding the relative effect of the two treatments and accounting for the patient-to-patient (or subject-to-subject) variation may be easier under these circumstances.

Another example of the within-patient design is the *crossover design*. Again, each subject receives each of the treatments but now sequentially in time with some subjects receiving the treatments in the order A followed by B and some in the order B followed by A.

In both the paired design and the crossover design, there is, of course, randomisation; in the second paired design example earlier, it is according to which forearm receives A and which forearm receives B, and randomisation is to treatment order, A/B or B/A, in the crossover design.

1.7 Crossover trials

The crossover trial was mentioned in the previous section as one example of a within-patient design. In order to discuss some issues associated with these designs, we will consider the simplest form of crossover trial – two treatments A and B and two treatment periods I and II.

The main problem with the use of this design is the possible presence of the so-called carry-over effect. This is the residual effect of one of the treatments in period I influencing the outcome on the other treatment in period II. An extreme example of this would be the situation where one of the treatments, say, A, was very efficacious, so much so that many of the patients receiving treatment A were cured of their disease, while B was ineffective and had no impact on the underlying disease. As a consequence, many of the subjects following the A/B sequence would give a good response at the end of period I (an outcome ascribed to A) but would also give a good response at the end of period II (an outcome ascribed to B) because they were cured by A. These data would give a false impression of the A versus B difference. In this situation, the B data obtained from period II is contaminated and the data coming out of such a trial are virtually useless.

It is important therefore to only use these designs when you can be sure that carry-over effects will not be seen. Introducing a washout period between period I and period II can help to eliminate carry-over so that when the subject enters period II, their disease condition is similar to what it was at the start of period I. Crossover designs should not be used where there is the potential to affect the underlying disease state. ICH E9 is very clear on the use of these designs.

ICH E9 (1998): 'Note for Guidance on Statistical Principles for Clinical Trials'

'Crossover designs have a number of problems that can invalidate their results. The chief difficulty concerns carryover, that is, the residual influence of treatments in subsequent treatment periods… When the crossover design is used it is therefore important to avoid carryover. This is best done by selective and careful use of the design on the basis of adequate knowledge of both the disease area and the new medication. The disease under study should be chronic and stable. The relevant effects of the medication should develop fully within the treatment period. The washout periods should be sufficiently long for complete reversibility of drug effect. The fact that these conditions are likely to be met should be established in advance of the trial by means of prior information and data'.

The crossover design is used extensively in phase I trials in healthy volunteers to compare different formulations in terms of their bioequivalence (where there is no underlying disease to affect). They can also be considered in diseases, for example, asthma, where the treatments are being used simply to relieve symptoms; once the treatments are removed, the symptoms return to their earlier level.

1.8 Signal, noise and evidence

1.8.1 Signal

Consider the example in Section 1.6 comparing treatments A and B in a parallel-group trial. The purpose of this investigation is to detect differences in the mean reductions in diastolic blood pressure between the two groups. The observed difference between $\bar{x}_1 = 4.6\,\text{mmHg}$ and $\bar{x}_2 = 7.1\,\text{mmHg}$ is 2.5 mmHg. We will refer to this difference as the *signal*, and this captures in part the evidence that the treatments truly are different. Clearly, if the observed difference was larger, we would likely be more inclined to conclude differences. Large differences give strong signals, while small differences give weak signals.

1.8.2 Noise

The signal, however, is not the only aspect of the data that plays a part in our conclusions. If we were to see a large amount of patient-to-patient variation, then we would be less inclined to conclude differences than if all the patients

I: A small amount of patient-to-patient variation

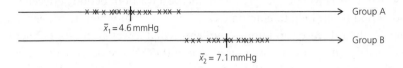

II: A large amount of patient-to-patient variation

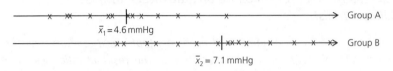

Figure 1.2 Differing degrees of patient-to-patient variation

in treatment group A had reductions tightly clustered around 4.6 mmHg, while those in treatment group B had values tightly clustered around 7.1 mmHg. As can be seen in Figure 1.2, the evidence for a real treatment difference in situation I is much stronger than the evidence seen in situation II although the mean values for both groups are actually the same in each case. We refer to the patient-to-patient variation as the *noise,* and clearly the extent of the noise will influence our willingness to declare differences between the treatments. An observed difference of 2.5 mmHg based on a small amount of noise is much stronger evidence for a true treatment difference than an observed difference of 2.5 mmHg in the presence of a large amount of noise.

The sample size plays an additional role in our willingness to conclude treatment differences and in a sense serves to compensate for the extent of the noise. If there is a large amount of patient-to-patient variation (a large amount of noise), then a large sample size is needed before we are able to *see what is happening on average* and conclude that the true means are indeed separated. In contrast, with a small amount of patient-to-patient variation, it is somewhat easier to recognise that the means truly are different, even with a small sample size.

1.8.3 Signal-to-noise ratio

These concepts of signal and noise provide a way of thinking for statistical experiments. In declaring differences, we look for strong signals and small amounts of noise, that is, a large *signal-to-noise ratio*. If either the signal is weak or the noise is large or both, then this ratio will be small and we will have little evidence on which to *declare* differences. The sample size can then be added into this mix. The value of a signal-to-noise ratio based on a small sample size is less reliable than the value of a signal-to-noise ratio based on a large sample size, and clearly this is also going to influence our willingness to declare treatment differences.

In one sense, the signal is out of our control; it will depend entirely on what the true treatment difference is. Similarly, there is little we can do about the patient-to-patient variability, although we can reduce this by having, for example, precise measures of outcome or a more homogeneous group of patients. The sample size however is very much under our control, and common sense tells us that increasing this will provide a more reliable comparison and make it easier for us to detect treatment differences when they exist.

Later, in Chapter 8, we will discuss power and sample size and see how to choose sample size in order to meet our objectives. We will also see in Section 3.3 how, in many circumstances, the calculation of the p-value is based on the signal-to-noise ratio, which when combined with the sample size allows us to numerically calculate the *evidence* in favour of treatment differences. We will see in that section, for example, that when comparing two treatment means with n subjects per group, the *evidence* for treatment differences is captured by the square root of $n/2$ multiplied by the signal-to-noise ratio.

1.9 Confirmatory and exploratory trials

ICH E9 makes a very clear distinction between *confirmatory* and *exploratory* trials. From a statistical perspective, this is an important distinction as certain aspects of the design and analysis of data depend upon this confirmatory/exploratory distinction.

ICH E9 (1998): 'Note for Guidance on Statistical Principles for Clinical Trials'

'A confirmatory trial is an adequately controlled trial in which the hypotheses are stated in advance and evaluated. As a rule, confirmatory trials are needed to provide firm evidence of efficacy or safety'.

ICH E9 (1998): 'Note for Guidance on Statistical Principles for Clinical Trials'

'The rationale and design of confirmatory trials nearly always rests on earlier clinical work carried out in a series of exploratory studies. Like all clinical trials, these exploratory studies should have clear and precise objectives. However, in contrast to confirmatory trials, their objectives may not always lead to simple tests of pre-defined hypotheses'.

Typically, later phase trials tend to contain the confirmatory elements, while the earlier phase studies – proof of concept, dose finding, etc. – are viewed as exploratory. Indeed, an alternative word for confirmatory is pivotal. It is the confirmatory elements of our trials that provide the pivotal information from a regulatory perspective.

ICH E9 (1998): 'Note for Guidance on Statistical Principles for Clinical Trials'

'Any individual trial may have both confirmatory and exploratory aspects'.

Usually, it is the primary and secondary endpoints that provide the basis of the confirmatory claims. Additional endpoints may then provide the basis for exploratory investigations.

1.10 Superiority, equivalence and non-inferiority trials

A clear distinction needs to be made between superiority, equivalence and non-inferiority trials.

In a *superiority* trial, our objective is to demonstrate either that our treatment works by demonstrating superiority over placebo or that we are superior to some reference or standard treatment.

In an *equivalence* trial, we are looking to show that we are similar to some reference treatment; bioequivalence trials are the most common examples of this type of trial.

Finally, in a *non-inferiority* trial, we are trying to demonstrate that we are no more than a certain, pre-specified, usually small amount worse than (*at least as good as*) some active reference treatment.

In therapeutic equivalence trials and in non-inferiority trials, we are often looking to demonstrate efficacy of our test treatment indirectly. It may be that for ethical or practical reasons, it is not feasible to show efficacy by undertaking a superiority trial against placebo. In such a case, we compare our test treatment to a control treatment that is known to be efficacious and demonstrate either strict equivalence or *at least as good as* (non-inferiority). If we are successful, then we can be confident that our test treatment works.

Alternatively, there may be commercial reasons why we want to demonstrate the non-inferiority of our treatment against an active control. Maybe our treatment potentially has fewer side effects than the active control, and we are prepared to pay a small price for this safety advantage in relation to efficacy. If this were the case, then of course we would need to show advantages in terms of a reduction in side effects, but we would also need to demonstrate that we do not lose much with regard to efficacy.

Non-inferiority trials are becoming more and more common as time goes on. This in part is due to the constraints imposed by the revised Helsinki Declaration (2004) and the increasing concern in some circles regarding the ethics of placebo use. These trials however require very careful design and conduct, and we will discuss this whole area in Chapter 12.

1.11 Data and endpoint types

It is useful to classify the types of data and endpoints that we see in our clinical investigations.

The most common kind of data that we see is *continuous* data. Examples include cholesterol level, exercise duration, blood pressure, FEV_1 and so on. Each of these quantities is based on a continuum of potential values. In some cases, of course, our measurement technique may only enable us to record to the nearest whole number (e.g. blood pressure), but that does not alter the basic fact that the underlying scale is continuous.

Probably, the second most common data type is *binary*. Examples of binary data include cured/not cured, responder/non-responder and died/survived. Here, the measure is based on a dichotomy.

Moving up from binary is *categorical* data where there are more than two categories that form the basis of the *measurement*. The following are examples of categorical variables:

• Death from cancer causes/death from cardiovascular causes/death from respiratory causes/death from other causes/survival
• Pain: none/mild/moderate/severe/very severe

The categories are non-overlapping and each patient is placed into one and only one of the outcome categories. Binary data is a special case where the number of categories is just two.

These two examples however are different; in the first example, the categories are unordered, while in the second example, there is a complete ordering across the defined categories. In the latter case, we term the data/endpoint type either *ordered categorical* or *ordinal*.

Ordinal data arises in many situations. In oncology (solid tumours), the RECIST criteria record outcome in one of four response categories (National Cancer Institute, www.cancer.gov):

• Complete response (CR) = disappearance of all target lesions
• Partial response (PR) = 30 per cent decrease in the sum of the longest diameter of target lesions
• Progressive disease (PD) = 20 per cent increase in the sum of the longest diameter of target lesions
• Stable disease (SD) = small changes that do not meet the aforementioned criteria

When analysing data, it is important of course that we clearly specify the appropriate order, and in this case, it is CR, PR, SD and PD.

Other data arise as *scores*. These are frequently as a result of the need to provide a measure of some clinical condition such as depression or anxiety. The Hamilton Depression (HAMD) Scale and the Hamilton Anxiety (HAMA) Scale provide measures in these cases. These scales contain distinct items that are scored individually, and then the total score is obtained as the sum of the

Table 1.2 Categorisation

Group	Cigarettes per day
1	0
2	1–5
3	6–20
4	>20

individual scores. For the HAMD Scale, there are usually 17 items – depressed mood, self-depreciation, guilt feelings, etc. – each scored on a three-point to five-point scale. The five-point scales are typically scored 0 = absent, 1 = doubtful to mild, 2 = mild to moderate, 3 = moderate to severe and 4 = very severe, while the three-point scales are typically 0 = absent, 1 = probable or mild and 2 = definite.

Finally, data can arise as *counts* of items or events; number of epileptic seizures in a 12-month period, number of asthma attacks in a 3-month period and number of lesions are just a few examples.

As we shall see later, the endpoint type to a large extent determines the class of statistical tests that we undertake. Commonly for continuous data, we use the t-tests and their extensions – analysis of variance and analysis of covariance. For binary, categorical and ordinal data, we use the class of chi-square tests (Pearson chi-square for categorical data and the Mantel–Haenszel chi-square for ordinal data) and their extension, logistic regression.

Note also that we can move between data types depending on the circumstances. In hypertension, we might be interested in:
- The fall in diastolic blood pressure (continuous)
- Success/failure with success defined as a reduction of at least 10 mmHg in diastolic blood pressure and diastolic below 90 mmHg (binary)
- Complete success/partial success/failure with complete success = reduction of at least 10 mmHg and diastolic below 90 mmHg, partial success =reduction of at least 10 mmHg but diastolic 90 mmHg or above and failure = everything else (ordinal)

There are further links across the data types. For example, from time to time, we group continuous, score or count data into ordered categories and analyse using techniques for ordinal data. For example, in a smoking cessation study, we may reduce the basic data on cigarette consumption to just four groups (Table 1.2), accepting that there is little reliable information beyond that.

We will continue this discussion in the next section on endpoints.

1.12 Choice of endpoint

1.12.1 Primary variables

Choosing a single primary endpoint is part of a strategy to reduce multiplicity in statistical testing. We will leave discussion of the problems arising with multiplicity until Chapter 10 and focus here on the nature of endpoints both from a statistical and a clinical point of view.

Generally, the primary endpoint should be that endpoint that is the clinically most relevant endpoint from the patients' perspective.

ICH E9 (1998): 'Note for Guidance on Statistical Principles for Clinical Trials'

'The primary variable ("target" variable, primary endpoint) should be that variable capable of providing the most clinically relevant and convincing evidence directly related to the primary objective of the trial'.

This choice should allow, among other things, a clear quantitative measure of benefit at the individual patient level. As we will see, identifying new treatments is not just about statistical significance, but it is also about clinical importance, and the importance of the clinical finding can only ever be evaluated if we can quantify the clinical benefit for patients.

Usually, the primary variable will relate to efficacy, but not always. If the primary objective of the trial concerns safety or quality of life, then a primary variable(s) relating to these issues would be needed.

The primary endpoint should not be confused with a summary measure of the benefit. For example, the primary endpoint may be a binary endpoint, survival beyond two years/death within two years, while the primary evaluation is based upon a comparison of two-year survival rates between two treatments. The primary endpoint *is not* the proportion surviving two years, but it is the binary outcome survival beyond two years/death within two years, the variable measured at the patient level.

The primary endpoint must be pre-specified in a confirmatory trial as specification after unblinding could clearly lead to bias. Generally, there would be only one primary endpoint, but in some circumstances, more than one primary endpoint may be needed in order to study the different effects of a new treatment. For example, in acute stroke, it is generally accepted that two primary endpoints are used – one relating to survival free of disability and a second relating to improvement in neurological outcome. See CPMP (2001) 'Note for Guidance on Clinical Investigation of Medicinal Products for the Treatment of Acute Stroke' for further details on this.

1.12.2 Secondary variables

Secondary variables may be defined that support a more detailed evaluation of the primary endpoint(s), or alternatively, such endpoints may relate to secondary objectives. These variables may not be critical to a claim but may help in understanding the nature of the way the treatment works. In addition, data on secondary endpoints may help to embellish a marketing position for the new treatment.

If the primary endpoint gives a negative result, then the secondary endpoints cannot generally recover a claim. If, however, the primary endpoint has given a positive result, then additional claims can be based on the secondary endpoints provided these have been structured correctly within the confirmatory strategy. In Chapter 10, we will discuss hierarchical testing as a basis for such a strategy.

1.12.3 Surrogate variables

Surrogate endpoints are usually used when it is not possible within the timeframe of the trial to measure true clinical benefit. Many examples exist as seen in Table 1.3.

Unfortunately, many treatments that have shown promise in terms of surrogate endpoints have been shown not to provide subsequent improvement in terms of the clinical outcome. Fleming and DeMets (1996) provide a number of examples where we have been disappointed by surrogate endpoints and provide in each of these cases possible explanations for this failure of the surrogate. One common issue in particular is that a treatment may have an effect on a surrogate through a particular pathway that is unrelated to the underlying disease process or the clinical outcome.

Treatment effects on surrogate endpoints therefore do not necessarily translate into treatment effects on clinical endpoints, and the validity of the surrogate depends not only on the variable itself but also on the disease area and the mode of action of the treatment. Establishing new valid surrogates is very difficult. Fleming and DeMets conclude that surrogates are extremely valuable in phase II *proof-of-concept* studies, but they question their general use in phase III confirmatory trials.

Table 1.3 Surrogate variable and clinical endpoints

Disease	Surrogate variable	Clinical endpoint
Congestive heart failure	Exercise tolerance	Mortality
Osteoporosis	Bone mineral density	Fractures
HIV	CD4 cell count	Mortality
Hypercholesterolemia	Cholesterol level	Coronary heart disease

---

Example 1.2 Bone mineral density and fracture risk in osteoporosis

Li, Chines and Meredith (2004) quote three clinical trials evaluating the effectiveness of alendronate, risedronate and raloxifene in increasing bone mineral density (BMD) and reducing fracture risk in osteoporosis. These treatments are seen to reduce fracture risk by similar amounts (47 per cent, 49 per cent and 46 per cent, respectively), yet their effects on increasing BMD are somewhat different (6.2 per cent, 5.8 per cent and 2.7 per cent, respectively). Drawing conclusions on the relative effectiveness of these treatments based solely in terms of the surrogate BMD would clearly be misleading.

1.12.4 Global assessment variables

Global assessment variables involve an investigator's overall impression of improvement or benefit. Usually, this is done in terms of an ordinal scale of categories. While the guidelines allow such variables, experience shows that they must at the very least be accompanied by objective measures of benefit. Indeed, both the FDA and the European regulators tend to prefer the use of the objective measures only, certainly at the primary endpoint level.

ICH E9 (1998): 'Note for Guidance on Statistical Principles for Clinical Trials'

'If objective variables are considered by the investigator when making a global assessment, then those objective variables should be considered as additional primary, or at least important secondary, variables'.

1.12.5 Composite variables

In some circumstances, it may be necessary to combine several events/endpoints to produce a combined or composite endpoint. The main purpose for doing so is to avoid multiple testing, and more will be said about this in Chapter 10. In addition, combining endpoints/events will increase the absolute numbers of events observed, and this can increase sensitivity (power) for the detection of treatment effects.

1.12.6 Categorisation

In general, a variable measured on a continuous scale contains more information and is a better reflection of the effect of treatment than a categorisation of such a scale. For example, in hypertension, the clinical goal may be to reduce diastolic blood to below 90 mmHg; that is not to say that a reduction down to 91 mmHg is totally unacceptable, while a reduction down to 89 mmHg is a perfect outcome. Having a binary outcome that relates to achieving 90 mmHg is clearly only a somewhat crude measure of treatment benefit. The CHMP recognise that the original variable contains more information, and although they support the presentation of the proportion of responders in order to gauge clinical benefit, they suggest that statistical testing be undertaken on the original scale.

CPMP (2002) 'Points to Consider on Multiplicity Issues in Clinical Trials'

'When used in this manner, the test of the null hypothesis of no treatment effect is better carried out on the original primary variable than on the proportion of responders'.

Nonetheless, categorisation can be of benefit under some circumstances. In an earlier section, we discussed the categorisation of number of cigarettes to a four-point ordinal scale, accepting that measures on the original scale may be subject to substantial error and misreporting; the additional information contained in the number of cigarettes smoked is in a sense spurious precision.

There may also be circumstances where a categorisation combines responses measured on different measurement domains, for example, to give a single dichotomous responder/non-responder outcome. There are connections here with global assessment variables. This approach is taken in Alzheimer's disease where the effect of treatment is in part expressed in terms of the 'proportion of patients who achieve a meaningful benefit (response)'; see the CHMP (2007) 'Draft Guideline on Medicinal Products in the Treatment of Alzheimer's Disease and Other Dementias'. In oncology, the RECIST criteria may be used simply to give the proportion of patients who achieve a CR or PR. This reduces the sensitivity of the complete scale but may make it easier to quantify the clinical benefit in what is often termed a *responder analysis*. For an interesting exchange on the value of dichotomisation, see Senn (2003) and Lewis (2004). Royston, Altman and Sauerbrei (2006) are against categorisation for data analysis as this tends to waste information and consequently is less able to detect treatment differences should they exist. Both these sets of authors however recognise that such analyses can be beneficial in terms of data presentation and communication.

Finally, a few words about the use of the visual analogue scale (VAS). A value on this 10 mm line gives a continuous measure (the distance between the left-hand end and the marked value), and these are used successfully in a number of therapeutic settings. Their advantage over an ordinal four- or five-point scale, however, is questionable as again there is an argument that the additional *precision* provided by VAS is of no value. A study by Jensen *et al.* (1989) in the measurement of post-operative pain showed that information relating to pain was best captured using an 11-point scoring scale (0, 1, 2, ..., 10) – sometimes referred to as a *Likert scale* – or a verbal rating scale with five points (mild, discomforting, distressing, horrible, excruciating). In addition, around 10 per cent of the patients were unable to understand the requirement for completion of the VAS for pain. These ordered categorical scales may well be as precise or more precise than the VAS and at the same time prove to be more effective because patients understand them better.

CHAPTER 2

Sampling and inferential statistics

2.1 Sample and population

Consider the comparison of a new treatment A to an existing treatment B for lowering blood pressure in mild to moderate hypertension in the context of a clinical trial conducted across Europe. The characteristics of the *population* of mild to moderate hypertensive patients to be studied will be defined by the inclusion (and exclusion) criteria and may well contain several millions of individuals. In another sense, this population will be infinite if we also include those patients satisfying the same inclusion/exclusion criteria in the future. Our clinical trial will, for example, involve selecting a *sample* of say 200 individuals from this population and randomly assigning 100 to treatment group A and 100 to the treatment group B.

Each subject in the sample will be observed and provide a value for the fall in diastolic blood pressure, the primary endpoint. The mean falls in blood pressure in groups A and B will then be computed and compared. Suppose that the group A and group B means are, respectively,

$\bar{x}_1 = 8.6$ mmHg

$\bar{x}_2 = 3.9$ mmHg

The conclusion we draw will be based on a comparison of these means, and in general, there are three possibilities in relation to what we conclude:
- Treatment A is better than treatment B.
- Treatment B is better than treatment A.
- There are no differences.

Suppose in this case we conclude on the basis of the data that treatment A is better than treatment B. This statement of course is correct in terms of what we have seen on average in the sample data, but the statement we are making is in fact stronger than that; it is a statement about the complete population. On the basis of the data, we are concluding that treatment A will, on average, work better than treatment B in this population; we are extrapolating from the sample to the population. Statisticians talk in terms of making *inferences*. On the basis of the sample data, we are inferring things about the complete population.

Statistical Thinking for Non-Statisticians in Drug Regulation, Second Edition. Richard Kay.
© 2015 John Wiley & Sons, Ltd. Published 2015 by John Wiley & Sons, Ltd.

In one sense, moving from the sample to the population in this way is a leap of faith! However, it should work provided the sample is representative of the population. If it is not representative, but if we can assume that the treatment difference is homogeneous across the population as a whole, then we would still obtain a valid estimate of that treatment difference.

In order to make any progress in understanding how inferential statistics works, we need to understand what happens when we take a sample from a population. In a later section, we will explore this through a computer simulation and see how all of this comes together in practical applications.

2.2 Sample statistics and population parameters

2.2.1 Sample and population distribution

The *sample histogram* in Figure 2.1 provides a visual summary of the distribution of total cholesterol in a group of 100 patients at baseline (artificial data). The x-axis is divided up into intervals of width 0.5 mmol/l, and the y-axis counts the number of individuals with values within those intervals.

We will sometimes refer to the sample histogram as the *sample distribution*.

These data form the sample and they have been taken from a well-defined population, which sits in the background. We can also envisage a corresponding histogram for the complete population, and this will have a smooth shape as a result of the size of that population; we use the terms *population histogram* or *population distribution* for this. Figure 2.2 shows the population histogram superimposed onto the sample histogram. Provided the sample is representative of the population, then the sample and population histograms should be similar. In practice, remember that we only see the sample histogram and the population histogram is hidden from us; indeed, we want to use the sample distribution to tell us about the distribution in the population.

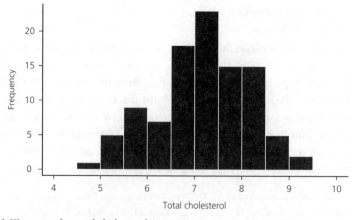

Figure 2.1 Histogram for total cholesterol ($n = 100$)

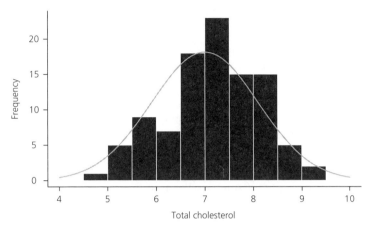

Figure 2.2 Sample histogram ($n = 100$) and population histogram

There are usually two aspects of these histograms that we are interested in, what is happening on average and the patient-to-patient variation or spread of the data values. The average will be used as a basis for measuring the signal, and in particular, we will be looking at differences between two averages for that, while the patient-to-patient variation relates directly to the noise as discussed in Section 1.8.2.

The measures of average that we commonly use are the mean and the median, while the standard deviation provides us with our measure of patient-to-patient variation.

2.2.2 Median and mean

The *median* (denoted by $\tilde{x}$) is the middle value when the data values are ordered from smallest to largest. The median can only be defined in this way when there are an odd number of values (subjects). When the number of subjects is even, we define the median to be the average of the middle two values. For the data in Figure 2.1, $n = 100$ and the median $\tilde{x} = 7.20$ mmol/l. The *mean* (denoted by $\bar{x}$) is the arithmetic average; $\bar{x} = \frac{1}{n}\sum x$. For the data in Figure 2.1, $n = 100$ and $\bar{x} = 7.16$ mmol/l.

2.2.3 Standard deviation

The *standard deviation* (denoted s or sd) is a measure of patient-to-patient variation and provides our measure of noise when we are dealing with parallel-group studies. There are other potential measures, but this quantity is used as it possesses a number of desirable mathematical properties and appropriately captures the overall amount of variability within the sample of patients.

It is related to another quantity called the *variance* and

Variance = (standard deviation)^2

So if the standard deviation is 3, the variance is 9, and if the variance is 25, then the standard deviation is 5.

The method of calculation of the standard deviation seems, at least at face value, to have some arbitrary elements to it. There are several steps:

- Calculate the mean of all values.
- Calculate the difference between each individual value and the mean, and square each of those differences.
- Take the average of these squared differences but with the *average* calculated by dividing by $n-1$, not n; the resulting quantity is called the variance (with units mmol/l^2 for the data in our example).
- Take the square root of the variance to revert to the original units, mmol/l; this is the standard deviation.

For the example data, $n=100$ and $s=0.98$ mmol/l.

People often ask, why divide by $n-1$ rather than n? Well, the answer is a fairly technical one. It can be shown mathematically that dividing by n gives a quantity that, on average, underestimates the true standard deviation, particularly in small samples and dividing by $n-1$ rather than n corrects for this underestimation. Of course for a large sample size, it makes very little difference – dividing by 99 is much the same as dividing by 100.

Another frequent question is, why square, average and then square root, and why not simply take the average distance of each point from the mean without bothering about the squaring? Well, you could do this, and yes, you would end up with a measure of patient-to-patient variability; this quantity is actually referred to as the *mean absolute deviation* and is indeed sometimes used as a measure of spread. The standard deviation, however, has several strong theoretical properties that we will need in our subsequent development and therefore, we will go with that as our measure of variation.

2.2.4 Notation

In order to distinguish between quantities measured in the sample and corresponding quantities in the population, we use different symbols:

The mean in the sample is denoted $\bar{x}$.
The mean in the population is denoted μ.
The standard deviation in the sample is denoted s or sd.
The standard deviation in the population is denoted σ.

Remember, $\bar{x}$ and s are quantities that we calculate from our data, while μ and σ are theoretical quantities (parameters) that are unknown to us but nonetheless exist in the context of the broader population from which the sample (and therefore the data) is taken. If we had access to every single subject in the population, then yes, we could compute μ and σ, but this is never going to be the case. We can also think of μ and σ as the *true* mean and *true* standard deviation, respectively, in the population as a whole.

The calculation of mean and standard deviation only really makes sense when we are dealing with continuous, score or count data. These quantities have little relevance when we are looking at binary or ordinal data. In such situations, we would tend to use proportions in the various categories as our summary statistics and population parameters of interest.

For binary data:

The sample proportion is denoted r.
The population proportion is denoted θ.

2.2.5 Box plots

The *box plot* is a useful way to display the distribution of data in a sample. Figure 2.3 displays a box plot for some artificial data where the 11 observations have values as follows:

32 15 22 31 32 23 19 51 37 24 25

When ordered from the smallest to largest, the observations are

15 19 22 23 24 25 31 32 32 37 51

The median value is 25. The *upper quartile* is the value in general that cuts off the largest 25 per cent of the observations, while the *lower quartile* in general is the value that cuts off the smallest 25 per cent of the observations. The easiest way to obtain the upper quartile in this small data set is to look firstly at the values above the median and to cut this group of observations into two further halves. The values above the median are 31 32 32 37 51, and it is the value 32 that cuts these into two halves, so 32 is the upper quartile. The calculation for the lower quartile is similar but looks at the data below the median. The lower quartile for these data is 22. The *interquartile (IQ) range* is the difference between the upper and lower

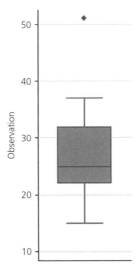

Figure 2.3 Box plot for artificial data

quartiles, 10 (=32 – 22) in this case. *Whiskers* are then placed at the furthest observed values in the data that are within 1.5*IQ range of the median. In the example, 1.5*IQ range = 15, and we look to find the largest value in the data that is just within 40 (=median + 15), which is 37, and the smallest value that is just within 10 (=median – 15), which is 15. The whiskers are then placed, respectively, at 15 and 37. All values outside of the whiskers are then marked individually.

These plots give a good visual impression about what is happening on average through the median, while the lower and upper quartiles show the spread of the *middle* 50 per cent of the data. The positioning of the whiskers helps us to identify if the distribution of the data is skewed rather than symmetric. It is not infrequently the case that we see the upper whisker further away from the median than the lower whisker, indicating what we refer to as *positively skew* data. We refer to the opposite setting, the lower whisker further away from the median than the upper whisker as *negatively skew.* Values outside of the whiskers can be considered as outlying values. We will discuss *outliers*, and action to be taken when we see such values, in Section 11.7.

2.3 The normal distribution

The *normal* or *Gaussian* distribution was in fact first discovered by de Moivre, a French mathematician, in 1733. Gauss came upon it somewhat later, just after 1800, but from a completely different start point. Nonetheless, it is Gauss who has his name attached to this distribution.

The normal distribution is a particular form for a population histogram. It is symmetric around the mean μ and is bell shaped. It has been noted empirically that in many situations, data, particularly when collected from random systems, gives a histogram with this *normal distribution* shape. In fact, there is a very powerful theorem called the *central limit theorem*, which looks at the behaviour of data and says that under certain general conditions data behave according to this distribution. An example of a normal distribution is given in Figure 2.4.

The normal distribution is all about the behaviour of averages. I am going to make a very bold philosophical statement at this point and that is, 'at the helicopter level, randomness is entirely predictable'. To explain, consider a lottery. In the UK, our national lottery involves choosing six numbers in the range 1–49, and draws take place on Wednesdays and Saturdays. The mechanism for choosing the six winning numbers involves a revolving drum containing the 49 numbered balls with the chosen balls (numbers) rolling down a tube and coming to rest. If you have the ticket containing the six chosen numbers, then you win an obscene amount of money, something close to a senior banker's bonus! It has been shown by looking at the data over the 18 years that the lottery has been running that the process for choosing the numbers is an entirely random process. However, if we look at all of the draws over the 18-year period and plot

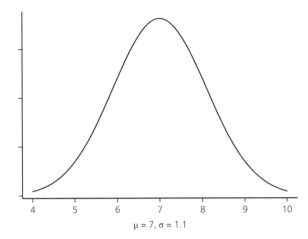

4   5   6   7   8   9   10

$\mu = 7, \sigma = 1.1$

Figure 2.4 Normal distribution for total cholesterol at baseline ($\mu = 7$ mmol/l, $\sigma = 1.1$ mmol/l)

the frequency distribution according to the numbers 1–49, it can be seen that 1 has occurred almost the same number of times as 2 and 2 has occurred almost the same number of times as 3 and so on. This is precisely what you would expect, and in the long term with a completely random process, the frequency for all of the numbers will be exactly the same – 'randomness is entirely predictable'. If these frequencies were not the same, then the process would not be random. You might ask, well, where does the normal distribution fit into this? Well, suppose on each occasion that the lottery numbers are drawn we calculate the numerical average of the six numbers that are chosen and then plot the histogram for all of these average values over the 18-year period. The histogram will look exactly like a normal distribution with mean value at 25. The reason why the mean will be 25 is because that is the average of the numbers 1–49, and the normal shape will occur because that is exactly how averages behave in a random system; this behaviour is completely predictable. The central limit theorem is in fact a very sophisticated law of averages. To extend this argument, it is invariably the case that each clinical outcome measure that we record, for example, blood pressure or cholesterol level, is the result of the influence or averaging of a number of different but interrelated physiological processes, and these considerations lead us to consider the normal distribution as a suitable distribution that can summarise the behaviour of such outcomes for a population of individuals.

As a consequence of both this theoretical base and the empirical evidence, we often assume that the data we are collecting have been drawn from a distribution with a normal shape; we assume that our data are *normally distributed*.

One further point relating to the normal distribution in the population is that, because of the symmetry, the median and the mean take the same value. This is in fact a property of any population distribution for data that is symmetric.

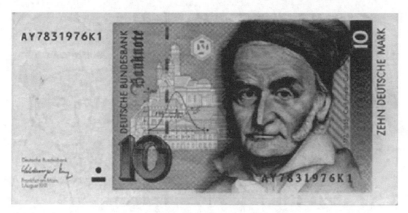

Figure 2.5 Gauss on the Deutsche 10 Mark note

Table 2.1 Probabilities for the normal distribution

Range	Percentage of patients
$\mu-2\sigma$ to $\mu+2\sigma$	95.4
$\mu-3\sigma$ to $\mu+3\sigma$	99.7
$\mu-1.645\sigma$ to $\mu+1.645\sigma$	90
$\mu-1.960\sigma$ to $\mu+1.960\sigma$	95
$\mu-2.576\sigma$ to $\mu+2.576\sigma$	99

Briefly returning to Gauss, one can gauge the importance of *his* discovery by observing the old German 10 Mark banknote in Figure 2.5. Here, we have Gauss, and just above the *10* and to the right, we can also see the normal distribution and its mathematical equation.

When the population does indeed follow this distribution, then the standard deviation, σ, has a more specific interpretation. If we move σ units below the mean to $\mu-\sigma$ and σ units above the mean to $\mu+\sigma$, then that interval $(\mu-\sigma, \mu+\sigma)$ will capture 68.3 per cent of the population values. This is true whatever we are considering, diastolic blood pressure, fall in diastolic blood pressure over a six-month period, cholesterol level, FEV_1 etc., and whatever the values of μ and σ; in all cases, 68.3 per cent of the patients will have data values in the range $\mu-\sigma$ to $\mu+\sigma$ provided the data are normally distributed.

Several further properties hold as shown in Table 2.1.

Note that the normal distribution curve has a mathematical equation and integrating the equation of this curve, for example, between $\mu-2\sigma$ and $\mu+2\sigma$, irrespective of the values of μ and σ, will always give the answer 0.954. So 95.4 per cent of the area under the normal curve is contained between $\mu-2\sigma$ and $\mu+2\sigma$, and it is this area calculation that also tells us that 95.4 per cent of the individuals within the population will have data values in that range.

Example 2.1 Normal distribution (Figure 2.4)

A population of patients in a cholesterol lowering study have total cholesterol measured at baseline. Assume that total cholesterol is normally distributed with mean of 7.0 mmol/l and standard deviation of 1.1 mmol/l so that the variance is 1.21 (=1.1²). We write this as N(7.0, 1.21). For historical reasons, we put the variance as the second parameter here. Under these assumptions, the following results hold:
- 68.3 per cent of the patients have total cholesterol in the range 5.9 mmol/l to 8.1 mmol/l.
- 90 per cent of the patients will have values in the range 5.19 mmol/l to 8.81 mmol/l.
- 95.4 per cent of the patients will have values in the range 4.8 mmol/l to 9.2 mmol/l.

2.4 Sampling and the standard error of the mean

Earlier in this chapter, we spoke about the essence of inferential statistics, drawing conclusions about a population based upon a sample taken from that population. In order to understand how we do this, we need to understand what happens when we take a sample from the population:
- Do we always reach the correct conclusion about the population?
- Are we sometimes misled by the sample data?
- How big a sample do we need to be confident that we will end up with a correct conclusion?

In order to gain an understanding of the sampling process, we have undertaken a computer simulation. For this simulation, we have set up, on the computer, a very large population of patients whose diastolic blood pressures have been recorded. The population has been structured to be normally distributed with mean of 80 mmHg and standard deviation of 4 mmHg, N(80, 16), as shown in Figure 2.6.

Imagine that this is a real clinical trial setting and our objective is to find out the value of the mean diastolic blood pressure in the population

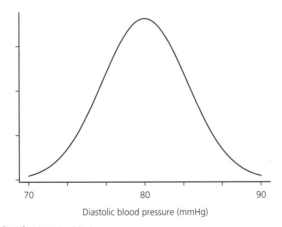

Diastolic blood pressure (mmHg)

Figure 2.6 Normal distribution, N(80, 16)

Table 2.2 Mean values $\bar{x}$ from 100 samples of size 50 from N(80, 16). Units are mmHg

1	80.218	26	79.894	51	79.308	76	80.821
2	80.767	27	79.629	52	79.620	77	80.498
3	78.985	28	80.233	53	80.012	78	79.579
4	81.580	29	79.738	54	80.678	79	81.051
5	79.799	30	80.358	55	80.185	80	80.786
6	80.302	31	79.617	56	79.901	81	79.780
7	79.094	32	79.784	57	79.778	82	79.802
8	80.660	33	79.099	58	79.597	83	80.510
9	79.455	34	79.779	59	79.320	84	79.592
10	79.275	35	81.438	60	79.076	85	79.617
11	80.732	36	80.066	61	80.580	86	79.587
12	79.713	37	79.591	62	79.878	87	79.124
13	79.314	38	80.254	63	79.656	88	79.520
14	80.010	39	80.494	64	79.302	89	79.587
15	79.481	40	79.259	65	80.242	90	79.544
16	79.674	41	80.452	66	78.344	91	80.054
17	80.049	42	80.957	67	80.653	92	80.458
18	79.156	43	80.113	68	79.848	93	79.895
19	80.826	44	80.043	69	80.294	94	79.293
20	80.321	45	80.436	70	80.797	95	79.376
21	79.476	46	81.220	71	79.226	96	80.296
22	80.155	47	79.391	72	78.883	97	79.722
23	79.429	48	80.552	73	79.871	98	78.464
24	80.775	49	80.422	74	80.291	99	78.695
25	80.490	50	80.265	75	79.544	100	79.692

(but remember that because this is a computer simulation, we know the answer!). So let's take a sample of size 50.

The mean, $\bar{x}$, from this sample turned out to be 80.218 mmHg. The one thing you will notice about this value is that it is not equal to μ, which is 80 mmHg, so we see immediately that the sampling process does not necessarily hit the absolute truth. So let's take a second sample. The second sample gave a mean of 80.767 mmHg; again, this value is not equal to the true mean. Not only that, the second sample has given a different answer to the first sample. We repeated this sampling process 100 times, going back to the population and taking further samples of size 50. The complete set of mean values is given in Table 2.2.

There are two things you will notice about this list of means. Firstly, not one of them has hit the true mean value of 80 mmHg. Secondly, all the values are different. The implication of this is as follows. Whenever you get an answer in a clinical trial, the only thing you know for certain is that it is the wrong answer! Not only that, if you were to repeat the trial under identical circumstances, same protocol, same investigator and so on, but with a new set of patients, then you would get a different answer. These are simply aspects of the sampling process; it is by no means a perfect process and we need to understand it more. This

so-called sampling variation is fundamentally a result of patient-to-patient variation; patients behave differently, and successive samples of 50 patients are going
to give different results. In order to be able to work in this uncertain environment,
we need to quantify the extent of the sampling variation.

The standard deviation of this list of $\bar{x}$ values can be calculated using the method
described earlier and give a measure of the inherent variability in the sampling process. A large value for this standard deviation would indicate that the $\bar{x}$ values are all
over the place and we are in an unreliable situation in terms of estimating where the
true mean (μ) lies; a small value for this standard deviation would indicate that the
$\bar{x}$ values are closely bunched together and the sampling process is giving a consistent, reliable value. This standard deviation for the list of $\bar{x}$ values was calculated to
be 0.626 and provides a measure of the variation inherent in the sampling process.

In practice, we will never have the luxury of seeing the behaviour of the sampling process in this way; remember, this is a computer simulation. However, there
is a way of estimating the standard deviation associated with the sampling process
through a mathematical expression applied to the data from a single sample. This
formula is given by $s/\sqrt{n}$, where s is the *sd* from the sample and n is the sample size.

So, in practice, we calculate the mean from a sample (size n) of data plus the
corresponding standard deviation, s. We then divide the standard deviation by
$\sqrt{n}$, and the resulting numerical value gives an estimate of the standard deviation
associated with the sampling process, the standard deviation for the repeat $\bar{x}$
values had we undertaken the sampling many times.
One potentially confusing issue here is that there are two standard deviations:

Example 2.2 Sampling variation

In the first computer simulation, $n=50$, $\bar{x} = 80.218$, and $s=4.329$, the standard deviation of
the 50 patient diastolic blood pressures in that sample.
  The estimated standard deviation associated with the repeat $\bar{x}$ values is then given by

$$\frac{s}{\sqrt{n}} = \frac{4.329}{\sqrt{50}} = 0.612$$

In other words, were we to repeat the sampling process, getting a list of $\bar{x}$ values by repeatedly
going back to the population and sampling 50 subjects, then 0.612 gives us an estimate of the
standard deviation associated with these $\bar{x}$ values.

---

one measures the patient-to-patient variability from the single sample/trial,
while the second estimates the mean-to-mean variation that you would get by
repeating the sampling exercise. To help distinguish the two, we reserve the term
standard deviation for the first of these (patient-to-patient variation), and we
call the second *the standard error* (se) of $\bar{x}$ (mean-to-mean variation). Thus in the
earlier example, 0.612 is the standard error of $\bar{x}$ from the first computer

simulation sample, an estimate of the standard deviation of mean values under repeated sampling. Note that this value is close to 0.626, the *standard error* calculated via the computer simulation through repetition of the sampling process.

Small standard error tell us that we are in a reliable sampling situation where the repeat mean values are very likely to be closely bunched together; a large standard error tells us we are in an unreliable situation where the mean values are varying considerably.

It is not possible at this stage to say precisely what we mean by small and large in this context; we need the concept of the confidence interval to be able to say more in this regard, and we will cover this topic in the next chapter. For the moment, just look upon the standard error as an informal measure of precision: high values mean low precision, and low values mean high precision. Further, if the standard error is small, it is likely that our estimate $\bar{x}$ will be close to the true mean, μ. This is because the $\bar{x}$ values will be bunched together, as a consequence of a small standard error, and as they will vary symmetrically around the true mean, they will all be *close* to that true mean. If the standard error is large, however, there is no guarantee that we will be close to the true mean, as we do not have that close bunching of the $\bar{x}$ values even though on average they will centre on the true mean.

Figure 2.7 shows histograms of $\bar{x}$ values for sample sizes of 20, 50 and 200 from 100 simulations (samples) in each case. It is clear that for $n=20$ there is considerable variation; there is no guarantee that the mean from a particular sample will be close to μ. For $n=50$, things are not quite so bad, although the sample mean could still be out at 82.0 or at 78.2. For the sample size of 200, there is only a small amount of variability; over 250 of the 1000 mean values are within 0.1 units of the true mean. These histograms/distributions are referred to as *sampling distributions*. They are the distributions of $\bar{x}$ from the sampling process. Remember, when you conduct a trial and get a mean value, it is just one realisation of such a sampling process. The standard error are the estimated standard deviations of the $\bar{x}$ values in these histograms and measure their spread.

2.5 Standard errors more generally

The standard error concept can be extended in relation to any *statistic* (quantity) calculated from the data.

2.5.1 The standard error for the difference between two means

As a further example, imagine a placebo-controlled cholesterol lowering trial. Generally in such trials, patients in each of the groups will receive lifestyle and dietary advice plus medication, either active or placebo, according to the randomisation scheme. Let μ_1 be the true mean reduction in total cholesterol in the active treatment group, and let μ_2 be the corresponding true mean reduction in the placebo

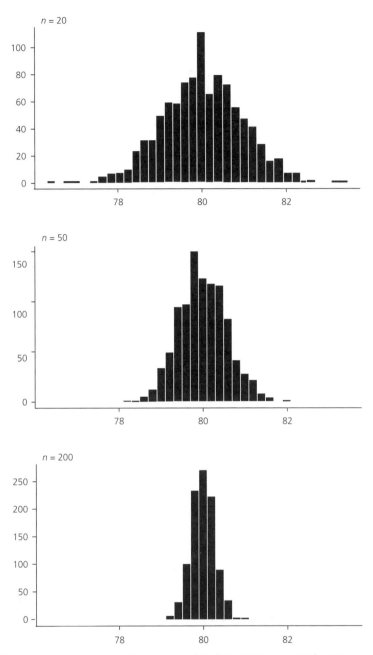

Figure 2.7 Sampling distribution of the mean $\bar{x}$; data from N(80, 16), sample size n

group. So μ_1 is the mean reduction you would get if all patients in the population were given active treatment, and μ_2 is the mean you would get if all patients were given placebo. The lifestyle and dietary advice will, of itself, have a positive effect, and coupled with the *placebo effect*, we will most likely see a mean reduction in each of the two treatment groups. The issue is, are we seeing a larger reduction in the active group compared to the placebo group? With this in mind, our main interest lies not in the individual means, but in their difference $\mu_1 - \mu_2$, the *treatment effect*.

Our best guess for the value of $\mu_1 - \mu_2$ is the observed difference in the sample means $\bar{x}_1 - \bar{x}_2$ from the trial.

Suppose that the value of $\bar{x}_1 - \bar{x}_2$ turns out to be 1.4 mmol/l. We know full well that this will not be equal to the true difference in the means, $\mu_1 - \mu_2$. We also know that if we were to repeat the trial under identical circumstances, same protocol, same investigator and so on, but of course with a different sample of patients, then we would come up with a different value for $\bar{x}_1 - \bar{x}_2$.

So we need to have some measure of precision and reliability, and this is provided by the standard error of $\bar{x}_1 - \bar{x}_2$. Again, we have a formula for this:

$$\sqrt{\left(\frac{1}{n_1} + \frac{1}{n_2}\right) \times \frac{(n_1 - 1)s_1^2 + (n_2 - 1)s_2^2}{n_1 + n_2 - 2}}$$

Here n_1 and n_2 are the numbers of patients in each of the two treatment groups and s_1 and s_1 are the standard deviations in each of those groups. This expression allows us to estimate the standard deviation of the $\bar{x}_1 - \bar{x}_2$ values that we would get were we to repeat the trial.

Example 2.3 Standard error for the difference between two means

In a placebo-controlled trial in cholesterol lowering, Table 2.3 contains the data for the two treatment groups..

The standard error for the difference in the means, $\bar{x}_1 - \bar{x}_2$, is

$$\sqrt{\left(\frac{1}{24} + \frac{1}{23}\right) \times \frac{(24 - 1) \times 0.92 \times 0.92 + (23 - 1) \times 1.05 \times 1.05}{24 + 23 - 2}} = 0.29$$

Table 2.3 Cholesterol lowering data (artificial)

	n	Mean (mmol/l)	sd (mmol/l)
Active	24	2.7	0.92
Placebo	23	1.3	1.05

Small values of this standard error indicate high reliability; it is likely that the observed value, $\bar{x}_1 - \bar{x}_2$, for the treatment effect is close to the true treatment effect, $\mu_1 - \mu_2$. In contrast, a large value for the standard error tells us that $\bar{x}_1 - \bar{x}_2$ is not a reliable estimate of $\mu_1 - \mu_2$. Again we will not discuss specifically what is meant by *small* and *large* in this context but we will come back to this in Chapter 3.

2.5.2 Standard errors for proportions

So far, we have considered standard error associated with means and differences between means. When dealing with binary data and proportions, different formulas apply.

In Section 2.2.4, we let r denote a proportion in the sample and θ the corresponding proportion in the population. For a single proportion r, the standard error formula is $\sqrt{r(1-r)/n}$ where n is the number of subjects in the sample.

For the difference between two proportions, for example, if we are looking at the difference $r_1 - r_2$ between the cure rate in the active group (group 1) and the cure rate in the placebo group (group 2), the standard error formula is $\sqrt{r_1(1-r_1)/n_1 + r_2(1-r_2)/n_2}$ where n_1 and n_2 are the numbers of subjects in groups 1 and 2, respectively.

2.5.3 The general setting

More generally, whatever statistic we are interested in, there is usually a formula that allows us to calculate its standard error. The formulas change but their interpretation always remains the same; a small standard error is indicative of high precision and high reliability. Conversely, a large standard error means that the observed value of the statistic is an unreliable estimate of the true (population) value. It is also always the case that the standard error is an estimate of the standard deviation of the list of repeat values of the statistic that we would get were we to repeat the sampling process, a measure of the inherent sampling variability.

As discussed in the previous section, the standard error simply provides indirect information about reliability; it is not something we can use in any specific way, as yet, to tell us where the truth lies. We also have no way of saying what is large and what is small in standard error terms. We will, however, in the next chapter, cover the concept of the confidence interval, and we will see how this provides a methodology for making use of the standard error to enable us to make statements about where we think the true (population) value lies.

CHAPTER 3

Confidence intervals and *p*-values

3.1 Confidence intervals for a single mean

3.1.1 The 95 per cent confidence interval

We have seen in the previous chapter that it is not possible to make a precise statement about the exact value of a population parameter, based on sample data, and that this is a consequence of the inherent variation in the sampling process. The confidence interval (CI) provides us with a compromise, rather than trying to pin down precisely the value of the mean μ or the difference between two means, $\mu_1 - \mu_2$, for example, we give a range of values, within which we are fairly certain that the true value lies.

We will first look at the way we calculate the confidence interval for a single mean μ and then talk about its interpretation. Later in this chapter, we will extend the methodology to deal with $\mu_1 - \mu_2$ and other parameters of interest.

In the computer simulation in Chapter 2, the first sample ($n = 50$) gave summary statistics (to 2 decimal places) as follows:

$\bar{x} = 80.22\,\text{mmHg}$ and $s = 4.33\,\text{mmHg}$

The lower end of the confidence interval, the *lower confidence limit*, is then given by

$$\bar{x} - 1.96\frac{s}{\sqrt{n}} = 80.22 - \left(1.96 \times \frac{4.33}{\sqrt{50}}\right) = 79.02$$

The upper end of the confidence interval, the *upper confidence limit*, is given by

$$\bar{x} + 1.96\frac{s}{\sqrt{n}} = 80.22 + \left(1.96 \times \frac{4.33}{\sqrt{50}}\right) = 81.42$$

The interval, (79.02, 81.42), then forms the *95 per cent confidence interval*.

These data arose from a computer simulation where, of course, we know that the true mean μ is 80 mmHg, so we can see that the method has worked in the sense that μ is contained within the range 79.02 to 81.42

The second sample in the computer simulation gave the following summary statistics: $\bar{x} = 80.77\,\text{mmHg}$ and $s = 4.50\text{mmHg}$ – and this results in the 95 per cent confidence interval as (79.52, 82.02). Again, we see that the interval has captured the true mean.

Statistical Thinking for Non-Statisticians in Drug Regulation, Second Edition. Richard Kay.
© 2015 John Wiley & Sons, Ltd. Published 2015 by John Wiley & Sons, Ltd.

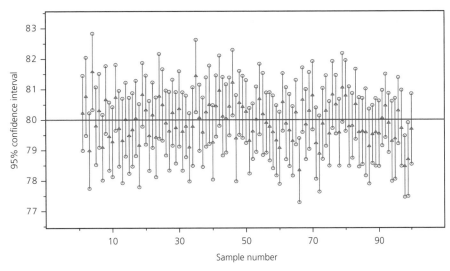

Figure 3.1 Computer simulation, 95 per cent confidence intervals, n = 50, mean = 80 mmHg

Now, look at all 100 samples taken from the normal population with μ = 80 mmHg. Figure 3.1 shows the 95 per cent confidence intervals plotted for each of the 100 simulations. A horizontal line has been placed at 80 mmHg to allow the confidence intervals to be judged in terms of capturing the true mean.

Most of the 95 per cent confidence intervals do contain the true mean of 80 mmHg, but not all. Sample number 4 gave a mean value $\bar{x}$ = 81.58 mmHg with a 95 per cent confidence intervals (80.33, 82.83), which has missed the true mean at the lower end. Similarly, samples 35, 46, 66, 98 and 99 have given confidence intervals that do not contain μ = 80 mmHg. So we have a method that seems to work most of the time, but not all of the time. For this simulation, as a whole, we have a 94 per cent (94/100) success rate. If we were to extend the simulation and take many thousands of samples from this population, constructing 95 per cent confidence intervals each time, we would in fact see a success rate of 95 per cent; exactly 95 per cent of those intervals would contain the true (population) mean value. This provides us with the interpretation of a 95 per cent confidence interval in practice; when we construct a 95 per cent confidence intervals from data, we can be 95 per cent certain that the true mean lies within the calculated range. Why? Because 95 per cent of these interval will indeed contain μ in the long run. Of course, in any particular case, we do not know whether our confidence interval is one of those 95 per cent or whether we have been unlucky and got one of the 5 per cent that do not contain the truth. In such a case, we will have been misled by the data.

Just as an aside, look back at the formula for the 95 per cent confidence interval. Where does the 1.96 come from? It comes from the normal distribution; 1.96 is the number of standard deviations you need to move out to, in order to capture 95 per cent of the values in the population. The reason we get the so-called 95 per cent coverage for the confidence intervals is directly linked to this property of the normal distribution.

3.1.2 Changing the confidence coefficient

We now have a procedure that allows us to make a statement about the value of μ with 95 per cent confidence, but we have to accept that such intervals will mislead us 5 per cent of the time. You may feel that this is too risky and instead request a 99 per cent confidence interval, which will only mislead you 1 per cent of the time. That's fine, but the formula will change, and instead of using 1.96 to give 95 per cent coverage, we will need to use 2.576 to give us 99 per cent coverage. The formula for the 99 per cent confidence interval is then

$$\bar{x} - 2.576\frac{s}{\sqrt{n}} \text{ to } \bar{x} + 2.576\frac{s}{\sqrt{n}}$$

For the first sample in the computer simulation, the 99 per cent confidence interval is (78.64, 81.80). This is a wider interval than the 95 per cent interval; the more confidence we require, the more we have to hedge our bets. It is fairly standard to use 95 per cent confidence interval, and this links with the conventional use of 0.05 (or 5 per cent) for the cut-off for statistical significance. We will say more about this link in Section 9.1. Under some circumstances, we also use 90 per cent confidence intervals and we will mention one such situation later. In multiple testing, it is also sometimes the case that we use *confidence coefficients* larger than 95 per cent; again, we will discuss the circumstances where this might happen in a later chapter.

3.1.3 Changing the multiplying constant

The formula for the 95 per cent confidence interval (and also for the 99 per cent confidence interval) given previously is in fact not quite correct. It is correct up to a point, in that it will work for very large sample sizes. For smaller sample sizes, we need to change the multiplying constant according to the values in Table 3.1.

The reason for this is again a technical one but relates to the uncertainty associated with the use of the sample standard deviation (s) in place of the true population value (σ) in the formula for the standard error. When σ is known, the multiplying constants given earlier apply. When σ is not known (the usual case), we make the confidence interval slightly wider in order to account for this uncertainty. When n is large, of course, s will be close to σ, and so the earlier multiplying constants apply approximately.

Multiplying factors are given here for 90 per cent, 95 per cent and 99 per cent confidence intervals. Note that the constants 1.960 and 2.576, those used for 95 per cent and 99 per cent confidence intervals previously, appear at the foot of the final two columns. The column on the left-hand side, termed degrees of freedom, is closely linked to sample size. When calculating a confidence interval for a mean, as in this section, we use the row corresponding to sample size (=n) − 1, so degrees of freedom for a single sample = n − 1. Do not agonise over the label, degrees of freedom; just think in terms of getting the appropriate multiplying constant by going into the row, sample size −1. A more complete table can be found in many standard

Table 3.1 Multiplying constants for calculating confidence intervals

Degrees of freedom (df)	Confidence coefficient		
	90%	95%	99%
5	2.02	2.57	4.04
10	1.81	2.23	3.17
11	1.80	2.20	3.11
12	1.78	2.18	3.06
13	1.77	2.16	3.01
14	1.76	2.15	2.98
15	1.75	2.13	2.95
16	1.75	2.12	2.92
17	1.74	2.11	2.90
18	1.73	2.10	2.88
19	1.73	2.09	2.86
20	1.73	2.09	2.85
25	1.71	2.06	2.79
30	1.70	2.04	2.75
35	1.69	2.03	2.72
40	1.68	2.02	2.70
45	1.68	2.01	2.69
50	1.68	2.01	2.68
100	1.66	1.99	2.63
200	1.65	1.97	2.60
∞	1.645	1.960	2.576

statistics textbooks. Alternatively, most statistics packages will contain a function that will give the multiplying constants for any value of degrees of freedom.

So if we were calculating a confidence interval for a mean μ from a sample of size 16, then we would look in row 15 for the multiplying constant and use 2.13 in place of 1.96 in the calculation of the 95 per cent confidence interval and 2.95 in place of 2.576 for the 99 per cent confidence interval.

3.1.4 The role of the standard error

Note the role played by the standard error in the formula for the confidence interval. We have previously seen that the standard error of the mean provides an indirect measure of the precision with which we have estimated a value for the true mean. The confidence interval has now translated the numerical value for the standard error into something useful in terms of being able to make a statement about where μ lies. A large standard error will lead to a wide confidence interval reflecting the imprecision and resulting poor information about the value of μ. In contrast, a small standard error will produce a narrow confidence interval, giving us a very definite statement about the value of μ.

For sample sizes beyond about 30, the multiplying constant for the 95 per cent confidence interval is $\cong 2$. Sometimes, for reasonably large sample sizes, we do not agonise over the value of the multiplying constant and simply use the value 2 as a good approximation. This gives us an approximate formula for the 95 per cent confidence interval as $(\bar{x} - 2se, \ \bar{x} + 2se)$.

Finally, returning again to the formula for the standard error, $s/\sqrt{n}$, we can, at least in principle, see how we could make the standard error smaller, increase the sample size n and reduce the patient-to-patient variability. These actions will translate into narrower confidence interval.

Example 3.1 Confidence interval for a single mean

In an asthma trial comparing two short-acting treatments, the following (hypothetical) data were obtained for the increase in FEV$_1$ (Table 3.2).

Table 3.2 Asthma data

Treatment	n	$\bar{x}$	s
A	18	54.6	14.6
B	21	48.8	12.9

95 per cent and 99 per cent confidence interval for μ_1 and μ_2, the population mean increases in FEV$_1$ in treatment groups A and B, are calculated as follows (Table 3.3).

Table 3.3 Confidence intervals for asthma data

Treatment	Multiplying constants (95%/99%)	$\dfrac{s}{\sqrt{n}}$	95% CI	99% CI
A	2.11/2.90	3.44	(47.3, 61.9)	(44.6, 64.6)
B	2.09/2.85	2.82	(42.9, 54.9)	(40.8, 56.8)

3.2 Confidence intervals for other parameters

3.2.1 Difference between two means

At the end of the previous chapter, we saw how to extend the idea of a standard error for a single mean to a standard error for the difference between two means. The extension of the confidence interval is similarly straightforward. Consider the placebo controlled trial in cholesterol lowering described in Example 2.3 in Chapter 2. We had an observed difference in the sample means $\bar{x}_1 - \bar{x}_2$ of 1.4 mmol/l and a standard error of 0.29 mmol/l. The formula for the 95 per cent confidence interval for the difference between two means $(\mu_1 - \mu_2)$ is

$$\bar{x}_1 - \bar{x}_2 - (\text{constant} \times se) \text{ to } \bar{x}_1 - \bar{x}_2 + (\text{constant} \times se)$$

This expression is essentially the same as that for a single mean: statistic $\pm$ (constant $\times$ se). The rules for obtaining the multiplying constant however are slightly different. For the difference between two means, we use Table 3.1 as before, but now, we go into that table at the row $n_1 + n_2 - 2$, where n_1 and n_2 are the sample sizes for treatment groups 1 and 2, respectively.

So for our data ($n_1 = 24$ and $n_2 = 23$), the multiplying constant (from row 45) is 2.01 and the calculation of the 95 per cent confidence interval is as follows:

Lower confidence limit $= 1.4 - 2.01 \times 0.29 = 0.8$ mmol/l

Upper confidence limit $= 1.4 + 2.01 \times 0.29 = 2.0$ mmol/l

The interpretation of this interval is essentially as before; we can be 95 per cent confident that the true difference in the (population) means, $\mu_1 - \mu_2$, is between 0.8 and 2.0. In other words, these data are telling us with 95 per cent confidence that the mean reduction μ_1 in the active group is greater than the corresponding mean reduction μ_2 in the placebo group by between 0.8 mmol/l and 2.0 mmol/l.

3.2.2 Confidence interval for proportions

The previous sections in this chapter are applicable when we are dealing with means. As noted earlier, these parameters are relevant when we have continuous, count or score data. With binary data, we will be looking to construct confidence intervals for rates or proportions plus differences between those rates.

Example 3.2 Trastuzumab in HER2-positive breast cancer

The following data (Table 3.4) are taken from Piccart-Gebhart *et al.* (2005) who compared trastuzumab after adjuvant chemotherapy in HER2-positive breast cancer with observation-only. The binary outcome here is one or more serious adverse events (SAEs) versus no SAEs during the one-year trial. The rate in the observation-only group provides the background incidence of SAEs.

Table 3.4 Trastuzumab data

	≥1 SAE	No SAEs	Total
Trastuzumab	117	1560	1677
Observation	81	1629	1710
Total	198	3189	3387

This display is termed a 2 × 2 *contingency table*.

The incidence rates in the test treatment and control groups respectively are

$$r_1 = \frac{117}{1677} = 0.070 \quad r_2 = \frac{81}{1710} = 0.047$$

For Example 3.2, if we label the true SAE incidence rates in the population as a whole as θ_1 (assuming all patients in the population received trastuzumab) and θ_2 (assuming all patients were only observed), then we would be interested in the confidence intervals for the individual rates θ_1 and θ_2 and also the difference in those rates, $\theta_1 - \theta_2$.

In Section 2.5.2, we set down the formulas for the standard error for both individual rates and the difference between two rates. These lead naturally to expressions for the confidence interval.

For the trastuzumab group, the 95 per cent confidence interval for θ_1 is given by

$$0.070 \pm 1.96\sqrt{\frac{0.070(1-0.070)}{1677}} = (0.058,\ 0.082)$$

The 95 per cent confidence interval for $\theta_1 - \theta_2$, the difference in the SAE rates, is given by

$$(r_1 - r_2) \pm 1.96\sqrt{\frac{r_1(1-r_1)}{n_1} + \frac{r_2(1-r_2)}{n_2}}$$

$$= (0.070 - 0.047) \pm 1.96\sqrt{\frac{0.070(1-0.070)}{1677} + \frac{0.047(1-0.047)}{1710}}$$

$$= (0.007,\ 0.039)$$

So with 95 per cent confidence, we can say that the absolute difference in SAE rates between trastuzumab and observation-only is between 0.7 per cent and 3.9 per cent.

Note that for binary data and proportions, the multiplying constant is 1.96, the value used previously when we first introduced the confidence interval idea. Again, this provides an approximation, but in this case, the approximation works well except in the case of very small sample sizes.

3.2.3 General case

In general, the calculation of the confidence interval for any statistic, be it a single mean, the difference between two means, a median, a proportion, the difference between two proportions and so on, always has the same structure:

$$\text{statistic} \pm (\text{constant} \times se)$$

where the *se* is the standard error for the statistic under consideration.

There are invariably rules for how to obtain the multiplying constant for a specific confidence coefficient, but as a good approximation and provided the sample sizes are not too small, using the value 2 for the 95 per cent confidence interval and 2.6 for the 99 per cent confidence interval would get you very close.

This methodology applies whenever we are looking at statistics based on single-treatment groups or those relating to differences between treatment groups. When we are dealing with ratios, such as the odds ratio or the hazard ratio, the methodology is changed slightly. We will cover these issues in a later chapter (see Chapter 4.5.5, for example for confidence intervals for the odds ratio).

3.2.4 Bootstrap confidence interval

The methods covered so far in Section 3.2 are applicable whenever we have a mathematical formula for the standard error. There are some complex situations however where a formula does not exist and we need to use a technique known as *bootstrapping* to obtain firstly the *standard error* and then the confidence interval.

Suppose that we have two treatment groups, A and B, including, respectively, 450 and 460 patients and we are looking to obtain the standard error of the difference between the two medians. We do in fact have a formula for calculating the standard error for the difference in the two medians, but for the purposes of this discussion, let's suppose we do not. Step 1 is to take a sample of patients at random (with replacement) of size 450 from group A. By replacement here, we mean that once we have chosen the first patient to go into our sample at random, we choose the second patient at random from the complete group of 450 patients; in other words, we put that patient back into the mix. So in the sample of 450 patients, each patient can appear more than once. We repeat this for group B, giving us what we call a *bootstrap sample* that contains 450 group A patients and 460 group B patients. In step 2, we calculate the difference in the medians from this bootstrap sample. In step 3, we repeat this sampling exercise a large number of times, typically 1000, so that we end up with 1000 bootstrap samples and 1000 values for the difference in the medians. The final step involves calculating the standard deviation of these 1000 median difference values. This gives us a value for the standard error for the difference in the medians, and our bootstrap confidence interval is then simply the observed difference in the medians plus/minus the usual multiple of the standard error. For a 95 per cent confidence interval, this multiple will be around 2, and for a 99 per cent confidence interval, this will be close to 2.6.

Note how this approach mimics the sampling process that we went through in Section 2.4.

3.3 Hypothesis testing

In our clinical trials, we generally have some very simple questions:
- Does the drug work?
- Is treatment A better than treatment B?
- Is there a dose response?
- Are treatments A and B clinically equivalent?

In order to evaluate the truth or otherwise of these statements, we begin by formulating the questions of interest in terms of hypotheses. The simplest (and most common) situation is the comparison of two treatments, for example, in a placebo controlled trial, where we are trying to detect differences and demonstrate that the drug works.

Assume that we are dealing with a continuous endpoint, for example, fall in diastolic blood pressure, and we are comparing means. If μ_1 and μ_2 denote the mean reductions in groups 1 and 2, respectively, then our basic question is as follows:

is $\mu_1 = \mu_2$ or is $\mu_1 \neq \mu_2$?

We formulate this question in terms of two competing hypotheses:

$H_0 : \mu_1 = \mu_2$,   termed the *null hypothesis*

and

$H_1 : \mu_1 \neq \mu_2$,   termed the *alternative hypothesis*

We base our conclusion regarding which of these two statements (hypotheses) we *prefer* on data, and the method that we use to make this choice is the *p*-value.

3.3.1 Interpreting the *p*-value

The '*p*' in *p*-value stands for probability, and as such, it lies between 0 and 1. I am sure we all know that if the *p*-value falls below 0.05, we declare statistical significance and conclude that the treatments are different, that is, $\mu_1 \neq \mu_2$. In contrast, if the *p*-value is above 0.05, then we talk in terms of non-significant differences. We will now explore just how this *p*-value is defined, and later, we will see the principles behind its calculation.

In the context of the comparison of an active treatment (A) with a placebo treatment (B) in lowering diastolic blood pressure, assume that we have the following summary statistics:

$\bar{x}_1 = 9.6$mmHg (active)

$\bar{x}_2 = 4.2$ mmHg (placebo)

with a difference, $\bar{x}_1 - \bar{x}_2 = 5.4$ mmHg.

Suppose that the *p*-value turns out to be 0.042. What does this *p*-value actually measure? We can see of course that it is ≤0.05, and so we would have statistical significance, but what does the probability 0.042 refer to? What is it the probability of?

Usually, people give one of two responses to this question:
- Proposed definition 1: *There is a 4.2 per cent probability that* $\mu_1 = \mu_2$.
- Proposed definition 2: *There is a 4.2 per cent probability that the observed difference of 5.4mmHg is due to chance.*

One of these definitions is correct and one is incorrect? Which way round is it?

Well, the second definition is the correct one. The first definition is not only incorrect, but it is also the common mistake that many people make. We will explore later in Section 9.3.1 why this definition causes so many problems and misunderstandings. For the moment, however, we will explore in more detail the correct definition. It is worthwhile expanding on the various components of the definition:

- There is a 4.2 per cent probability that
- the observed difference *or a bigger difference in either direction (A better than B or B better than A)*
- is a chance finding *that has occurred with equal treatments ($\mu_1 = \mu_2$ or when the null hypothesis is true)*

Commit this definition to memory, it is important!

To complete the logic, we consider this statement and argue as follows: there is only a 4.2 per cent chance of seeing a difference as big as the one observed with equal treatments. This is a small probability, and it is telling us that these data are not at all likely to have occurred with equal treatments, and it is on this basis that we do not believe that the treatments are equal. We declare statistically significant differences between the treatment means.

In contrast, if the *p*-value had been, say, 0.65, then the definition says that there is a 65 per cent probability of seeing a difference as big (or bigger) than the one observed with equal treatments. Now, 65 per cent is quite a high probability, and what we are seeing in this case is a difference that is entirely consistent with $\mu_1 = \mu_2$; it is the kind of difference you would expect to see with equal treatments, and therefore, we have no reason to doubt the equality of the population means.

Another way of thinking about the *p*-value is as a measure of how consistent the difference is with equal treatments (or equivalently with the null hypothesis). A low *p*-value says that the difference is not consistent with equal treatments, while a high value says that the difference is consistent with equal treatments. The conventional cut-off between *low* and *high* is 0.05.

Many people ask at this stage: why 0.05? Well, it is in one sense an arbitrary choice – the cut-off could easily have been 0.04 or 0.075, but 0.05 has become the agreed value, the convention. We will explore the implications of this choice later when we look at type I and type II errors.

The way that the hypotheses are set up is that we always structure H_1 to be our *objective*. H_1 represents the desirable outcome; we want to come out of the clinical trial concluding in favour of H_1. The *p*-value measures how consistent the data are with H_0, and if the *p*-value is small, the data are not consistent with H_0, and we declare statistical significance and decide in favour of H_1. In this way, we are essentially trying to disprove H_0. This is the *scientific method* with its roots in philosophical reasoning; the way science advances is by disproving things rather than by proving them. For example, proving that *all swans are white* is very difficult, but you only have to see one black swan to disprove that statement.

3.3.2 Calculating the *p*-value

We will start with a very simple situation to see how we actually calculate *p*-values. Suppose we want to know whether a coin is a fair coin; by that, we mean that when we flip the coin, it has an equal chance of coming down heads (H) or tails (T).

Let pr(H) denote the probability of the coin coming down heads. We can then formulate null and alternative hypotheses as follows:

$$H_0 : pr(H) = \frac{1}{2} \text{(fair coin)} \quad H_1 : pr(H) \neq \frac{1}{2} \text{(unfair coin)}$$

We now need some data on which to evaluate the hypotheses. Suppose we flip the coin 20 times and end up with 15 heads and 5 tails. Without thinking too much about probabilities and *p*-values, what would your intuition lead you to conclude? Would you say that the data provide evidence that the coin is not fair, or are the data consistent with the coin being fair?

We will now be a little more structured about this. Because this is such a simple situation, we can write down everything that could have happened in this experiment and fairly easily calculate the probabilities associated with each of those outcomes *under the assumption that the coin is fair*. These outcomes and probabilities are contained in Table 3.5.

Note that we have included a column H − T; this is the number of heads minus the number of tails. This is done in order to link with what we do when we are comparing treatments where we use *differences* to measure treatment effects.

So with a fair coin, getting 12 heads and 8 tails, for example, will happen on 0.120 (12 per cent) of occasions. The most likely outcome with a fair coin, not surprisingly, is 10 heads and 10 tails, and this will happen 17.6 per cent of the time. The extreme outcomes are not at all likely, but even 20 heads and 0 tails can still occur, and we will see this outcome 0.000095 per cent of the time!

Our data were 15 heads and 5 tails, so how do we calculate the *p*-value? Well, remember the earlier definition and translate that into the current setting: *the probability of getting the observed difference or a bigger difference in either direction with a fair coin*. To get the *p*-value, we add up the probabilities (calculated when the null hypothesis is true; coin fair) associated with our *difference* (15 heads and 5 tails gives a difference of H − T = 10) or a bigger difference H − T in either direction. This is given by

$$= (0.00000095 + 0.000019 + 0.00018 + 0.0011 + 0.0046 + 0.015) \times 2$$
$$= 0.0417998 \text{ or } 0.0418 = p$$

This means that there is only a 4.18 per cent probability of seeing the 15/5 split or a more extreme split (either way) with a fair coin. This probability is below the magical 5 per cent, we have a statistically significant result, and the evidence suggests that the coin is not fair.

Had we seen the 14/6 split, however, the *p*-value would have increased to 0.0417998 + 2 × 0.037 = 0.1157998, a non-significant result; the 14/6 split is not sufficiently extreme for us to be able to reject the null hypothesis (according to the conventional cut-off at 5 per cent). The 15/5 split (H − T = 10 or − 10) therefore is the smallest split that just achieves statistical significance.

Table 3.5 Outcomes and probabilities for 20 flips of a fair coin (see below for the method of calculation for the probabilities)

Heads (H)	Tails (T)	H − T	Probability (when coin fair)
20	0	20	0.00000095
19	1	18	0.000019
18	2	16	0.00018
17	3	14	0.0011
16	4	12	0.0046
15	5	10	0.015
14	6	8	0.037
13	7	6	0.074
12	8	4	0.120
11	9	2	0.160
10	10	0	0.176
9	11	−2	0.160
8	12	−4	0.120
7	13	−6	0.074
6	14	−8	0.037
5	15	−10	0.015
4	16	−12	0.0046
3	17	−14	0.0011
2	18	−16	0.00018
1	19	−18	0.000019
0	20	−20	0.00000095

Calculating the probabilities for a fair coin:

Suppose we flip the coin just three times. The possible combinations are written below. Because the coin is fair, these are all equally likely. And so each has probability $(1/2^3) = 0.125$ of occurring.

	Probability
H H H	0.125
H H T	0.125
H T H	0.125
T H H	0.125
T T H	0.125
T H T	0.125
H T T	0.125
T T T	0.125

In terms of numbers of heads (H) and numbers of tails (T), there are just four possibilities, and we simply add up the probabilities corresponding to the individual combinations.

Heads (H)	Tails (T)	Probability (when coin fair)
3	0	$0.125 = 1 \times 1/2^3$
2	1	$0.375 = 3 \times 1/2^3$
1	2	$0.375 = 3 \times 1/2^3$
0	3	$0.125 = 1 \times 1/2^3$

For 20 flips, we get the probabilities by multiplying $1/2^{20}$ by the number of combinations that give rise to that particular outcome, so, for example, with 12 heads and 8 tails, this is $20! \div 12! \times 8!$ where $n!$ denotes $n \times n - 1 \times \ldots \times 2 \times 1$.

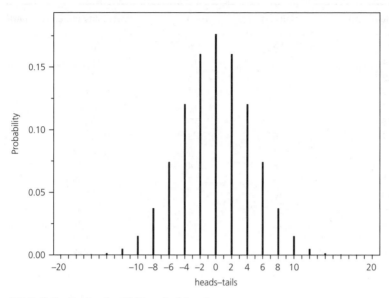

Figure 3.2 Null distribution for 20 flips of a fair coin

It is useful to look at this visually. Figure 3.2 plots each of the outcomes on the *x*-axis with the corresponding probabilities, calculated when the null hypothesis (under the null hypothesis) is true, on the *y*-axis. Note that the *x*-axis has been labelled according to *heads – tails* (H − T), the number of heads minus the number of tails. This identifies each outcome uniquely and allows us to express each data value as a difference. More generally, we will label this the *test statistic*; it is the statistic on which the *p*-value calculation is based. The graph and the associated table of probabilities are labelled the *null distribution (of the test statistic)*.

Using the plot, we calculate the *p*-value firstly by identifying the outcome we saw in our data and secondly by adding up all those probabilities associated with that outcome and more extreme outcomes (*bigger* differences in terms of the test statistic) in both directions (positive and negative). Returning to the H − T difference of 10 or −10 (the 15/5 split), this outcome is at the boundary between $p \leq 0.05$ and $p > 0.05$ and just achieves statistical significance. We call this value for the test statistic the *critical value*.

3.3.3 A common process

In the previous section, we have calculated the *p*-value in a very simple situation. Nonetheless, in more complex situations, the steps that are required to calculate *p* are basically the same. Just briefly returning to the coin, all possible outcomes were expressed in terms of the difference, H − T. This quantity is what we referred to in Section 1.8.1 as the signal. Large differences are giving strong signals, strong evidence that the coin is not fair, and small differences in contrast are giving weak signals.

We will develop the methodology for calculating p-values in relation to the comparison of two independent means for a between-patient design. The resulting statistical test is known as the unpaired or two-sample t-test. The evidence for differences will depend on the strength of the signal together with the extent of the noise and the sample size.

The null and alternative hypotheses are specified as follows:

$$H_0 : \mu_1 = \mu_2 \quad H_1 : \mu_1 \neq \mu_2$$

The signal is measured by the observed difference $\bar{x}_1 - \bar{x}_2$, and the noise is captured by the standard deviations s_1 and s_2 observed in treatment groups 1 and 2, respectively, and finally, we also need to factor in the sample sizes n_1 and n_2.

Consider the earlier example comparing two treatments for the reduction of blood pressure. The sample sizes in the two treatment groups were $n_1 = 20$ and $n_2 = 20$, and the sample means were

$$\bar{x}_1 = 9.6 \text{ mmHg (active)}$$
$$\bar{x}_2 = 4.2 \text{ mmHg (placebo)}$$

The observed difference $\bar{x}_1 - \bar{x}_2 = 5.4 \text{mmHg}$ is the signal, and in order to calculate the p-value, we need to calculate the probability of seeing a difference between the treatment means at least as large as 5.4 when in fact the true treatment means are the same. There is a mathematical trick that allows us to do this in a fairly straightforward way by considering the signal divided by the standard error. The reason for doing this is that when the null hypothesis is true ($\mu_1 = \mu_2$), this ratio, $\left(\dfrac{\bar{x}_1 - \bar{x}_2}{se} \right)$, has a predictable behaviour and we can calculate probabilities associated with its values. Remember *randomness is entirely predictable*, and when the null hypothesis is true, any differences seen between the two sample means are just due to chance (random variation). We can calculate the required probabilities under those circumstances.

Applying the formula, the standard error calculation (see Section 2.5.1) gives $se = 2.57$, and the numerical value of the difference between the means divided by the standard error (=5.4/2.57) is then 2.10. In this example, this is what we will call the *test statistic*, and it is going to be the statistic on which the test is based. This ratio is also known as the *z-score*, and we will use these two terms interchangeably at various points in our development.

Seeing a signal >5.4 mmHg is equivalent to seeing a signal/se ratio >2.10, assuming that the noise is fixed, and it is this ratio that will lead to the p-value.

The probabilities associated with values of this signal/se ratio, under the assumption that the two population means are the same, are given by a particular distribution, the t-distribution. Figure 3.3 displays these probabilities for the example we are considering. Note that we have labelled this the t-distribution on 38 degrees of freedom (df); we will say more about where the 38 comes from in the next chapter.

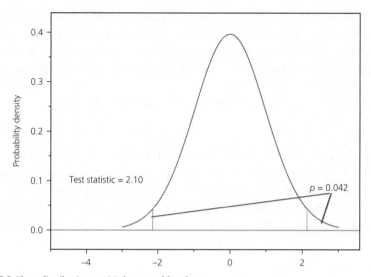

Figure 3.3 The t-distribution on 38 degrees of freedom
Probability density on the y-axis is actually the probability per unit on the x-axis. This makes the total area under the curve equal to 1 or 100%.

Using computer programs, we can add up all the probabilities associated with the observed value 2.10 of the test statistic and more extreme values in both directions (A better than B and B better than A) as seen in the identified areas under the t-distribution to give the *p*-value, 0.042.

This calculation of the *p*-value comes from the probabilities associated with these signal/se ratios (z-scores), and this forms a common theme across many statistical test procedures. To reiterate, the signal/se ratio is also referred to as the test statistic. The distribution of the test statistic when the null hypothesis is true (equal treatments) is termed the *null distribution*.

In general, we can think of the *p*-value calculation as a series of five steps as follows:

1 Formulate null and alternative hypotheses. In all cases, the alternative hypothesis represents the *desirable* outcome. In a superiority trial, this means that the null hypothesis is equality (or no effect/no change/no dependence), while the alternative hypothesis is inequality (there is an effect/a change/a dependence).

2 Calculate the value of the test statistic (usually = signal/se = z-score). The formula for the test statistic will be based on a standard approach determined by the data type, the design of the trial (between or within patient) and the hypotheses of interest. Mathematics has provided us with optimum procedures for all the common (and not so common) situations, and we will see numerous examples in subsequent sections.

3 Determine the null distribution of the chosen test statistic, that is, what are the probabilities associated with all the potential values of the test statistic when the null hypothesis is true? Again, mathematical theory (*randomness is*

entirely predictable) has provided us with solutions to this, and all of these null distributions are known; we simply have to look them up.

4 Obtain the *p*-value by adding up the probabilities associated with the calculated value of the test statistic and more extreme values when the null hypothesis is true. This will correspond to adding up the probabilities associated with the observed value or more extreme values of that signal (treatment difference).

Finally, *step 5* is to draw conclusions; if $p \leq 0.05$, then declare statistical significance; if $p > 0.05$, then the differences are not statistically significant.

There is another way to think about the test statistic in terms of *evidence* for true differences. If the signal is strong (large differences) and the standard error is small, indicating that we have a reliable estimate of the true difference, then the ratio of the signal and the standard error (the test statistic) will be numerically large, either in a positive or a negative direction depending on the direction of the treatment effect. When this happens, we will have a value of the test statistic that is well away from zero and in what we call the tails of the null distribution. Figure 3.3 indicates a situation where that has happened, and this is precisely the setting where we end up with small, statistically significant *p*-values. The ratio of the signal to the standard error or z-score can therefore be thought of as a measure of evidence for differences, where large values allow us to conclude in favour of such differences.

Finally, what we are talking about here links back to our discussion on the signal-to-noise ratio, sample size and evidence in Chapter 1. We said then that a large value of the signal-to-noise ratio points towards treatment difference, whereas a small value of the signal-to-noise ratio does not. We also added that a large sample size tells us that this ratio is reliable, while a small sample size tells us this the ratio is unreliable. The sample size combines with the signal-to-noise ratio to produce the signal/se ratio to give us our measure of evidence. In particular for the difference between two means with an equal number (n) of patients per group and an assumed common standard deviation, it is easy to show that the signal/se ratio is equal to the square root of $n/2$ multiplied by the signal-to-noise ratio as mentioned at the end of Section 1.8.3.

3.3.4 The language of statistical significance

There is a fair amount of language that we wrap around this process. We talk in terms of a *test of significance*. If $p \leq 0.05$, we declare statistical significance and *reject the null hypothesis at the 5 per cent level*. We call 5 per cent the *significance level* – it is the level at which we declare statistical significance. If $p > 0.05$, then we say that we have a non-significant difference and we are *unable to reject the null hypothesis at the 5 per cent level*.

Our conventional cut-off for statistical significance is 5 per cent, but we also use other levels, notably 1 per cent and 0.1 per cent. If $p \leq 0.01$, then the evidence is even stronger that there are differences and we have highly significant differences. If $p \leq 0.001$, then the evidence is even stronger still and we have very highly significant differences.

There is often quite a bit of discussion when we see $0.05 < p \leq 0.10$: *almost significant, a trend towards significance, approaching significance* and other imaginative phrases! I have some sympathy with such comments. One thing we have to remember is that the *p*-value scale is a continuum, and to have a strict cut-off at 0.05 is in a sense unrealistic. There really is little difference, from a strength of evidence point of view, between $p = 0.048$ and $p = 0.053$, yet one gives statistical significance and one does not. Unfortunately, many practitioners (including regulators) seem to have a strict demarcation at 0.05. In one sense, this is understandable; having a strict cut-off at 0.05 removes any ambiguity.

3.3.5 One-sided and two-sided tests

The *p*-value calculation detailed in the previous section gives what we call a *two-sided* or a *two-tailed test* since we calculate *p* by taking into account values of the test statistic equal to, or more extreme, than that observed, in both directions. So, for example, with the coin, we look for movement away from *coin fair* both in terms of *heads more likely than tails* and *tails more likely than heads*.

In part, this is because of the way we set up the hypotheses; in our earlier discussion, we asked, 'is the coin fair?' or 'is the coin not fair?' We could have asked a different question – 'is the coin fair?' or 'are heads more likely than tails?' – in which case, we could have been justified in calculating the *p*-value only in the direction corresponding to *heads more likely than tails*. This would have given us a *one-sided (or a one-tailed) p-value*. Under these circumstances, had we seen 17 tails and 3 heads, then this would not have led to a significant *p*-value, and we would have discounted that outcome as of no interest; it is not in the direction that we are looking for.

Clearly, one-sided *p*-values are of interest to sponsors: firstly, they are smaller and more likely to give a positive result, and, secondly, many sponsors would argue that they are only interested in departures from the null hypothesis in one particular direction, the one that favours their drug. While this may be an argument a sponsor might use, the regulators (and the scientific community more generally) unfortunately would not support it. Regulators are interested in differences both ways and insist that generally *p*-values are two-sided. It must be said though that in many cases they are also comfortable with one-sided *p*-values, but when this is the case, they also state that the significance level used is 0.025 rather than 0.05. Now, because most situations are symmetric, the two-sided *p* is usually equal to 2 × the one-sided *p*, so it actually makes no difference operationally whether we use one-sided or two-sided *p*-values in terms of detecting a positive outcome for the experimental treatment!

ICH E9 (1998): 'Note for Guidance on Statistical Principles for Clinical Trials'

'It is important to clarify whether one- or two-sided tests of statistical significance will be used, and in particular to justify prospectively the use of one-sided tests … The approach of setting type I errors for one-sided tests at half the conventional type I error used in two-sided tests is preferable in regulatory settings'.

CHAPTER 4

Tests for simple treatment comparisons

4.1 The unpaired t-test

In Section 3.3.3, we introduced the general structure for a significance test with the comparison of two means in a parallel-group trial. This resulted in a procedure that goes under the general heading of the two-sample (or unpaired) t-test. This test was developed for continuous data, although it is applicable more widely and, in particular, is frequently used for score and count data.

The test was developed almost 100 years ago by William Sealy Gosset. Gosset was in fact a chemist by training and was employed by the Guinness brewery, initially in Dublin, Ireland, but subsequently at the Guinness brewery in London. He became interested in statistics and in particular in the application of statistics to the improvement of quality within the brewing process. Gosset's work was based on a combination of mathematics and empirical experience (trial and error), but the procedures he came up with have certainly stood the test of time; the unpaired t-test is undoubtedly the most commonly used (although not always appropriately) statistical test of them all.

The calculation of the p-value in the example in Section 3.3.3 consisted of adding up the probabilities, associated with values of the signal/se ratio greater than the observed value of 2.10, given by the t-distribution. It turns out that these probabilities depend upon the number of patients included in the trial. There are an infinite number of t-distributions (t_1, t_2, t_3, ...), and the one we choose is based on calculating the total sample size (both groups combined) and subtracting two. We will see that this t-distribution is used in other settings where the rule for choosing the particular distribution is different, but the rule for the unpaired t-test is $n_1 + n_2 - 2$. This quantity, the index to identify which particular t-distribution to use, as noted in Section 3.3.3 is called the *degrees of freedom*.

There is a connection with what we are seeing here and the calculation of the confidence interval in Chapter 3. Recall Table 3.1 within Section 3.1.3, *Changing the multiplying constant*. It turns out that p-values and confidence intervals are linked, and we will explore this further in a later chapter. The multiplying constants for df = 38 are 2.02 for 95 per cent confidence and 2.71 for 99 per cent confidence. If we were to look at the t_{38} distribution, we would see

---

Statistical Thinking for Non-Statisticians in Drug Regulation, Second Edition. Richard Kay.
© 2015 John Wiley & Sons, Ltd. Published 2015 by John Wiley & Sons, Ltd.

that ±2.02 cuts off the outer 5 per cent probability, while ±2.71 cuts off the outer 1 per cent probability.

Having calculated the p-value, we would also calculate the 95 per cent confidence interval for the difference $\mu_1 - \mu_2$ to give us information about the magnitude of the treatment effect. For the data in the example in Section 3.3.3, this confidence interval is given by

$$(5.4 \pm 2.02 \times 2.57) = (0.2,\ 10.6)$$

So with 95 per cent confidence, we can say that the true treatment effect $(\mu_1 - \mu_2)$ is somewhere in the interval 0.2 mmHg to 10.6 mmHg.

4.2 The paired t-test

The *paired t-test* also known as the *one-sample t-test* was also developed by Gosset. This test is primarily used for the analysis of data arising from within-patient designs, although we also see it applied when comparing a baseline value with a final value within the same treatment group.

Consider a two-period, two-treatment crossover trial in asthma comparing an active treatment (A) and a placebo treatment (B) in which the following PEF (l/min) data, in terms of the value at the end of each period, were obtained (Table 4.1).

Patients 1–16 received treatment A followed by treatment B, while patients 17–32 received treatment B first followed by treatment A.

The final column above has calculated the A–B differences, and as we shall see, the paired t-test works entirely on the column of differences. Again, we will follow through several steps for the calculation of the p-value for the A versus B comparison:

1 Let μ be the population mean value for the column of differences. The null and alternative hypotheses are expressed in terms of this quantity:

$$H_0 : \mu = 0 \qquad H_1 : \mu \neq 0$$

Table 4.1 Data from a crossover trial in asthma (hypothetical)

Patient	A	B	Difference (A–B)
1	395	362	33
2	404	385	19
3	382	386	−4
.			
.			
.			
32	398	344	54

A non-zero value for μ will reflect treatment differences; a positive value in particular is telling us that the active treatment is effective.

2 Again, the test will be based on the signal/se ratio. In this case, the signal is the observed mean $\bar{x}$ of the column of differences, and se is the standard error associated with that mean. For these data,

$$\bar{x} = 28.4 \text{l/min} \quad se(\text{of } \bar{x}) = 11.7 \text{l/min}$$

The se here is obtained from the standard deviation of the differences divided by the square root of 32, the number of differences in that final column.

The test statistic = signal/se = 28.4/11.7 = 2.43 captures the evidence for treatment differences. Larger values, either positive or negative, are an indication of treatment differences.

3 The probabilities associated with the values that this signal/se ratio can take when the treatments are the same ($\mu = 0$) are again given by the t shape; in this case, the appropriate t-distribution is t_{31}, the t-distribution on 31 df. Why t_{31}? The appropriate t-distribution is indexed by the number of patients or number of differences -1.

4 Our computer programs now calculate the p-value, the probability associated with getting a value for the signal/se ratio at least as large as 2.43, in either direction, when the null hypothesis is true. This value turns out to be 0.021 (see Figure 4.1). This value also reflects, assuming that the se is fixed, the probability of seeing a mean difference at least as big as 28.4l/min by chance (with equal treatments). This signal is sufficiently strong for us to conclude a real treatment effect.

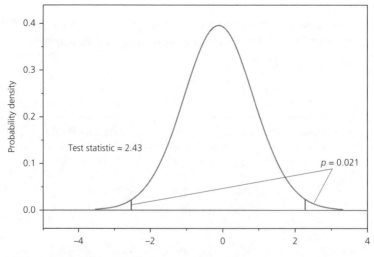

Figure 4.1 The t-distribution on 31 df

The p-value is <0.05, giving statistical significance at the 5 per cent level, and we conclude, on the basis of the evidence, that treatment A (active) is more efficacious than treatment B (placebo); the active treatment works.

This test is based entirely on the column of differences; once the column of differences is calculated, the original data are no longer used. An alternative approach might have been to simply calculate the mean value on A and the mean value on B and to compare the two using the unpaired t-test. Would this have worked? In fact, no, using the unpaired t-test in this way would have been incorrect; the unpaired t-test is used to compare means across two independent samples. The paired t-test uses the data in the most efficient way; forming the column of differences links the observations on the same patient and is effectively using each patient as their own control. Calculating the A and B means separately and taking their difference would in fact have given the same signal as the mean of the column of differences, but the se would have been different. It would not reflect the patient-to-patient variability in the A − B differences, but would be based on the patient-to-patient (within-group) variability in the value of the endpoint itself.

Does it matter which way round the differences are calculated, A−B or B−A? No, as long as we are consistent across all of the patients, it does not matter and will simply have the effect of changing the sign of the test statistic, but the two-sided p-value will remain unchanged.

As with the unpaired t-test, it would be useful to calculate a confidence interval for the treatment effect, μ. This is given by

$$\left(\bar{x} \pm 2.04 \times se\right) = \left(28.4 \pm 2.04 \times 11.7\right)$$
$$= \left(4.5, \ 52.3\right)$$

Here, 2.04 is the appropriate multiplication constant for 95 per cent confidence with 32 patients. So, we can be 95 per cent confident that the treatment difference (active treatment effect), μ, is between 4.5 l/min and 52.3 l/min.

Before we move on, it should be pointed out that the paired t-test provides a valid analysis for continuous data arising from a crossover trial only when the trial is balanced, that is, when the number of patients following the A/B sequence is the same as the number of patients following the B/A sequence. When this is not true, the analysis needs to be modified slightly. This is because in many settings there will also be a *period effect*, that is, irrespective of treatment, patients may respond differently in period I compared to period II. This could be caused, for example, by the temporal nature of the underlying disease, by external conditions that may be changing over time, or through a learning effect. If a period effect is present, but the trial is balanced, then there will be equal numbers of A and B patients giving responses in period I and also in period II, and under fairly general conditions, the period effect will cancel out in the paired t-test comparison of the treatments. When balance is not present, then this effect will not cancel out and there will be bias. The reader is referred to Senn (2002), Section 3.6 for details of how to deal with this.

4.3 Interpreting the t-tests

The following example illustrates several issues and problems associated with the interpretation of p-values arising out of the t-tests. The setting is a very common one where a variable is measured at baseline and then subsequently at the end of the treatment period and the analysis focuses on the relative effects of the two treatments.

Example 4.1 Comparison of two active treatments for the treatment of major depressive disorder in a randomised control trial

The primary endpoint in this trial was the 17-point Hamilton Depression Scale (HAMD-17), and the data presented in Table 4.2 correspond to mean (se).

Table 4.2 Data on HAMD-17 (hypothetical)

	Baseline	Final (week 8)	Change from baseline
Active A (n = 36)	27.4 (1.18)	15.3 (0.92)	12.1 (0.95)
Active B (n = 35)	26.8 (1.22)	11.8 (1.32)	15.0 (1.17)

There are a number of comparisons that we can undertake:
1 Unpaired t-test comparing treatment means at baseline, p = 0.73
2 Unpaired t-test comparing treatment means at week 8, p = 0.030
3 Unpaired t-test comparing the mean change from baseline in the active A group with that in the active B group, p = 0.055
4 Paired t-test of baseline with week 8 in the active A group, $p \ll 0.001$ (this means the p-value is very much less than 0.001)
5 Paired t-test of baseline with week 8 in the active B group, $p \ll 0.001$
Let us consider each of these tests in turn and their interpretation:
1 Test 1 is telling us that the treatment means are comparable at baseline, which is what we would expect to see given that this is a randomised trial. Of course, chance differences can sometimes occur. Indeed, in a randomised trial, we would expect to see $p \leq 0.05$ for such a baseline comparison 5 per cent of the time. See Section 6.9 for a further discussion on this point.
2 This test compares the treatment groups at week 8. The p-value suggests a treatment difference, but does this test necessarily provide an analysis of the data that uses all of the information? Is there a possibility that we are being misled? Note that even though the earlier comparison of baseline means gave a non-significant p-value, the mean in active A group at baseline is slightly higher than the mean in the B group. Could this have contributed to the observed difference at week 8?
3 Test 3 for the comparison of the mean change from baseline between the groups is marginally non-significant. It would appear that the difference seen in test 2 is, in part, caused by the differences already seen at baseline. Looking at change from baseline has accounted for the minor baseline imbalances and, in general, is the basis for a more appropriate and

sensitive analysis than simply looking at the week 8 means. It would be inappropriate to place too much emphasis on the fact that in test 3 the *p*-value is technically non-significant; recall that 0.05 is a somewhat arbitrary cut-off with regard to what we define as *statistical significance*. It is test 3 that provides the most appropriate information for evaluating the relative effects of the two treatments.

We will say quite a bit later, in the chapter on adjusting the analysis (Chapter 5) about additional improvements to this kind of analysis that increase sensitivity further and also avoid the so-called potential problem of regression towards the mean. For the moment though, it is test 3 that is the best way to compare the treatments.

4 Test 4 has given a very impressive *p*-value, but what is the correct interpretation of this test? The fall in HAMD score from 27.4 to 15.3 surely indicates that active A is an effective treatment! Well, actually it does not. The fall seen in this group could indeed have been caused by the medication, but equally, it could have been caused, for example, by the ancillary counselling that all patients will be receiving or as a result of the placebo effect (the psychological impact of being in the trial and receiving *treatment*), and we have no way of knowing which of these factors is having an effect and in what combination. The only way of identifying whether active drug A is efficacious is to have a parallel placebo group and undertake test 3; this would isolate the effect due to the specific medication from the other factors that could be causing the fall.

5 Test 5 should be interpreted in exactly the same way as test 4. The fall is impressive, but is it due to the active medication? We don't know and in the absence of a placebo group we will never know.

Suppose that test 4 had given $p = 0.07$ and test 5 had given $p = 0.02$. Would that therefore mean that active B is a better treatment than active A? No, in order to evaluate the relative effect of two treatments, we have to compare them! Directly that is, not indirectly through the test 4 and 5 comparisons back to baseline.

4.4 The chi-square test for binary data

4.4.1 Pearson chi-square

The previous sections have dealt with the t-tests, methods applicable to continuous data. We will now consider tests for binary data, where the outcome at the subject level is a simple dichotomy: success/failure. In a between-patient, parallel-group trial, our goal here is to compare two proportions or rates.

In Section 3.2.2, we presented data from a clinical trial comparing trastuzumab to observation only after adjuvant chemotherapy in HER2-positive breast cancer. The incidence rates in the test treatment and control groups were, respectively, 7.0 per cent and 4.7 per cent.

The proportion of patients suffering SAEs in the trastuzumab group (7.0 per cent) is clearly greater than the corresponding proportion in the observation-only group (4.7 per cent), but is this difference (signal) strong enough for us to conclude that there are real differences, or could this be a difference that is compatible with chance?

Table 4.3 Observed and expected $O(E)$ frequencies for the trastuzumab data

	≥1 SAE	No SAEs	Total
Trastuzumab	$O_1(E_1) = 117(98)$	$O_2(E_2) = 1560(1579)$	$n_1 = 1677$
Observation	$O_3(E_3) = 81(100)$	$O_4(E_4) = 1629(1610)$	$n_2 = 1710$
Total	198	3189	3387

The chi-square test for comparing two proportions or rates was developed by Karl Pearson around 1900 and predates the development of the t-tests. The steps involved in the *Pearson chi-square test* can be set down as follows:

1 The null and alternative hypotheses relate to the two true rates, θ_1 and θ_2:

$$H_0 : \theta_1 = \theta_2 \qquad H_1 : \theta_1 \neq \theta_2$$

2 In forming a test statistic, Pearson argued in the following way. In the data as a whole, we see a total of 198 patients suffering SAEs. Had there been no differences between the groups in terms of the rate of SAEs, then we would have seen equal proportions of patients suffering SAEs in the two groups. This would have meant seeing $198 \times (1677/3387) = 98$ patients with SAEs in the trastuzumab group and $198 \times (1710/3387) = 100$ in the observation-only group. Similarly, we should have seen 1579 patients not suffering SAEs in the trastuzumab group and 1610 such patients in the observation-only group. We term these values, the *expected frequencies*, and denote them by E; the *observed frequencies* are denoted by O. These observed and expected frequencies are set down in Table 4.3 where the entries in the 2×2 contingency table are $O(E)$.

We now need a measure of how far away we are from *equal treatments*. Clearly, if the Es (what we should have seen with equal treatments) are close to the Os (what we have actually seen), then we have little evidence of a real difference in the incidence rates between the groups. However, the further apart the Os are from the Es, the more we believe the true SAE rates are different. The test statistic is formed by looking at each of the four *cells* of the table and firstly calculating $(O - E)$. Some of these values will be positive and some negative, for example, $+19$ in the trastuzumab ≥1 SAE cell and -19 in the observation-only ≥1 SAE cell. We then square these values (this gets rid of the sign), divide by the corresponding E (we will say more of this later) and add up the resulting quantities across the four cells as shown below.

$$\sum \frac{(O - E)^2}{E}$$

$$= \frac{(117 - 98)^2}{98} + \frac{(1560 - 1579)^2}{1579} + \frac{(81 - 100)^2}{100} + \frac{(1629 - 1610)^2}{1610}$$

$$= 7.75$$

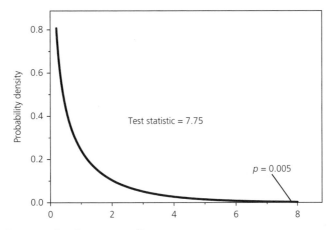

Figure 4.2 Chi-square distribution on 1 df

This value captures the evidence in support of treatment differences. If what we have seen (Os) is close to what we should have seen with *equal* treatments (Es), then this statistic will have a value close to zero. If, however, the Os and the Es are well separated, then this statistic will have a larger positive value; the more the Os and the Es disagree, the larger it will be. For the moment, this test statistic is not in the form of a signal/se ratio, but we will see later that it can also be formulated in that way.

3 Pearson calculated the probabilities associated with values of this test statistic when the treatments are the same, to produce the null distribution. This distribution is called the chi-square distribution on one df, denoted χ_1^2, and is displayed in Figure 4.2. Note that values close to zero have the highest probability. Values close to zero for the test statistic would only result when the Os and the Es agree closely, whereas large values for the test statistic are unlikely when the treatments are truly the same.

4 To obtain the p-value, we now need to add up all of the probabilities associated with values of the test statistic at least as big as the value observed, 7.75 in our data. As can be seen from Figure 4.2, this value is well out to the right of the distribution and gives, in fact, $p = 0.005$.

5 The p-value is ≤ 0.01, and so we have a highly significant result, a highly significant difference between the treatment groups in terms of SAE rates. Trastuzumab is associated with a significant increase in the SAE rate compared to observation only.

Several aspects of this p-value calculation deserve mention:

• The calculation of the test statistic involves division by E. This essentially weights the evidence from the different cells, so that a cell with a smaller expected frequency gets more weight and a cell with a larger expected frequency is down weighted. This makes sense since an $O - E$ difference of 19 in around 100 is a much more relevant *difference* than a difference of 19 in 1600 and the test statistic is more influenced by the former than the latter.

- The $(O-E)^2$ values are all equal to 361, so algebraically, the test statistic could be written as

$$(O-E)^2 \left[\frac{1}{E_1} + \frac{1}{E_2} + \frac{1}{E_3} + \frac{1}{E_4} \right] = 361 \times \left[\frac{1}{98} + \frac{1}{1579} + \frac{1}{100} + \frac{1}{1610} \right]$$

- The null distribution for the t-test depended on the number of subjects in the trial. For the chi-square test comparing two proportions, and providing the sample size is reasonably large, this is not the case; the null distribution is always χ_1^2. As a consequence, we become very familiar with χ_1^2. The *critical value* for 5 per cent significance is 3.841, while 6.635 cuts off the outer 1 per cent probability and 10.83 the outer 0.1 per cent.

4.4.2 The link to a ratio of the signal to the standard error

The formulation of the chi-square test procedure in the previous section, using observed and expected frequencies, is the standard way in which this particular test is developed and presented in most textbooks. It can be shown, however, that this procedure is akin to a development following the earlier signal/se ratio approach.

In comparing two rates, the signal is provided by the observed difference $r_1 - r_2$ in the rates. The standard error for that difference is given by the expression (see Section 2.5.2) $\sqrt{\frac{r_1(1-r_1)}{n_1} + \frac{r_2(1+-r_2)}{n_2}}$. The probabilities associated with the resulting signal/se ratio (the test statistic) when the true rates θ_1 and θ_2 are equal are provided by a special case of the normal distribution, $N(0, 1)$: the normal distribution with mean zero and standard deviation 1. For the trastuzumab example, the signal takes the value 0.023 and the value of the standard error is 0.0081. So to obtain the p-value based on this null distribution, we compare the value of our test statistic ($=0.023/0.0081=2.84$) with the $N(0, 1)$ distribution giving a p-value of 0.0046. The Pearson chi-square test had earlier given $p=0.0054$, a very similar value.

In general, it can be shown that the approach following the signal/se ratio method is mathematically very similar to the standard formulation of the chi-square test using observed and expected frequencies, and in practice, they will invariably give very similar results. Altman (1991) (Section 10.7.4) provides more detail on this connection.

4.5 Measures of treatment benefit

The chi-square test has given a p-value, and this provides the evidence, in general, in relation to the existence of a treatment difference. Through the confidence interval for the difference in the SAE rates calculated earlier in Section 3.2.2, we have some idea of the extent of the treatment effect in absolute terms. There are, however, other measures of treatment benefit/harm in common usage for binary data. Each of these measures – odds ratio (OR), relative risk (RR), relative risk reduction (RRR) and number needed to treat (NNT) – is a way of expressing the treatment benefit. They each have their advantages and their disadvantages, and I think it is fair to say that none of them is universally accepted as the *single best approach*. We will define each of them in turn and provide an interpretation and critique of their use. For further details and discussion, see Grieve (2003).

4.5.1 Odds ratio

In order to understand the odds ratio, you first of all need to understand odds. For the data of Example 3.3, consider each of the treatment groups separately.

For the trastuzumab group, the odds of a patient suffering one or more SAEs are $117/1560 = 0.075$; for every patient free from SAEs, there are 0.075 patients suffering one or more SAEs. For the observation-only group, the odds of a patient suffering one or more SAEs are $81/1629 = 0.050$. In this group, for every patient not suffering SAEs, there are 0.050 patients who do suffer one or more SAEs.

The *odds ratio* is then the ratio of the odds of a patient suffering one or more SAEs:

$$OR = 0.075/0.050 = 1.51$$

An odds ratio of one, or close to one, is telling us that the treatments are the same (or at least similar). An odds ratio greater than one tells us that you are worse off in the test treatment group, and vice versa, but over and above that, the interpretation is not straightforward. It is the definition itself that provides this; the value 1.51 for the odds ratio indicates that the odds of suffering at least one SAE in the trastuzumab group is 1.51 times the odds of suffering at least one SAE in the observation-only group or alternatively a 51 per cent increase in the odds of suffering at least one SAE. What makes this difficult to interpret is that these are statements on the *odds* scale and the odds scale is something that we find difficult to work with.

Usually, the odds relating to the test treatment group go on the top when calculating the ratio (the numerator), while the odds for the control group go on the bottom (the denominator). However, there is no real convention regarding whether it is the odds in favour of success or the odds in favour of failure that we calculate. Had we chosen to calculate the odds in favour of no SAE, the odds ratio would have been $\dfrac{1/0.075}{1/0.050}$, which has the value $0.66 (=1/1.51)$, so take care that when you see an odds ratio presented, you are clear how the calculation has been organised.

4.5.2 Relative risk

The relative risk is defined again as a ratio, this time in relation to the risks calculated for the two treatments. For the trastuzumab group, the *risk* is the proportion of patients suffering one or more SAEs that takes the value

117/1677=0.070, while for the observation-only group, this is 81/1710=0.047. The *relative risk* (sometimes called the *risk ratio*) is then the ratio of these risks:

RR = 0.070/0.047 = 1.47

An relative risk of one, or close to one, is again indicative of similar treatments. An relative risk above one, as here, is saying that the risk in the test treatment group is higher than the risk in the control group. The interpretation beyond that is a little simpler than the odds ratio. The relative risk of 1.47 is telling us that the risk in the trastuzumab group is 47 per cent higher than the risk in the observation-only group.

There are also conventions with relative risk. As with the odds ratio, we usually put the risk for the test treatment group as the numerator and the risk for the control group as the denominator. But now, because we are calculating risk, there should be no confusion with regard to what we view as the event; we tend to calculate relative risk and not relative benefit.

4.5.3 Relative risk reduction

Consider the data presented in Table 4.4 relating to the binary outcome died/survival in a parallel-group trial.

The relative risk is 0.20/0.35=0.57.

When the relative risk is less than one, as in this case, we often also calculate the reduction in the relative risk:

Relative risk reduction $(RRR) = 1 -$ relative risk

In the example relative risk reduction=0.43, there is a 43 per cent reduction in the risk (of death) in the active group compared to control.

We tend to use relative risk reduction where the intervention is having a benefit in reducing the risk. In the earlier example involving trastuzumab and the incidence of patients suffering one or more SAEs, the active treatment was associated with an increase in risk. We could speak in terms of a relative risk increase (RRI) of 0.47 (=1.47−1), a 47 per cent increase in the risk of suffering one or more SAEs, but this tends not to be done.

4.5.4 Number needed to treat

In the example of the previous section (Table 4.4), 80 per cent of patients in the active group survived compared to 65 per cent in the placebo group. So out of 100 patients, we would expect to see, on average, an additional 15 per cent

Table 4.4 Active/placebo comparison: Binary outcome survival (hypothetical)

	Died	Survived	Total
Active	20	80	100
Placebo	35	65	100
Total	55	145	200

(80 per cent − 65 per cent) surviving in the active group. The *number needed to treat* is then 100/15 or 6.7. We need to treat on average an additional 6.7 patients with the active treatment in order to save one additional life.

A convenient formula for number needed to treat is:

$$NNT = \frac{1}{(0.80 - 0.65)}$$

The denominator here is the difference in the survival proportions.

We usually round this up to the nearest integer, so NNT = 7. We need to treat seven patients with the active medication in order to see one extra patient survive compared to placebo.

There may be some situations where the test treatment is, in fact, harmful relative to the control treatment in terms of a particular endpoint. In these circumstances, it does not make sense to take talk about number needed to treat, and we refer instead to *number needed to harm (NNH)*. So, for the data in Example 3.3, the SAE rate in the trastuzumab group was 70 per cent compared to 47 per cent in the observation-only group, and the number needed to harm is equal to 1/(0.70 − 0.47), which rounds up to five.

4.5.5 Confidence intervals

We saw in the previous section methods for calculating confidence intervals for the difference in the SAE rates or the event rates themselves. We will now look at methods for calculating a confidence interval for the odds ratio.

Calculating confidence intervals for ratios is a little more tricky than calculating confidence intervals for differences. We saw in Chapter 3 that, in general, the formula for the confidence interval is

$$statistic \pm (constant \times se)$$

With a ratio, it is not possible to obtain a standard error formula directly; however, it is possible to obtain standard errors for log ratios. (Taking logs converts a ratio into a difference with log A/B = log A − log B.) So we first of all calculate confidence intervals on the log scale. It does not make any difference what base we use for the logs, but by convention, we usually use natural logarithms, denoted *ln*.

The standard error for the *ln* of the odds ratio is given by

$$\sqrt{\frac{1}{O_1} + \frac{1}{O_2} + \frac{1}{O_3} + \frac{1}{O_4}}$$

where the *O*s are the respective observed frequencies in the 2 × 2 contingency table (see Table 4.3). In the trastuzumab example, this is given by

$$\sqrt{\frac{1}{117} + \frac{1}{1560} + \frac{1}{81} + \frac{1}{1629}} = 0.149$$

The 95 per cent confidence interval for the *ln* of the odds ratio is then

$$\ell n 1.51 \pm (1.96 \times 0.149) = (0.120,\ 0.704)$$

Finally, we convert this back onto the odds ratio scale by taking antilogs of the ends of this interval to give a 95 per cent confidence interval for the odds ratio as (1.13, 2.02). We can be 95 per cent confident that the odds ratio lies within this range.

In a similar way, we can calculate a confidence interval for the RR. The method is the same as for the odds ratio but with a different formula for the standard error. The standard error for the log of the relative risk is given by

$$\sqrt{\frac{1}{O_1} + \frac{1}{O_3} - \frac{1}{n_1} - \frac{1}{n_2}}$$

In the trastuzumab example, this is given by

$$\sqrt{\frac{1}{117} + \frac{1}{81} - \frac{1}{1677} - \frac{1}{1710}} = 0.140$$

The 95 per cent confidence interval for the *ln* of the relative risk is then

$$ln\ 1.47 \pm (1.96 \times 0.140) = (0.110,\ 0.660)$$

Converting this back onto the relative risk scale gives a 95 per cent confidence interval for the relative risk as (1.12, 1.93), and we can be 95 per cent confident that the relative risk lies within this range.

Previously, when we had calculated a confidence interval, for example, for a difference in rates or for a difference in means, then the confidence interval was symmetric around the estimated difference; in other words, the estimated difference sat squarely in the middle of the interval, and the endpoints were obtained by adding and subtracting the same amount (2 × se). When we calculate a confidence interval for the odds ratio, that interval is symmetric only on the log scale. Once we convert back to the odds ratio scale by taking antilogs, that symmetry is lost. This is not a problem, but it is something that you will notice. It is a property of all standard confidence intervals calculated for ratios.

In similar ways to the aforementioned, we can obtain confidence intervals for a relative risk and for a relative risk reduction. Confidence intervals for NNT are a little more complicated; see Grieve (2003) and Altman (1998) for further details.

4.5.6 Interpretation

In large trials and with events that are rare, the odds ratio and relative risk give very similar values. In fact, we can see this in the trastuzumab example where the odds ratio was 1.51 and the relative risk was 1.47. In smaller trials and with more common events, however, this will not be the case. Comparable values for the odds ratio and the relative risk arise more frequently in cohort studies where generally the sample sizes are large and the events being investigated are often rare, and these measures tend to be used interchangeably. As a result, there seems to be some confusion as to the distinction, and it is my experience that the odds ratio and RR are occasionally labelled incorrectly in clinical research papers, so take care.

It is possible to convert from an odds ratio to an RR (and vice versa). The formula is

$$RR = \frac{OR}{1 - r_c + (r_c \times OR)}$$

where r_c is the absolute risk in the control group. When calculating an odds ratio, or alternatively taking a value for an odds ratio from a publication, the value for the absolute risk in the control group may not be available directly. It may be the case however that a value for this risk is available from an alternative source and an approximate value for the RR can then be calculated. Converting from an odds ratio to an RR can be useful since as discussed earlier the odds ratio can be difficult to interpret. The RR is much easier in this regard.

A question that is sometimes asked is, why do we use the odds ratios when they are such difficult quantities to interpret? Well, there are essentially two reasons. Firstly, in case–control studies in epidemiology, it is not possible to calculate a relative risk; it is only possible to calculate an odds ratio. It is usually the case however in such studies that we are dealing with rare events and the relative risk and the odds ratio are again numerically close together and the odds ratio can then interpreted as if it were a relative risk. I will say more about this issue in a later chapter (see Section 17.4.2). Secondly, we have developed a number of mathematical techniques, such as those relating to meta-analysis (see Chapter 18) and logistic regression (see Section 6.6), that revolve around the odds ratio, and consequently, it tends to dominate our way of thinking about binary data. In summary, although not ideal, the odds ratio is central to the way we analyse and report binary data. However, as pointed out by Grimes and Schulz (2008), 'For most clinicians, odds ratios will remain … well, odd'.

It is also worth mentioning that all of the measures – difference in event rates, OR, RR, RRR and NNT – expressed in isolation, have limitations. What we are trying to do with such quantities is to use a single measure to summarise the data. All of the information is actually contained in the two event proportions/ rates r_1 and r_2, and attempting to summarise two numbers by a single number is inevitably going to lead to problems in particular cases. Beware of those limitations and revert back to r_1 and r_2, if need be, to tell the full story.

4.6 Fisher's exact test

The Pearson chi-square test is what we refer to as a large sample test; this means that provided the sample sizes are fairly large, then it works well. Unfortunately, when the sample sizes in the treatment groups are not large, there can be problems. Under these circumstances, we have an alternative test, *Fisher's exact test*.

Table 4.5 Data for Fisher's exact test

	Success	Failure	Total
Group A	6	18	24
Group B	1	23	24
Total	7	41	48

Table 4.6 Probabilities for Fisher's exact test

Successes on A	Successes on B	Probability
7	0	0.0047
6	1	0.0439
5	2	0.1593
4	3	0.2921
3	4	0.2921
2	5	0.1593
1	6	0.0439
0	7	0.0047

The way this works is as follows. Consider Table 4.5.

Given there are only seven successes in total (and 41 failures), we can easily write down everything that could have happened (recall the way we looked at the flipping of the coin in Section 3.3.2) and calculate the probabilities associated with each of these outcomes when there really are no differences between the treatments (Table 4.6).

We observed the 6/1 split in terms of successes across the two treatment groups in our data, and we can calculate the two-sided p-value by adding up the probabilities associated with those outcomes, which are as extreme, or more extreme, than what we have observed, when the null hypothesis is true (equal treatments). This gives $p = 0.097$ (= $(0.0439 + 0.0047) \times 2$). The corresponding chi-square test applied (inappropriately) to these data would have given $p = 0.041$, and the conclusion would have been slightly different.

The rule of thumb for the use of Fisher's exact test is based on the expected frequencies (E) in the 2×2 contingency table; each of these should be at least five for the chi-square test to be applicable. In our example, the expected frequencies in each of the cells corresponding to *success* are 3.5, supporting the use of Fisher's exact test in this case.

In fact, Fisher's exact test could be used under all circumstances for the calculation of the p-value, even when the sample sizes are not small. Historically, however, we tend not to do this; Fisher's test requires some fairly hefty combinatorial calculations in large samples to get the null probabilities, and in the past, this was very difficult. For larger sample sizes, p-values calculated using either the chi-square test or Fisher's exact test will be similar, so we tend to reserve use of Fisher's exact test for only those cases where there is a problem and use the chi-square test outside of that.

4.7 Tests for categorical and ordinal data

4.7.1 Categorical data

The Pearson chi-square test extends in a straightforward way when there are more than two outcome categories.

Consider four outcome categories labelled A, B, C and D and the comparison of two treatments in terms of the distribution across these categories. Taking the example of categorical data from Chapter 1, we might have:

A = death from cancer causes

B = death from cardiovascular causes

C = death from other causes

D = survival

Consider the following hypothetical data (Table 4.7).

The chi-square test proceeds, as before, by calculating expected frequencies. These are given in Table 4.8.

As before, we compute

$$\sum \frac{(O-E)^2}{E}$$

with the sum being over all eight cells.

Table 4.7 Observed frequencies (O)

	A	B	C	D	Total
Group 1	15	13	20	52	100
Group 2	17	20	23	40	100
Total	32	33	43	92	200

Table 4.8 Expected frequencies (E)

	A	B	C	D	Total
Group 1	16	16.5	21.5	46	100
Group 2	16	16.5	21.5	46	100
Total	32	33	43	92	200

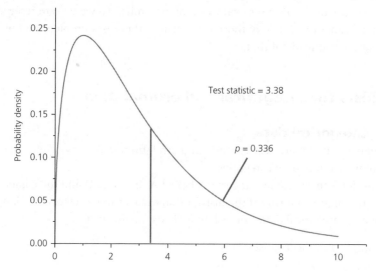

Figure 4.3 Chi-square distribution on 3 df

The resultant test statistic is then compared to the chi-square distribution but this time on three df, written χ_3^2. As we mentioned earlier, the particular chi-square shape that we use is not determined by the number of patients; rather, it depends upon the size of the contingency table. In this example, we have a 2×4 table (four outcome categories), and with two treatment groups, the df for the chi-square distribution are equal to the number of categories -1.

In the example, the test statistic value is 3.38, and Figure 4.3 illustrates the calculation of the p-value, which for these data turns out to be $p = 0.336$. This is a non-significant result.

Although this test provides a valid comparison of the treatment groups in relation to the outcome categories, it is not of any great value in providing a useful conclusion from a clinical perspective. The procedure provides a test of the null hypothesis:

$$H_0 : \theta_{1A} = \theta_{2A} \text{ and } \theta_{1B} = \theta_{2B} \text{ and } \theta_{1C} = \theta_{2C} \text{ and } \theta_{1D} = \theta_{2D}$$

where the suffices label both the treatment group and the outcome category, against what we call the *general alternative hypothesis:*

$$H_1 : \text{the opposite of } H_0$$

But suppose we see a significant p-value, what does it mean? Well, it simply means that there are some differences somewhere across the categories, but nothing more specific than that, and that is not particularly useful.

A further issue is that we very rarely see strictly categorical outcomes in practice in our clinical trials; it is much more common to have an ordering of the categories, giving us ordered categorical or ordinal data, and we will deal with this in the next section. Finally, the problem we discussed in the previous section regarding small sample sizes applies here, and Fisher's exact test should be used when this is the case. The rule of thumb again is that all the expected frequencies should be at least five for the chi-square test to be valid. Computer programs tend to give both p-values (chi-square test and Fisher's exact test) automatically, and it is no great problem therefore to pick the appropriate one depending on sample size and the rule of thumb.

4.7.2 Ordered categorical (ordinal) data

An endpoint that consists of a series of ordered categories is frequently used in our clinical trials in many different therapeutic settings.

The Pearson chi-square test is not appropriate for ordinal data as it does not take any account of the ordering of the outcome categories. The appropriate test is the *Mantel–Haenszel (MH) chi-square test* (Mantel and Haenszel, 1959). This test takes account of the ordering by scoring the ordered categories (e.g. improved = 1, no change = 2, worse = 3) and comparing the average score in one treatment group with the average score in the second treatment group. It is not quite as simple as this, but that is the general idea! In fact, the scores are chosen by the observed data patterns in the two groups combined.

The formula for the test statistic is somewhat complex, but again, this statistic provides the combined evidence in favour of treatment differences. When Mantel and Haenszel developed this procedure, they calculated that when the treatments are identical, the probabilities associated with the test statistic follow a χ_1^2 distribution. This is irrespective of the number of outcome categories, and the test is sometimes referred to as the *chi-square one degree of freedom test for trend*.

Example 4.2 Flutamide plus leuprolide compared to leuprolide alone in the treatment of prostate cancer

The following data (Table 4.9) are taken from a randomised controlled add-on trial (Crawford *et al.*, 1989) comparing leuprolide + placebo (L + P) with leuprolide + flutamide (L + F) in prostate cancer. The endpoint here is improvement in pain at week 4.

Table 4.9 Flutamide data

	Improved	No change	Worse	Total
L + P	50	180	33	263
L + F	73	174	20	267
Total	123	354	53	530

In this example comparison of the test statistic value with χ_1^2 gives $p = 0.006$, a very highly significant result.

A significant p-value coming out of this test is indicative of a shift or trend in one direction across these categories for one treatment compared to the other. It is illustrative to look at the percentages in the various categories as shown in Table 4.10.

Table 4.10 Flutamide data as percentages

	Improved	No change	Worse	Total
L + P	19%	68%	13%	263
L + F	27%	65%	7%	267

In the L + F treatment group, there has been a shift towards the improvement end of the scale compared to the L + P treatment group, and it is this trend that the MH chi-square test has picked up. The Pearson chi-square test does not look for such trends and would have simply compared the 19 per cent with the 27 per cent, the 68 per cent with the 65 per cent and the 13 per cent with the 7 per cent in an overall, average way. Had the ordering been ignored and the Pearson chi-square test applied (incorrectly), then the p-value would have been 0.023. Although this is still statistically significant indicating treatment differences, the p-value is very different from the correct p-value of 0.006, and in many cases, such differences would lead to incorrect conclusions.

As with binary and categorical data, is there an issue with small sample sizes? Well, in fact, no, there is not. The MH test is a different kind of chi-square test and is not built around expected frequencies. As a consequence, it is not affected by small expected frequencies and can be used in all cases for ordinal data. There are some pathological cases where it will break down, but these should not concern us in practical settings.

4.7.3 Measures of treatment benefit

Measures such as the difference in event rates, OR, RR, RRR and NNT do not easily translate into the categorical data context. If we want to construct such measures in these cases, we would collapse the outcome categories to two, the binary case, and proceed as before. In the categorical example covered earlier, this could involve collapsing categories A, B and C to produce a binary outcome death/survival. For example, if the categorical outcome was *Main Reason for Discontinuation*, which was classified as Adverse Event, Withdrawal of Consent, Protocol Violation or Others, there may be interest in expressing an odds ratio in relation to Adverse Event, in which case we would collapse the other three categories and proceed as in the binary case.

For ordinal data, we could follow the categorical data recommendations by collapsing adjacent outcomes, so, for example, by looking at *improved* versus *not improved* (=no change or worse). Another approach that is sometimes used is to work with the so-called common odds ratio. With three outcome categories, as in the example, this would involve forming two 2 × 2 contingency tables by firstly collapsing *improved* and *no change* and secondly collapsing *no change* and *worse*. In each of these two separate tables, we calculate the odds ratio; the common odds ratio is then obtained as an *average* of the two. In our example, the two odds ratios are 1.77 and 1.60, so the common odds ratio would be somewhere in the middle of these two values. The averaging process is a little complex, and we will not go into details here. The common odds ratio is then the odds in favour of success on average however you define success; *improved* or a combination of *improved* and *no change*.

4.8 Extensions for multiple treatment groups

In this section, we will discuss the extension of the t-tests for continuous data and the chi-square tests for binary, categorical and ordinal data to deal with more than two treatment arms.

4.8.1 Between-patient designs and continuous data

In this setting, there is a technique, termed *one-way analysis of variance (one-way ANOVA)*, which gives an overall *p*-value for the simultaneous comparison of all of the treatments. Suppose, for example, we have four treatment groups with means μ_1, μ_2, μ_3 and μ_4. This procedure gives a *p*-value for the null hypothesis:

$$H_0 : \mu_1 = \mu_2 = \mu_3 = \mu_4$$

against the general alternative hypothesis:

H_1 : the opposite of H_0, that there are differences somewhere

A significant *p*-value from this test would cause us to reject the null hypothesis, but the conclusion from this only tells us that there are some differences somewhere; at least two of the μs are different. At that point, we would want to look to identify where those differences lie, and this would lead us to pairwise comparisons of the treatment groups and reverting to a series of unpaired t-tests. It could be argued that the question posed by the one-way ANOVA technique is of little value and that it is more relevant to start directly with a set of structured questions relating to the comparisons of pairs of treatments.

For example, let us suppose that we have three treatment groups: test treatment (μ_1), active control (μ_2) and placebo (μ_3). In a superiority setting, there are two questions of interest:

1 Does the test treatment work?

$$H_0 : \mu_1 = \mu_3\, H_1 : \mu_1 \neq \mu_3$$

2 Is the test treatment better than the control treatment?

$$H_0 : \mu_1 = \mu_2\, H_1 : \mu_1 \neq \mu_2$$

Both of these questions are answered by the unpaired t-test.

One small advantage, however, of one-way ANOVA is that it uses all of the data from all of the treatment groups to give us a measure of noise, so even when we are comparing the test treatment group with the control treatment group, we are using information on the patient-to-patient variation in the placebo group to help estimate the noise; we work with a pooled estimate of the standard deviation. There are ways of adapting the unpaired t-test to incorporate this broader base of information, but even then the gains are small except in very small trials where information regarding the noise is at a premium. See Julious (2004) for further details.

In summary, there is not much to be gained in using one-way ANOVA with multiple treatment groups. A simpler analysis structuring the appropriate pairwise comparisons will more directly answer the questions of interest. One final word of caution though: undertaking multiple comparisons in this way raises another problem, that of multiplicity. For the time being, we will put that issue to one side; we will, however, return to it in Chapter 10.

4.8.2 Within-patient designs and continuous data

In this context, each patient would be receiving each of the multiple treatments. In the crossover trial with three treatments, this would likely be a three-period, three-treatment design, and patients would be randomised to one of the six sequences: ABC, ACB, BAC, BCA, CAB or CBA. Although there are again ways of asking a simultaneous question relating to the equality of the three treatment means through an ANOVA approach, this is unlikely to be of particular relevance; questions of real interest will concern pairwise comparisons.

Comments as previously mentioned for the between-patient designs apply also for the within-patient designs, and in many cases, the best approach will be to focus on a sequence of pairwise comparisons using the paired t-test.

In the context of within-patient designs, for example, the multi-period crossover, there could however be some additional considerations. Such designs are frequently used in phase I where sample sizes are small and the gains afforded by the common estimation of standard deviation could well be worthwhile, so we should not by any means dismiss these methods completely.

4.8.3 Binary, categorical and ordinal data

As with continuous data, the most relevant questions for binary, categorical and ordinal data will invariably relate to pairwise comparisons of treatments. We mentioned earlier for continuous data that one minor advantage was the ability to use information from all of the treatment groups to estimate patient-to-patient variation assuming a common standard deviation across the treatment groups. With binary, categorical and ordinal data, however, even this small advantage does not apply; there is no standard deviation of this kind with these data types. The recommendation again, therefore, is to focus on the chi-square procedures developed earlier in this chapter for pairwise treatment comparisons.

4.8.4 Dose-ranging studies

The discussion so far in this section has assumed that the treatment groups are unordered. There are, however, situations where these multiple treatment groups correspond to placebo and then increasing dose levels of a drug. It could still be in these circumstances that we are looking to compare each dose level with placebo in order to identify, for example, the minimum effective dose and again we are back to the pairwise comparisons.

There will be, however, some circumstances where we are just interested in trends; if we increase the dose, does the mean response increase?

For continuous data, there is a procedure within the one-way ANOVA methodology that is able to focus on this; we would be looking for a trend across the treatment groups.

For binary, categorical and ordinal data, there is also an approach that is a further form of the MH chi-square test. You will recall that the MH test is used for ordinal responses comparing two treatments. Well, this procedure generalises to allow ordering across the treatment groups in addition, for each of the binary, categorical and ordinal data types. More details for binary, categorical and ordinal data can be found in Stokes, Davis and Koch (2000).

4.8.5 Further discussion

For the remainder of this book, as we investigate further designs and methods of analysis, we will focus our developments on two treatment group comparisons. When we have more than two treatment groups, our questions are usually in relation to pairwise comparisons in any case, as discussed earlier, and these can be handled directly by reducing to those specific evaluations. For binary, categorical and ordinal data, this is precisely the approach. For continuous data, there are some advantages in efficiency in using a combined estimate of the standard deviation from the complete experiment, and this is what is usually done.

Specific mention will be made, however, in multiple treatment group settings where issues arise that require considerations outside of these.

CHAPTER 5

Adjusting the analysis

5.1 Objectives for adjusted analysis

The main reason why we might want to adjust the analysis is to account for imbalances in baseline factors. We have already discussed in Chapter 1 the importance of stratifying the randomisation to avoid baseline imbalances and confounding between treatment group and factors at baseline that are key determinants of outcome. However, even if the randomisation is stratified, there may still be minor imbalances that could influence our measures of treatment difference. Also, we cannot stratify for everything, and in addition, there may be factors that come to light while the trial is ongoing that are predictors of outcome that clearly were not able to be included in any stratified randomisation.

The methodology we will present in this section also provides a framework for evaluating the homogeneity of treatment effect in subgroups defined by the baseline factors. This is important in terms of underpinning our ability to generalise the results of the study to the population as a whole, something the regulators refer to as *generalisability*.

5.2 Comparing treatments for continuous data

Consider the following hypothetical situation comparing an active treatment+dietary advice with placebo+dietary advice in cholesterol lowering where the primary endpoint is the reduction (baseline minus final) in total cholesterol (mmol/l). Summary statistics are provided in Table 5.1, and these have been broken down by age group.

There are two particular features of these data that are worth noting at this stage. Firstly, there are imbalances in the distribution of age across the two treatment groups. The patients in the control group tend to be younger; the mean age in the active group was 57.8 years compared to 55.6 years in the control group. Secondly, irrespective of treatment group, the younger patients are on average performing better than the older patients, and the mean reduction in total cholesterol is greatest in both treatment groups in the patients aged <50 and smallest in the

Statistical Thinking for Non-Statisticians in Drug Regulation, Second Edition. Richard Kay.
© 2015 John Wiley & Sons, Ltd. Published 2015 by John Wiley & Sons, Ltd.

Table 5.1 Sample sizes and mean values for reduction in total cholesterol (mmol/l) in a (hypothetical) trial comparing an active treatment+dietary advice with placebo+dietary advice. Data Set 1

Age group	Placebo	Active
<50	$n=28$, mean$=0.36$	$n=21$, mean$=0.68$
≥50, <60	$n=17$, mean$=0.17$	$n=16$, mean$=0.39$
≥60	$n=33$, mean$=0.10$	$n=43$, mean$=0.36$

Table 5.2 Treatment differences by age category. Entries are sample size and mean value. Data Set 1

Age group	Placebo (P)	Active (A)	Difference (A–P) in means
<50	$n=28$, 0.36	$n=21$, 0.68	$n=49$, 0.32
≥50, <60	$n=17$, 0.17	$n=16$, 0.39	$n=33$, 0.22
≥60	$n=33$, 0.10	$n=43$, 0.36	$n=76$, 0.27

patients aged ≥60. Ignoring age category, the overall mean reduction in the active group was 0.45 mmol/l ($n=80$), while the overall mean reduction in the placebo group was 0.21 mmol/l ($n=78$) so that, to three decimal places, the treatment difference was 0.246 mmol/l. This results in a p-value from the unpaired t-test of 0.072, not quite statistically significant at the 5 per cent level. However, given the imbalance in age across the two treatment groups and also noticing that older patients don't do quite so well, we need to recognise that the active group has been penalised by having more than its fair share of older patients. Had we not had this imbalance, then we may well have seen statistically significant differences in favour of the active treatment.

Let's think about how we might adjust the analysis to correct for those base-line imbalances. The first step in this adjustment approach is to calculate the treatment difference within each age category. These differences are given in Table 5.2.

Having calculated the differences between the active mean and the placebo mean, we now average these three values, 0.32, 0.22 and 0.27, to give us our overall measure of treatment difference. This is the *adjusted treatment difference* and for these data takes the value 0.274. It is not the simple average of these three values but a weighted average, weighted according to the sample size in each of the age categories overall. We do this because averages based on larger sample sizes are more reliable and more precise than those based on smaller sample sizes, so we give them more weight. Don't worry too much about this weighting; it is a technical issue relating to optimising the statistical properties of the procedure. Had there been equal numbers of patients overall in the three age categories, there would not have been any weighting, and we would have taken just the straight numerical average, so think of it in those terms.

Note that the adjusted treatment difference of 0.274 is larger than the overall difference calculated earlier of 0.246, which was based on calculating the difference between the two raw means. The process of calculating treatment differences for each age group and then averaging those differences is not influenced by the imbalances between the treatment groups in terms of age. For example, the difference seen for the patients in the <50 group of 0.32 has simply been calculated from the individual treatment means of 0.68 and 0.36 and is not in any way affected by there being fewer patients <50, in the active group compared to the placebo group. The adjusted difference is then a better measure of the true treatment difference; it is comparing like with like in terms of two groups balanced according to the age distribution of the patients. The adjusted difference of 0.274 is the signal in this particular case, while the noise is a weighted combination of the individual standard deviations in each of the six cells of the table. The resulting p-value is 0.045, which now interestingly is statistically significant at the 5 per cent level.

Adjusting for baseline factors in this way provides a fair view of the treatment difference, something that would be lost if we simply compared the raw means in an unadjusted analysis. One common question is, if the treatment groups are perfectly balanced, isn't this adjusted analysis just a waste of time? The answer to that question is no – it is not a waste of time. Adjusting the analysis never harms you. If the treatment groups are perfectly balanced for baseline factors, then adjusting the analysis will make no difference, and the p-value for the adjusted analysis will agree with the p-value comparing the overall raw means. If the treatment groups are not perfectly balanced, then the adjusted analysis will correct for those imbalances. Of course, at the planning stage, you will never know whether or not you are going to see imbalances, so pre-specifying the adjusted analysis is an insurance policy just in case.

This method of analysis is referred to as *two-way analysis of variance (ANOVA)* or alternatively as a *stratified analysis*. The focus is to compare the treatment groups while recognising potential treatment group differences in the distribution of baseline factors. To enable this to happen, we allow the true treatment means μ_A and μ_B for groups A and B to be different for the different age groups as seen in Table 5.3.

The null hypothesis we evaluate is then

$$H_0 : \mu_{A1} = \mu_{B1} \text{ and } \mu_{A2} = \mu_{B2} \text{ and } \mu_{A3} = \mu_{B3}$$

against the general alternative hypothesis H_1 that there are differences somewhere.

This null hypothesis is saying that the treatment means are the same within each age group, but not necessarily across age groups. Two-way ANOVA gives us a p-value for the adjusted treatment difference that is evaluating this null

Table 5.3 True means according to age group

Age group	Treatment A	Treatment B	Difference
<50	μ_{A1}	μ_{B1}	$\mu_{A1} - \mu_{B1}$
≥50, <60	μ_{A2}	μ_{B2}	$\mu_{A2} - \mu_{B2}$
≥60	μ_{A3}	μ_{B3}	$\mu_{A3} - \mu_{B3}$

hypothesis. If that p-value is significant ($p \leq 0.05$), then we reject the null hypothesis, and there is evidence that the treatments are different.

This analysis implicitly assumes that the treatment effect is consistent across the various age categories. For the data being considered in this section, this seems a reasonable assumption, but we will return to a more formal evaluation of this assumption in a later section. The weighted average of the treatment differences provides the best estimate of the overall treatment effect. In our example, this was 0.274 mmol/l and we can construct confidence intervals around this value to allow an interpretation of the limits for the size of the true treatment difference.

There is a further advantage for this kind of analysis; it improves power, our ability to detect treatment differences if they truly exist. This is true irrespective of whether or not there are imbalances at baseline. The reason for this is that generally adjusting the analysis in this way reduces the noise. When we undertake an unadjusted analysis, the standard deviation is calculated as the *average* of the two standard deviations for the complete groups of patients in treatment groups A and B. With the adjusted analysis as discussed earlier, the standard deviation is calculated as the *average* of the six standard deviations in the six cells of the table, one for each treatment and age group combination. The latter will tend to be smaller than the former since in general there will be greater homogeneity within each treatment and age group combination than there would be taking each of the treatment groups as a whole.

In the next chapter, we will talk about adjusting the analysis for several factors simultaneously. We often call the factors we wish to adjust for *covariates*, and there is considerable regulatory guidance on adjustment for covariates. Adjusting in this way is frequently part of the primary analysis for certain endpoints, and as with all analyses, details should be set down in the protocol.

ICH E9 (1998): 'Note for Guidance on Statistical Principles for Clinical Trials'

'In some instances an adjustment for the influence of covariates or for subgroup effects is an integral part of the planned analysis and hence should be set out in the protocol'.

In the European *Points to Consider on Adjustment for Baseline Covariates* (2003) paper, there is the clear recommendation to use adjusted analyses to account for baseline imbalances.

CPMP (2003): 'Points to Consider on Adjustment for Baseline Covariates'

'When there is some imbalance between treatment groups in a baseline covariate that is solely due to chance then adjusted treatment effects may account for this observed imbalance when unadjusted analyses do not'.

One final point concerns the *requirement* to adjust for factors that were used as stratification factors at the randomisation stage. There are technical and statistical reasons why we need to do this.

CPMP (2003): 'Points to Consider on Adjustment for Baseline Covariates'

'The primary analysis should reflect the restriction on the randomization implied by the stratification. For this reason, stratification variables – regardless of their prognostic value – should usually be included as covariates in the primary analysis'.

5.3 Least squares means

In our example, the two overall (raw) treatment means were 0.45 in the active group and 0.21 in the placebo group. We recognise, because of the baseline age imbalances, that these means however are not directly comparable. In conjunction with adjusting the treatment comparison, it seems natural therefore to adjust the individual treatment means to also account for the baseline imbalances. The total sample size is 158, and had the groups been perfectly balanced for age, then we would have seen a proportion $0.31\left(=\dfrac{49}{158}\right)$ in the <50 category in each of the treatment groups, a proportion $0.21\left(=\dfrac{33}{158}\right)$ in each of the treatment groups in the middle age category and finally a proportion $0.48\left(=\dfrac{76}{158}\right)$

in each of the treatment groups in the ≥60 category. We can then reconstruct both the active and placebo means that would have been seen had we had this perfect balance. These reconstructed (adjusted) means are obtained as weighted combinations of the observed means across the three age categories as follows:

Active adjusted mean $= 0.31 \times 0.68 + 0.21 \times 0.39 + 0.48 \times 0.36 = 0.47$
Placebo adjusted mean $= 0.31 \times 0.36 + 0.21 \times 0.17 + 0.48 \times 0.10 = 0.20$

As we would expect, these adjusted means are slightly further apart than the original raw means, which were 0.45 for the active group and 0.21 for the placebo group. Had the groups been perfectly balanced, we would have observed a bigger treatment difference. This adjustment of the individual treatment means fits exactly with our adjusted method for comparing the treatments in that the difference $0.47 - 0.20 = 0.27$, which was the adjusted treatment difference we calculated previously; this is a mathematical connection. For reasons that we will explain in the next chapter, we usually refer to these adjusted means as *least squares (LS) means*.

5.4 Evaluating the homogeneity of the treatment effect

5.4.1 Treatment-by-factor interactions

The adjusted framework is based on calculating treatment differences within subgroups defined by the factor being adjusted for and then averaging those differences. As we have said, there is an implicit assumption within that framework that these differences are similar across the various levels of the factor. Evaluating whether this assumption is appropriate is an important next step as this could impact on the generalisability of the trial results. If the treatment effect is not homogeneous, then we will talk in terms of having *treatment-by-factor* or *treatment-by-covariate* interactions. The ICHE9 guideline is quite clear on the need to evaluate the homogeneity of the treatment effect.

ICH E9 (1998): 'Note for Guidance on Statistical Principles for Clinical Trials'

'The treatment effect itself may also vary with subgroup or covariate – for example, the effect may decrease with age or may be larger in a particular diagnostic category of subjects. In some cases such interactions are anticipated or are of particular prior interest (e.g. geriatrics), and hence a subgroup analysis, or a statistical model including interactions, is part of the planned confirmatory analysis'.

The CHMP (2003) *Points to Consider* paper reinforces this view:

CHMP (2003): 'Points to Consider on Adjustment for Baseline Covariates'

'However, treatment by covariate interactions should be explored, as recommended in the ICH E9 guideline'.

We will firstly discuss a significance test for the treatment-by-covariate interaction and then talk about graphical methods.

Table 5.4 Treatment differences by age category. Entries are sample size and mean value. Data Set 2

Age group	Placebo (P)	Active (A)	Difference (A – P) in means
<50	$n=28, 0.36$	$n=21, 0.68$	$n=49, 0.32$
≥50, <60	$n=17, 0.17$	$n=16, 0.29$	$n=33, 0.12$
≥60	$n=33, 0.10$	$n=43, 0.16$	$n=76, 0.06$

Consider again the (hypothetical) setting evaluating a treatment for lowering cholesterol with new summary statistics as set out in Table 5.4.

In these data, the active treatment is performing on average better than placebo, but now, the extent of the difference is not consistent. There is a large difference among the <50 age category, a smaller difference in the middle age category and an even smaller difference in the ≥60 age category.

To assess this inconsistency, two-way ANOVA additionally provides a p-value for the hypothesis

$$H_0 : \mu_{A1} - \mu_{B1} = \mu_{A2} - \mu_{B2} = \mu_{A3} - \mu_{B3}$$

against the general alternative hypothesis that the treatment differences are not all equal.

This null hypothesis is saying that the treatment difference/effect is consistent. If the p-value from this test is significant, then the data are supporting heterogeneity of treatment effect according to age, and we have a significant treatment-by-age (sometimes written as treatment×age) interaction.

Power and sample size calculations (see later chapter on this topic) will have focused on testing the main effect of treatment and not on the evaluation of the treatment-by-age interaction. As a consequence, this test for interaction will have low power and only pick up marked heterogeneity. To counter this to an extent, we normally evaluate the significance of the interaction test at a less strict significance level than is usual, so, for example, using $p \leq 0.10$ as a signal to reject the null hypothesis of homogeneity rather than when $p \leq 0.05$. In discussing the treatment-by-covariate significance test, the ICH states:

ICH E9 (1998): 'Note for Guidance on Statistical Principles for Clinical Trials'

'When using such a statistical significance test, it is important to recognise that this generally has low power in a trial designed to detect the main effect of treatment'.

It is important therefore not to rely overly on statistical significance when evaluating interactions and to use clinical judgment about what constitutes an important differential treatment effect numerically. Indeed, the CPMP *Points to Consider* paper, published several years after ICH E9, takes a fairly extreme view and cautions against the use of formal significance testing for interactions altogether.

CHMP (2003): 'Points to Consider on Adjustment for Baseline Covariates'

'Tests for interactions often lack statistical power and the absence of statistical evidence of an interaction is not evidence that there is no clinically relevant interaction. Conversely, an interaction cannot be considered as relevant on the sole basis of a significant test for interaction. Assessment of interaction terms based on statistical significance tests is therefore of little value'.

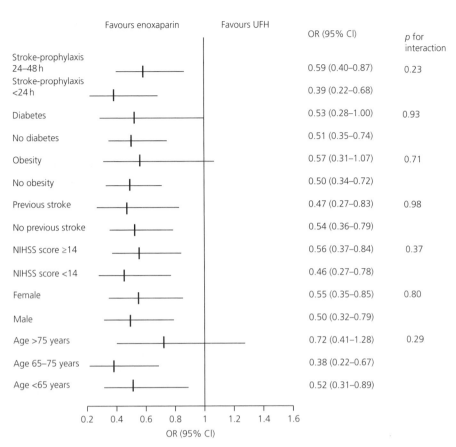

Figure 5.1 Forest plot for risk for venous thromboembolism in patients with acute ischaemic stroke by patient characteristics for enoxaparin and unfractionated heparin. NIHSS, National Institutes of Health Stroke Scale; OR, odds ratio; UFH, unfractionated. Source: Sherman DG, Albers GW, Bladin C, Fieschi C, Gabbai AA, Kase CS *et al.* (2007). The efficacy and safety of enoxaparin versus unfractionated heparin for the prevention of venous thromboembolism after acute ischaemic stroke (PREVAIL Study): an open-label randomized comparison. Lancet, 369, 1347-1355. Reproduced with permission from Elsevier.

The ICH guideline also mentions the use of graphical methods, and we will discuss these further in conjunction with subgroup evaluation in Section 10.8. Figure 5.1, taken from Sherman *et al.* (2007), is the kind of plot they are looking for. This *forest plot* displays treatment differences together with 95 per cent confidence intervals and also the *p*-value for interaction.

5.4.2 Quantitative and qualitative interactions

The ICH makes the distinction between quantitative and qualitative interactions. A *quantitative interaction* refers to the situation where the treatment difference is consistently in one direction (e.g. treatment A is always better than treatment B), but there are differences in terms of magnitude. A *qualitative interaction* is where the treatment difference is in a different direction for some level or levels of the factor (e.g. treatment A is better than treatment B for patients <50, but treatment B is better than treatment A for patients ≥50). All of the interactions seen in Figure 5.1 are quantitative interactions. Had the odds ratio for patients aged >75 years, for example, been >1, favouring UFH, then we would have had a qualitative interaction for that factor.

If heterogeneity of treatment effect is found, then this could possibly undermine the generalisability of the results. For example, with a qualitative interaction, one treatment is performing better on average in one or more subgroups but worse in other subgroups, and it will be difficult to draw a general conclusion of 'treatment A is a better treatment than treatment B'. Even a quantitative interaction will sometimes give problems in terms of estimating with confidence the magnitude of the treatment effect. We will further discuss the interpretation of these forest plots in Section 10.8 in relation to subgroup testing and multiplicity.

5.5 Methods for binary, categorical and ordinal data

The *Cochran–Mantel–Haenszel (CMH) tests* are a collection of procedures that extend the simple chi-squared tests introduced in Chapter 4 to allow adjustment for baseline factors when dealing with binary, categorical and ordinal data. Landis, Heyman and Koch (1978) provide further details.

When adjusting for a baseline factor with binary data, we will have a series of 2×2 tables, one for each level of the factor. For categorical and ordinal data with c categories, we will have a series of $2 \times c$ tables. The CMH test in the first instance provides a single p-value for the main effect of treatment.

In terms of summary statistics for binary data, we usually work with the odds ratio, and when we adjust for a baseline factor, these are averaged over the different levels of the factor. It is also possible to obtain, in a similar way, *average* values for both the reduction in event rates and for relative risk (RR) if these are needed. For ordinal data, we work with the common odds ratio in each of the $2 \times c$ tables averaged over the levels of the factor.

The same issues arise with the heterogeneity of the treatment effect as in the preceding text with continuous data, and indeed, the ICH and CHMP comments detailed there are relevant for all data types. For binary data, there is a significance test, the Breslow–Day test (Breslow and Day, 1994), which provides a p-value for the homogeneity of the treatment effect across levels of the factor. Again, graphical methods are also available and follow the approach seen earlier, plotting estimated odds ratios for each baseline factor and the subgroups defined by levels of those factors together with their corresponding 95 per cent confidence intervals. Indeed, the example displayed in Figure 5.1 is based on a binary outcome ratios.

5.6 Multi-centre trials

5.6.1 Adjusting for centre

As indicated in the ICH E9 guideline, there are two reasons why we conduct multi-centre trials:

- To recruit sufficient numbers of patients within an appropriate timeframe
- To evaluate the robustness of the treatment effect across a range of centres and provide a basis for generalisability

The first issue is of practical importance; there is probably no other way the required numbers of patients could be recruited. The second issue is very much in line with our discussions earlier in this chapter in relation to evaluation of the homogeneity of treatment effect according to levels of baseline factors. A multi-centre structure enables us to look at treatment differences in different centres or clusters of centres to assess whether what we are seeing is a consistent effect. Without this consistency, it would be difficult to draw conclusions about the value of the treatment across a broad patient population.

In some cases, a trial will have been set up to recruit from a small number of large centres and where the randomisation is stratified by centre. In this case, the analysis should be adjusted for centre. Following on from that, we can investigate the homogeneity of treatment effect across the different centres in the same way that we adjusted for baseline covariates in Section 5.4. Alternatively, some trials may be conducted across a large number of small centres, for example, GP studies. It is unlikely in these cases that the randomisation would be stratified by centre although it may be that groupings of centres have been defined at the design stage (e.g. by geographical region) and the randomisation is stratified by those centre groupings. Under these circumstances, the groupings form pseudo-centres, and these would be taken into account in the statistical analysis through an adjusted analysis.

5.6.2 Significant treatment-by-centre interactions

Suppose that in a particular setting there is some evidence of treatment-by-centre interactions. A simple interpretation of the data is then not straightforward.

In the section on multi-centre trials, the ICH E9 guideline makes the following point:

ICH E9 (1998): 'Note for Guidance on Statistical Principles for Clinical Trials'

'If heterogeneity of treatment is found, this should be interpreted with care and vigorous attempts should be made to find an explanation in terms of other features of trial management or subject characteristics … In the absence of an explanation, heterogeneity of treatment effect as evidenced, for example, by marked quantitative interactions implies that alternative estimates of the treatment effect may be required,

giving different weights to the centres, in order to substantiate the robustness of the estimates of treatment effect. It is even more important to understand the basis of any heterogeneity characterised by marked qualitative interactions, and failure to find an explanation may necessitate further clinical trials before the treatment effect can be reliably predicted'.

Work is needed therefore to find an explanation when interactions are seen. That explanation may come from looking, for example, at differential compliance within the centres or different characteristics of the patient sample recruited at the different centres. Inevitably, a treatment-by-centre interaction is simply a surrogate for some *hidden* explanation. It must also be said that the explanation may be *chance*! In a trial with a reasonable number of centres, where treatment A really is a better treatment than treatment B, seeing one treatment reversal (a centre in which treatment B is numerically superior to treatment A) would not be unlikely. Senn (2007, Section 14.2.6) investigates this and shows, under some fairly standard conditions, that the probability of seeing at least one reversal goes above 50 per cent with six or more centres, so be cautious with over-interpretation with regard to interactions.

5.6.3 Combining centres

The ideal situation in many multi-centre trials is to have a small number of large centres (or pre-defined pseudo-centres). This gives the necessary consistency and control yet still allows the evaluation of homogeneity. In practice, however, we do not always end up in this situation, and combining centres at the data analysis stage inevitably needs to be considered. From a statistical perspective, adjusting for small centres in the analysis is problematic and leads to unreliable estimates of treatment effect, so we generally have to combine.

There are no fixed rules for these combinations, but several points should be noted:

- Combining centres just because they are small or combining centres to produce centres of similar size has no scientific justification (see CPMP (2003) *Points to Consider on Adjustment for Baseline Covariates*).
- Combinations should be based on similarity (by region, by country, by type, etc.). For example, a trial in depression may be run across many centres with at most 10 patients being recruited at each centre; some of the centres will be GP centres, while others will be specialist psychiatric facilities. In this case, combining by centre type (GP or specialist psychiatrist facility) would make sense, and this would allow the homogeneity of treatment effect between GP centres and specialist psychiatric centres to be investigated.
- Ideally, rules for combining centres should be detailed in the statistical analysis plan.
- Any final decisions regarding combinations should be made at the blind review stage prior to breaking the blind.

We will discuss the decision-making process with regard to the statistical analysis plan and the blind review in Section 21.3.4.

CHAPTER 6

Regression and analysis of covariance

6.1 Adjusting for baseline factors

We saw in the previous chapter how to adjust for single factors in treatment comparisons using two-way ANOVA for continuous data and the CMH test for binary, categorical and ordinal data. Generally, it can be advantageous to adjust for several factors simultaneously. To a certain extent, this could be done using the methods of Chapter 5 by using combinations of levels of the different factors to define the strata. For example, suppose we wish to adjust for both age (<50 versus ≥50) and sex. We could do this by defining four strata as follows:

Males, <50 years
Males, ≥50 years
Females, <50 years
Females, ≥50 years

In one sense, this can work perfectly well although it is not easy to use such an analysis as a basis for investigating treatment-by-factor interactions. For example, if the treatment effect was different for males and females but was not influenced by age, then this would be difficult to identify within this structure.

Further as the number of baseline factors increases, this approach becomes a little unwieldy. The method of analysis of covariance (ANCOVA) is a more general methodology that can deal with the increase in complexity caused by wanting to adjust simultaneously for several factors and that can also give improved ways of exploring interactions. We will develop this methodology later in the chapter, but as a lead into that we will firstly discuss regression.

6.2 Simple linear regression

Regression provides a collection of methods that allow the investigation of dependence, how an outcome variable depends upon something that we measure at baseline.

As an example, suppose in an oncology study we wish to explore whether time to disease recurrence from entry (months) into the study depends upon the

Statistical Thinking for Non-Statisticians in Drug Regulation, Second Edition. Richard Kay.
© 2015 John Wiley & Sons, Ltd. Published 2015 by John Wiley & Sons, Ltd.

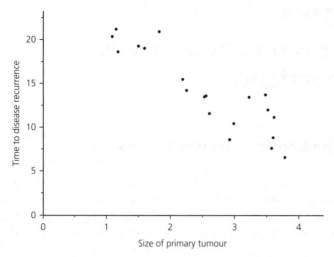

Figure 6.1 Scatter plot for dependence of time to disease recurrence on size of primary tumour

size of the primary tumour measured at baseline (diameter in cm). The scatter plot in Figure 6.1 represents (artificial) data on 20 subjects.

A visual inspection of the plot would suggest that there is some dependence, but in many cases, this will not be quite so clear-cut. We explore the dependence from a statistical point of view by fitting a straight line to the data.

The equation of a straight line is

$$y = a + bx$$

where a is the intercept (the value of y where the line crosses the y-axis) and b is the slope (the amount by which y increases when x increases by one unit).

The value of b is of greatest importance. If b is positive, then there is a positive dependence; as x increases, then so does y. If b is negative, then there is a negative dependence; as x increases, then y decreases. Finally, if $b=0$, then there is no dependence; as x increases, nothing happens to y.

The method that we use to fit the straight line so that it describes the data in the best possible way is called *least squares*. This involves measuring the vertical distance of each point from a line placed on the plot as shown in Figure 6.2, squaring each of those distances (this among other things gets rid of the sign) and choosing that line that makes the average of these squared distances as small as possible. In our example, this *least squares regression line* has the equation

$$y = 25.5 - 4.48x$$

The value of the slope is −4.48 and this estimates the average increase in time to disease recurrence as the tumour size at baseline increases by 1 cm. The primary question of interest here is 'does time to disease recurrence depend upon tumour

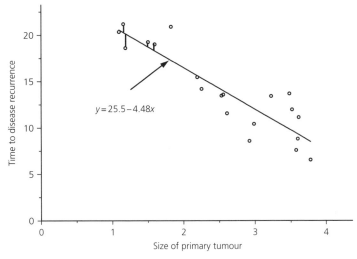

Figure 6.2 Least-squares regression line

size at baseline?' To address this question, we, as usual, formulate null and alternative hypotheses

$$H_0 : b = 0 \quad H_1 : b \neq 0$$

and construct an appropriate test. This involves the signal, which is the estimate of b from the data, and a measure for the noise, which is actually equal to the standard deviation of the vertical distances of the points from the fitted line. The standard error (se) of the estimate of b involves this standard deviation and there is a formula for the calculation of this. Finally, the test statistic is as before, the signal is divided by the associated standard error, and the null distribution is t_{n-2}, where n is the number of subjects. A significant p-value ($p \leq 0.05$) from this test is telling us that b is significantly different from zero, indicating dependence. A non-significant p-value is telling us that there is insufficient evidence to conclude dependence. In fact, for these data, $p \ll 0.001$, a very highly significant dependence of time to disease recurrence on the size of the primary tumour at baseline. The slope of -4.48 indicates that on average, for each 1 cm increase in the diameter of the primary tumour, there is a 4.48-month decrease in the time to disease recurrence.

This technique of *simple linear regression* therefore provides a straightforward way to evaluate whether a particular baseline variable is predictive of outcome. We will extend these ideas in the next section to evaluate several baseline variables/factors simultaneously.

6.3 Multiple regression

In Section 6.2, we saw how to study the dependence of an outcome variable on a variable measured at baseline. It could well be that there are several baseline variables that predict outcome, and in this section, we will see how to incorporate these variables simultaneously through a methodology termed *multiple (linear) regression.*

Taking up the example from the previous section, it may be that time to disease progression depends potentially not just on size of the primary tumour but also on age and sex, and we would like to explore the nature of that dependence. Clearly, size of primary tumour and age are both numerical, while sex is not; we incorporate qualitative variables of this kind by using so-called indicator variables. Generally, these take the values zero and one according to the *value* of the variable. It also does not matter which way round they are coded. Switching the codes would simply result in the coefficient of that variable changing sign:

Let x_1 = size of primary tumour
x_2 = age
x_3 = 0 male
     1 female

The extension of simple linear regression to deal with multiple baseline variables is somewhat difficult to visualise, but algebraically it is simply a matter of adding terms to the equation

$$y = a + b_1 x_1 + b_2 x_2 + b_3 x_3$$

Now, b_1 measures the effect of size on time to disease recurrence, while the coefficients b_2 and b_3 measure the effects of age and sex, respectively. More specifically, b_1 and b_2 are the changes in the average time to disease recurrence as size and age each increase by one unit, respectively, while b_3 measures the sex effect, the average time to disease recurrence for females minus that for males. Each of these quantities, which we can estimate from the data again using the method of least squares, represents the contribution of each of the variables separately in the presence of the other variables.

The questions of interest revolve around the values of the b coefficients. Do age and size of primary tumour predict time to disease recurrence? Is there a sex effect? We address these questions by formulating hypotheses:

$H_{01} : b_1 = 0$ $H_{11} : b_1 \neq 0$
$H_{02} : b_2 = 0$ $H_{12} : b_2 \neq 0$
$H_{03} : b_3 = 0$ $H_{13} : b_3 \neq 0$

Each of these is evaluated by dividing the estimate of the corresponding b value by its standard error and comparing it to the t_{n-4} distribution (the degree of freedom for the appropriate t shape is the number of subjects minus [1 + the number of x variables in the model]). Note that multiple regression with just a single variable reduces to simple linear regression.

Suppose that the fitted equation turns out to be

$$y = 23.8 - 3.51\ x_1 - 1.74\ x_2 + 0.47x_3$$

Therefore, for a 1 cm increase in the tumour size, time to disease recurrence reduces by on average an estimated 3.51 months; for each additional year in age, there is on average an estimated 1.74-month reduction in time to disease recurrence; and finally, the time to disease recurrence is estimated to be slightly higher for females by on average 0.47 months. It is also fairly straightforward to construct confidence intervals around these estimates.

The p-values associated with each term in this model were

$$H_{01} : b_1 = 0\quad p = 0.007$$
$$H_{02} : b_2 = 0\quad p = 0.02$$
$$H_{03} : b_3 = 0\quad p = 0.48$$

This suggests that size of primary tumour and age are important predictors of time to disease recurrence, while sex appears to be unimportant.

Note that this approach is not the same as conducting three linear regression analyses on the baseline variables separately. In fact, such an approach could give a confused picture if the baseline variables being considered were correlated. For example, suppose that age and size of primary tumour are correlated with older patients tending to present with larger tumours. Also, suppose that it is size of primary tumour that is the driver in terms of time to disease recurrence and that age has no effect additional to that. The separate linear regressions would indicate that both size of primary tumour and age predict outcome; age would be identified as a predictor of outcome only as a result of its correlation with size. Multiple regression, however, would give the correct interpretation. Size of primary tumour would be seen as a predictor of outcome, but once that effect is accounted for, age would add nothing to this prediction.

There is sometimes discussion about whether to use categories for a continuous variable, for example, having a binary age variable taking the value 0 for patients aged <50 years and taking the value 1 for patients aged ≥ 50, or whether to include the continuous variable itself in the modelling. Categorisation will generally waste information and is not recommended; it is much better to retain the variable in its continuous form. See Royston, Altman and Sauerbrei (2006) for a detailed discussion on this point. Similar comments will apply later in this chapter when looking at covariates in ANCOVA.

With a large number of potential baseline variables, it may be of interest to select those variables that are impacting on outcome, and methods (*stepwise regression*) are available for doing this. Using this methodology, the unimportant variables are eliminated, leaving a final equation containing just the important predictive factors. This methodology is often used to construct *prognostic indices*.

6.4 Logistic regression

Multiple regression as presented so far is for continuous outcome variables y. For binary, categorical and ordinal outcomes, the corresponding technique is called *logistic regression*. Suppose that in our earlier example we defined success to be *disease-free for five years*, then we might be interested in identifying those variables/factors at baseline that were predictive of the probability of success.

Define y now to take the value one for a success and zero for a failure. For mathematical reasons, rather than modelling y as we did for continuous outcome variables, we now model the probability that $y=1$, written $pr(y=1)$.

This probability, by definition, will lie between zero and one, so to avoid numerical problems, we do not model $pr(y=1)$ directly but a transformation of $pr(y=1)$, the so-called logit or logistic transform:

$$\ln\left\{\frac{pr(y=1)}{[1-pr(y=1)]}\right\} = a + b_1 x_1 + b_2 x_2 + b_3 x_3$$

Computer packages such as SAS can fit these models, provide estimates of the values of the b coefficients together with standard errors and give p-values associated with the hypothesis tests of interest. The null hypotheses will be exactly as H_{01}, H_{02} and H_{03} in Section 6.3.

Methods of stepwise regression are also available for the identification of a subset of the baseline variables/factors that are predictive of outcome in this case. A good example of the application of logistic regression, identifying the clinical signs that predict severe illness in neonatals in countries of low or middle income, is provided by The Young Infants Clinical Signs Study Group (2008). The logistic regression model extends both to categorical data using the *polychotomous logistic model* and to ordinal data using the *ordinal logistic model*. For an example of the former, see Marshall and Chisholm (1985) in the area of diagnosis.

6.5 Analysis of covariance for continuous data

6.5.1 Main effect of treatment

We will return to the example where we have just a single baseline variable, size of primary tumour, predicting the outcome time to disease recurrence, but now in addition, we have randomised the patients to one of two treatment groups, test treatment and placebo.

Figure 6.3 displays a possible pattern for the results. Note firstly that as before there appears to be a dependence of time to disease recurrence on the size of the primary tumour. In addition, it also seems that the patients receiving the test treatment have longer times to disease recurrence compared to those receiving the control treatment, irrespective of the size of the primary tumour.

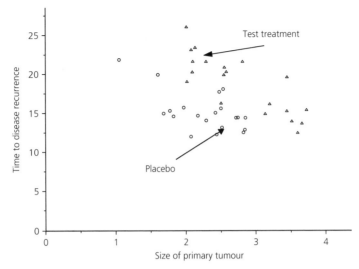

Figure 6.3 Scatter plot for two treatment groups

A formal comparison of the two treatments could be based on the unpaired t-test, comparing the mean time to disease recurrence in the test treatment group with the mean time to disease recurrence in the control group. While this is a valid test, it may not be particularly sensitive. The separation between the two groups is clear, but if we now simply read off the times to disease recurrence on the y-axis, we will see considerable overlap between the groups; we will have lost some sensitivity by ignoring the size of the primary tumour variable.

Consider an alternative approach, fitting simple linear regression lines to the data from these two groups of patients. The equations of these lines can be written as

$y = a_1 + bx$ test treatment
$y = a_2 + bx$ placebo

Figure 6.4 shows these lines fitted to the data. Note that we have constrained the slopes of these lines to be the same; we will return to this point later. The intercepts, a_1 and a_2, are the points where the lines cross the y-axis.

Had the treatments been equally effective, then the points in the placebo group would not have been, in general, below the points in the test treatment group; the lines would be coincidental with $a_1 = a_2$. Indeed, the larger the treatment difference, the bigger the difference between the two intercepts, a_1 and a_2. Our main interest is to compare the treatments, and within this framework, we compare the values of a_1 and a_2 through the null hypothesis $H_0 : a_1 = a_2$ and the alternative hypothesis $H_1 : a_1 \neq a_2$. The signal is provided by the estimate of $a_1 - a_2$ and there is an associated standard error for that estimate; we compare the signal/se ratio to t_{n-3} to give the p-value.

The quantity $a_1 - a_2$ is the vertical distance between the lines and represents the (adjusted) difference in the mean time to recurrence in the test treatment group minus the mean time to recurrence in the control group, the treatment effect. It is

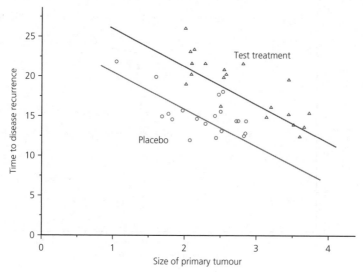

Figure 6.4 Scatter plot and fitted lines for two treatment groups

straightforward also to obtain a confidence interval around this adjusted treatment effect to capture the true difference.

This technique is called *analysis of covariance* and size of the primary tumour is the covariate. Taking account of the covariate here has led to a much more powerful analysis than that provided by the simple unpaired t-test. Of course, the main reason why we are seeing such an improvement in sensitivity is that the covariate is such a strong predictor of outcome. These improvements will not be quite so great with weaker predictors.

It is also possible to include more than one covariate in the analysis in cases where several are thought to be influential for the outcome by simply adding on terms to the earlier equations as with multiple regression. That is,

$$y = a_1 + b_1 x_1 + b_2 x_2 + b_3 x_3 \quad \text{test treatment}$$
$$y = a_2 + b_1 x_1 + b_2 x_2 + b_3 x_3 \quad \text{placebo}$$

Again, we test the hypothesis $H_0 : a_1 = a_2$. The estimate of $a_1 - a_2$ is used as the signal, and the ratio of this estimate divided by its standard error (the test statistic) is compared to t_{n-q}, where n is the number of subjects and q is the number of covariates +2 to give a p-value.

We call these equations (or models) *main effects models*. In the next subsection, we will be adding to the main effects (of treatment and the covariates) treatment-by-covariate interaction terms.

6.5.2 Treatment-by-covariate interactions
Returning to the case with a single covariate, we have assumed that the two lines are parallel. This may not be the case. Figure 6.5 shows a situation where it would not be appropriate to assume parallel lines. Here, patients presenting

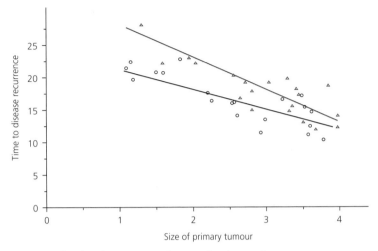

Figure 6.5 Scatter plot showing treatment by covariate interaction

with small tumours do much better in the test treatment group compared to the placebo group, but there are virtually no differences between the treatments for those patients presenting with large tumours.

We have previously in Chapter 5 discussed treatment-by-factor interactions, where the treatment effect is seen to be different for the different levels of the factor. More generally, we can consider treatment-by-covariate interactions, where the treatment effect depends on the value of the covariate. We can investigate this by considering a model where we allow the lines to have different slopes as well as different intercepts:

$y = a_1 + b_1 x$ test treatment
$y = a_2 + b_2 x$ placebo

This now gives us the opportunity to assess whether there are any interactions by fitting these two lines to the data and formulating a test of the hypothesis $H_0 : b_1 = b_2$ against the alternative $H_1 : b_1 \neq b_2$. A significant p-value, and as with treatment-by-factor interactions we would be looking at $p < 0.10$ as *a guideline for statistical significance*, would indicate the presence of an interaction. In this case, talking in terms of the *treatment effect* makes little sense as a consistent treatment effect does not exist. A non-significant p-value would suggest that it is safe to assume that the treatment effect is fairly constant across the levels of the covariate, and the model, with a common slope b, provides an adequate description of the data.

If a significant treatment-by-covariate interaction is found, then it could be useful to divide the patients into subgroups in terms of the size of the primary tumour, say, small, medium and large, and look at the treatment difference within those subgroups to try to better understand the nature of the interaction.

In the presence of several covariates, there will be a series of b coefficients, two for each covariate as follows:

$$y = a_1 + b_{11}x_1 + b_{12}x_2 + b_{13}x_3 \quad \text{test treatment}$$
$$y = a_2 + b_{21}x_1 + b_{22}x_2 + b_{23}x_3 \quad \text{placebo}$$

Assessing the treatment-by-covariate interactions is then based on comparing the bs: b_{11} with b_{21}, b_{12} with b_{22} and b_{13} with b_{23} in separate hypothesis tests.

6.5.3 A single model

These models can be written in a more precise form by defining a binary indicator to denote treatment. Let $z=0$ for patients randomised to the placebo group and let $z=1$ for patients randomised to the test treatment. The model with a single covariate and assuming a common slope can then be written as

$$y = a + cz + bx$$

Now, when $z=0$ (placebo group), $y=a+bx$ and when $z=1$ (test treatment group), $y=(a+c)+bx$.

The b in this model is as previously, but now, $a=a_1$ and $c=a_2-a_1$. We refer to this in mathematics as a re-parameterisation; don't be put off by it! The hypothesis $H_0: a_1=a_2$ is now replaced by the hypothesis $H_1: c=0$. None of this changes the analysis in any sense; it is just a more convenient way to write down the model and will be useful later when we bring together the ideas of ANOVA and ANCOVA.

Although conceptually it is useful to think of fitting straight lines to each of the treatment groups separately, this is not in practice how it is done. We simply fit this single equation. This also allows us to use the information on the noise from the two groups combined to obtain standard error. Finally, we build in the interaction terms by adding on to this common equation a *cross-product term, $z \times x$,* and using another re-parameterisation:

$$y = a + cz + bx + dzx$$

so when $z=0$ (placebo group), $y=a+bx$ and when $z=1$ (test treatment group), $y=(a+c)+(b+d)x$.

b_1 in the previous model in Section 6.5.2 is now b in this common model, while $d=b_2-b_1$. Assessing the presence of a treatment-by-covariate interaction (common slope) is then done through the hypothesis that $d=0$.

For several covariates, we simply introduce a cross-product term for each covariate with corresponding coefficients d_1, d_2 and d_3 to investigate interactions. The presence of treatment-by-covariate interactions can then be investigated through these coefficients.

6.5.4 Connection with adjusted analyses

ANCOVA is a form of adjusted analysis; we are providing an adjusted treatment effect in the presence of covariates. This is very much like the adjusted analysis we presented in the previous chapter. For the single covariate example, had we defined strata according to the size of the primary tumour, say, small, medium and large, and then undertaken two-way ANOVA to compare the treatments, then we would have got very similar results to those seen here through ANCOVA. This applies to the *p*-values for the assessment of treatment difference, the estimated (adjusted) treatment difference, the associated confidence intervals and the *p*-values for studying the homogeneity of the treatment effect, which is simply looking for treatment-by-covariate interactions.

6.5.5 Advantages of ANCOVA

ANCOVA offers a number of advantages over simple two treatment group comparisons:

- Produces improvements in efficiency (smaller standard errors, narrower confidence intervals, increased power).
- Corrects for baseline imbalances. Randomisation will, on average, produce groups that are comparable in terms of baseline characteristics. It is inevitable, however, that small differences will still exist, and if these are differences in important prognostic factors, then they could have an impact on the treatment comparisons. By chance, there will be occasions also when substantial imbalance exists. In fact, in Figures 6.3 and 6.4, we have such imbalances and these imbalances could cause bias in our evaluation of a treatment effect. Here, purely by chance, we have ended up with a predominance of patients with large tumours in the test treatment group and a predominance of small and medium tumours in the control treatment group. A simple unpaired t-test would possibly fail to detect a treatment difference or even conclude a difference in the wrong direction as a result of this baseline imbalance. ANCOVA helps correct for those baseline imbalances; once the two regression lines are estimated, then ANCOVA *ignores* the data (and therefore the imbalance) and simply works with the distance between the lines for the treatment effect.
- Allows assessment of prognostic factors. Fitting the ANCOVA model provides coefficients for the covariates, and although this is not the primary focus of the analysis, these coefficients and associated confidence intervals provide information on the effect of the baseline covariates on outcome. This information can be useful for trial planning, for example choosing factors on which to stratify the randomisation for the future.
- Provides a convenient framework for the evaluation of treatment-by-covariate interactions; in some cases, such interactions are anticipated, while in other cases such analyses are exploratory.

ICH E9 (1998): 'Note for Guidance on Statistical Principles for Clinical Trials'

'In most parts, however, subgroup or interaction analyses are exploratory and should be clearly identified as such; they should explore the uniformity of any treatment effects found overall.'

The adjusted analyses discussed in Chapter 5 also share some of these advantages and provide improvements in efficiency, can also account for baseline imbalances and allow the evaluation of the homogeneity of the treatment effect. On this final point, however, and as discussed in Section 6.1, simple adjusted analyses looking at combinations of factors are less able to identify the nature of those interactions. With ANCOVA, it is possible to say which particular covariates are causing such interactions. A further point to note here and, as mentioned earlier, is that simple adjusted analyses become more difficult as the number of covariates increases, although some would argue that including more than a small number of covariates is not needed (see Section 6.7).

Should treatment-by-covariate interactions be found, either through a test of homogeneity in an adjusted analysis or through ANCOVA, then analysis usually proceeds by looking at treatment differences within subgroups. Plots of treatment effects with associated confidence intervals within these subgroups are useful in this regard.

One disadvantage of ANCOVA is that the modelling does involve a number of assumptions and if those assumptions are not valid, then the approach could mislead. For example, it is assumed (usually) that the covariates affect outcome in a linear way; there is invariably too little information in the data to be able to assess this assumption in any effective way. In contrast, with an adjusted analysis, assumptions about the way in which covariates affect outcome are not made, and in that sense, it can be seen as a more robust approach. In some regulatory circles, simple adjusted analyses are preferred to ANCOVA for these reasons.

6.5.6 Least squares means

The method we use to fit ANVOCA models is again least squares, measuring the vertical distances of the points from the regression lines and choosing values for the parameters in the model that make the average of the resulting squared distances as small as possible.

We discussed in the previous section how ANCOVA can correct for baseline imbalances in the covariate and suppose again that those imbalances were present. The mean values for time to disease recurrence calculated from the data, and the numerical difference between those means, would give us a misleading impression of the true treatment benefit; we somehow need to correct those mean values for the baseline imbalance in tumour size. A straightforward way to do this would be to take the average tumour size for the two treatment groups combined and then use the fitted regression equations with the common slope to predict the time to disease recurrence for this *average* patient in each of the two treatment groups. Figure 6.6 shows this construction diagrammatically.

We refer to these *fitted* values as the *least squares means*; the mathematics here is very much in line with what we did in Section 5.3 when we were looking at simple methods for adjusting the analysis. They provide a better summary of the average effectiveness of the two treatments in an absolute sense, but maybe

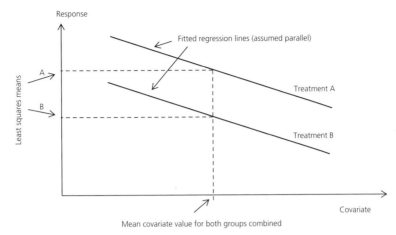

Figure 6.6 Calculating least squares means

more importantly, their difference provides a better estimate of the relative effectiveness of the two treatments. The difference between these least squares means is also the vertical distance between the two fitted lines and is numerically equal to $a_1 - a_2$, the difference in the intercepts. We discussed the use of this adjusted treatment difference in Section 6.5.1 and argued that it provided an appropriate measure of the true treatment difference.

6.6 Binary, categorical and ordinal data

Analysis of covariance for these data types is based on logistic regression. With continuous data, although we developed the concepts by looking at separate lines for the different treatment groups, we ended up writing down a single equation. This is really the start point with binary, categorical and ordinal data and logistic regression. We will focus this discussion on the most common setting, the binary case; extensions for ordinal data are straightforward.

Again, let $z=0$ for patients in the control group and $z=1$ for patients in the test treatment group and assume that we have several covariates, say, x_1, x_2 and x_3. The main effects model looks at the dependence of $\text{pr}(y=1)$ on treatment and the covariates:

$$\ell n \left\{ \frac{\text{pr}(y=1)}{[1 - \text{pr}(y=1)]} \right\} = a + cz + b_1 x_1 + b_2 x_2 + b_3 x_3 \quad .$$

The coefficient c measures the impact that treatment has on $\text{pr}(y=1)$. If $c=0$, then $\text{pr}(y=1)$ is unaffected by which treatment group the patients are in; there is no treatment effect. Having fitted this model to the data and in particular obtained an estimate of c and its standard error, then we can test the hypothesis $H_0: c=0$ in the usual way through the signal/se ratio.

The quantity c is very closely related to the odds ratio (OR); in fact, c is the log of the OR, adjusted for the covariates. The antilog of c (given by e^c) gives the adjusted OR. Confidence intervals in relation to this OR can be constructed initially by obtaining a confidence interval for c itself and then taking the antilog of the lower and upper confidence limits for c.

Example 6.1 Effect of betamethasone on incidence of neonatal respiratory distress

This randomised trial (Stutchfield *et al.*, 2005) investigated the effect of betamethasone on the incidence of neonatal respiratory distress after elective caesarean section. Of the 503 women randomised to the active treatment, 11 babies were subsequently admitted to the special baby unit with respiratory distress compared to 24 babies out of 495 women randomised to the control group. A total of 492 women in the active treatment group were included in the primary analysis together with 471 of the women in the control group.

The OR for the binary outcome (baby admitted to the special baby unit for respiratory distress) is then 11/492 divided by 24/471, giving a value 0.439. The chi-square test comparing the treatments with regard to the rates of admission gave $p=0.02$.

A logistic regression analysis was undertaken with

$z = 0$ if mother randomised to control

$z = 1$ if mother randomised to betamethasone

The analysis was adjusted for gestational age and involved two indicator variables; the standard gestational age was 39 weeks and

$x_1 = 1$ if gest. age = 37 weeks

    0 if otherwise

$x_2 = 1$ if gest. age = 38 weeks

    0 if otherwise

The coefficient of the treatment indicator z was −0.840 giving an (adjusted) OR for the treatment effect of 0.432 ($e^{-0.840}=0.432$). The coefficient b_1 of x_1 was 2.139 and the coefficient b_2 of x_2 was 1.472. So a value of $x_1=1$ (gestational age = 37 weeks) gives an increase of 2.139 on the log odds scale or, equivalently, an increase of 8.5 ($e^{2.139}=8.5$) on the odds of being admitted to the special baby unit compared to the standard 39 weeks' gestational age. For 38 weeks' gestational age, the increase to the odds of being admitted is 4.4 ($e^{1.472}=4.4$) compared to a gestational age of 39 weeks.

We can also investigate the presence of treatment-by-covariate interactions by including cross-product terms:

$$\ell n\left\{\frac{\mathrm{pr}(y=1)}{\left[1-\mathrm{pr}(y=1)\right]}\right\} = a + cz + b_1x_1 + b_2x_2 + d_1zx_1 + d_2zx_2$$

Questions relating to those interaction terms are addressed through the d coefficients as before for continuous data. In Example 6.1, looking for treatment-by-covariate interactions would be asking whether the treatment benefit, in terms of a reduction in the likelihood of the baby suffering respiratory distress, was the same for babies delivered at 37, 38 and 39 weeks.

Logistic regression offers similar advantages as ANCOVA for continuous data: correcting for baseline imbalances, allowing the evaluation of the effects of the covariates and providing a convenient framework for the identification of treatment-by-covariate interactions. With regard to efficiency, the issues are slightly different. It is important with logistic regression to identify and include those covariates that are predictive of outcome in the modelling; otherwise, the treatment effects could be biased. See Ford, Norrie and Ahmedi (1995) for discussion on this point.

6.7 Regulatory aspects of the use of covariates

ICH E9 and the CPMP (2003) *Points to Consider on Adjustment for Baseline Covariates* make a number of useful points. These are in addition to those already set down in Chapter 5:

- Pre-planning. It is important that the covariates to be included are decided in advance.

CPMP (2003): 'Points to Consider on Adjustment for Baseline Covariates'

'Covariates to be included in the analysis must be pre-specified in the protocol or in the statistical analysis plan.'

If new knowledge becomes available regarding important covariates after completion of the statistical analysis plan, then *modify* the plan at the blind review stage.

- Baseline imbalances

CPMP (2003): 'Points to Consider on Adjustment for Baseline Covariates'

'Baseline imbalance in itself should not be considered an appropriate reason to include a baseline measure as a covariate.'

In the final section of this chapter, we will say more about baseline imbalances and how to deal with them.

- Covariates affected by treatment allocation. Variables measured after randomisation (e.g. compliance, duration of treatment) should not be used as covariates in a model for evaluation of the treatment effect as these may be influenced by the treatment received. A similar issue concerns *late baselines*, that is, covariate measures that are based on data captured after randomisation. The term *time-dependent covariate* is sometimes used in relation to these considerations.

ICH E9 (1998): 'Note for Guidance on Statistical Principles for Clinical Trials'

'It is not advisable to adjust the main analyses for covariates measured after randomisation because they may be affected by the treatments.'

CPMP (2003): 'Points to Consider on Adjustment for Baseline Covariates'

'A covariate that may be affected by the treatment allocation (for example, a covariate measured after randomisation such as duration of treatment, level of compliance or use of rescue medication) should not normally be included in the primary analysis of a confirmatory trial. When a covariate is affected by the treatment either through direct causation or through association with another factor, the adjustment may hide or exaggerate the treatment effect. It therefore makes the treatment effect difficult to interpret.'

- It is good practice for continuous outcome variables recording change from baseline to adjust the analysis or include the baseline value of the outcome variable in the analysis as a covariate. When this is done, including the outcome variable itself or the change from baseline in that variable makes no difference mathematically to the analysis; the same *p*-values and estimates of treatment effect will be obtained, so the choice is one of interpretability. If the baseline value is not included in this way, then there could be problems with regression towards the mean.

  Regression towards the mean is a phenomenon that frequently occurs with data and in a wide variety of situations. For example, in a chronic condition like asthma, patients will often enter a trial because they have recently suffered a number of exacerbations and are having a particularly bad time with their condition. Almost irrespective of treatment, they will likely improve because asthma severity is cyclical and intervention has occurred at a low point. If change from baseline was then used as the variable to measure the effectiveness of a treatment, the mean change from baseline in each of the two treatment groups would undoubtedly overestimate the benefit of treatment in each of the treatment groups; part of those improvements would be due to *regression towards the mean*. Further, in a randomised comparison, if one treatment group, by chance, contained patients with poorer baseline values, then comparing the mean change from baseline in one group with the mean change from baseline in the other group could give a biased conclusion. Of course, randomisation should protect against this, but in particular cases, imbalances can be present and including the baseline value as a covariate in ANCOVA or adjusting through ANOVA will correct for this bias.

CPMP (2003): 'Points to Consider on Adjustment for Baseline Covariates'

'When the analysis is based on a continuous outcome there is commonly the choice of whether to use the raw outcome variable or the change from baseline as the primary endpoint. Whichever of these endpoints is chosen, the baseline value should be included as a covariate in the primary analysis. The use of change from baseline without adjusting for baseline does not generally constitute an appropriate covariate adjustment. Note that when the baseline is included as a covariate in the model, the estimated treatment effects are identical for both "change from baseline" and the "raw outcome" analysis.'

- How many covariates? It is usually not appropriate to include lots of covariates in an analysis.

CPMP (2003): 'Points to Consider on Adjustment for Baseline Covariates'

'No more than a few covariates should be included in the primary analysis.'

Remember however that variables used to stratify the randomisation should be included. It is also not usually appropriate to select covariates within ANCOVA models using stepwise (or indeed any other) techniques. The main purpose of the analysis is to compare the treatment groups, not to select covariates.

CPMP (2003): 'Points to Consider on Adjustment for Baseline Covariates'

'Methods that select covariates by choosing those that are most strongly associated with the primary outcome (often called "variable selection methods") should be avoided. The clinical and statistical relevance of a covariate should be assessed and justified from a source other than the current dataset.'

Finally, including covariates that are highly correlated adds little to the analysis and should be avoided. Clinical knowledge of such correlations should help to prevent this from happening.

6.8 Baseline testing

It is generally accepted among statisticians that baseline testing, that is, producing p-values for comparisons between the treatment groups at baseline, is of little value. If randomisation has been performed correctly, then 5 per cent of significance test comparisons at baseline will give statistically significant results; any imbalances seen at baseline must be due to chance. The only value to such testing is to evaluate whether the randomisation has been performed correctly, for example, in the detection of fraud. Altman (1991), Section 15.4, provides an extensive discussion on the issue of baseline testing.

CPMP (2003): 'Points to Consider on Adjustment for Baseline Covariates'

'Statistical testing for baseline imbalance has no role in a trial where the handling of randomisation and blinding has been fully satisfactory.'

It is nonetheless appropriate to produce baseline tables of summary statistics for each of the treatment groups. These should be looked at from a clinical perspective and imbalances in variables that are potentially predictive of outcome noted. Good practice hopefully will have ensured that the randomisation has been stratified for important baseline prognostic factors and/or the important prognostic factors have been included in some kind of adjusted analysis, for example, ANCOVA. If this is not the case, then sensitivity analyses should be undertaken through ANOVA or ANCOVA to make sure that those imbalances are not the sole cause of an observed positive (or negative) treatment difference.

CPMP (2003): 'Points to Consider on Adjustment for Baseline Covariates'

'When there is some imbalance between the treatment groups in a baseline covariate that is solely due to chance then adjusted treatment effects may account for this observed imbalance when unadjusted analyses may not. If the imbalance is such that the experimental group has a better prognosis than the control group, then adjusting for the imbalance is particularly important. Sensitivity analyses should be provided to demonstrate that any observed positive treatment effect is not solely explained by imbalances at baseline in any of the covariates.'

CHAPTER 7

Intention-to-treat and analysis sets

7.1 The principle of intention-to-treat

When we analyse data, there are inevitably questions that arise regarding how to deal with patients who withdraw, with patients who have violated the protocol, with patients who have taken a banned concomitant medication and so on. The principle of intention-to-treat (ITT) helps guide our actions. We will firstly explain the principle through two examples and then discuss various aspects of its interpretation before addressing the application of the principle in practice.

Example 7.1 Surgery compared to radiotherapy in operable lung cancer

Consider a (hypothetical) trial comparing surgery and radiotherapy in the treatment of operable lung cancer. Assume that a total of 200 patients were randomised to one of these two groups as shown in Figure 7.1.

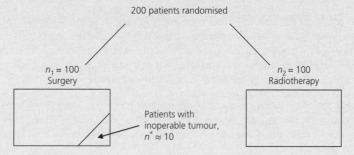

Figure 7.1 Randomised trial comparing surgery and radiotherapy

Unfortunately some of the patients randomised to the surgery group were found on the operating table not to have operable tumours. The intended operative procedure could not be undertaken for these patients and they were simply closed up and in fact given the radiotherapy regimen defined for the radiotherapy group. Assume that there were 10 such patients. The primary endpoint was survival time and all 200 patients were followed up until death. At the analysis stage, we have to decide how to deal with the 10 patients who were assigned to surgery, but who did not receive the intended surgery. Several possibilities exist for the analysis and we will consider the following three:

Statistical Thinking for Non-Statisticians in Drug Regulation, Second Edition. Richard Kay.
© 2015 John Wiley & Sons, Ltd. Published 2015 by John Wiley & Sons, Ltd.

Option 1: compare the mean survival time of the 90 who received the intended surgery with the mean survival time of the 100 who were assigned to radiotherapy.

Remember that all 200 patients provide data on the primary endpoint so this analysis ignores the data on 10 of those patients, those who were assigned to surgery but did not receive the intended operative procedure. Perhaps we can think of ways of including those data. Options 2 and 3 include these patients.

Option 2: compare the mean survival time of the 90 patients who received the intended surgery with the mean survival time of the 100 + 10 patients who ended up getting radiotherapy.

The argument here is that the 10 patients who *switched* from surgery to radiotherapy are most likely to behave like the 100 patients initially assigned to the radiotherapy group.

Option 3: compare the groups according to the randomisation scheme, that is, the mean survival time of the 100 patients initially assigned to surgery with the mean survival time of the 100 patients initially assigned to radiotherapy.

These three options differ merely in the way the 10 patients who were assigned to surgery but did not receive the intended surgery are handled. Option 1 ignores them, option 2 puts them in the radiotherapy *group*, while option 3 leaves them in the surgery *group*.

There are two things to note immediately. Firstly, the 10 patients in the surgery group who do not have operable tumours are likely to have very poor prognoses. These are the patients who have advanced tumours, maybe multiple tumours, that cannot easily be excised. Secondly, randomisation will have given us balanced groups so equally there will be approximately 10 patients in the radiotherapy group who also do not have operable tumours and similarly have very poor prognosis, but these patients remain unseen and unidentified.

Now, consider the implications arising out of each of these options.

Option 1: this option removes 10 very poor prognosis patients from the surgery group but leaves a similar group of very poor prognosis patients in the radiotherapy group. This clearly introduces bias as it is not comparing like with like. The radiotherapy group will, because of the omission of 10 very specific poor patients in the surgery group, be on average a better prognosis group than the surgery group to which they are being compared.

Option 2: this option is twice as bad! The 10 very poor prognosis patients from the surgery group have been transferred to the radiotherapy group to give a total of 20 very poor prognosis patients in that group. The bias in the resulting analysis is likely to be even bigger than the bias under option 1.

Option 3: this is the only valid option. It is the only option that compares groups that are alike in terms of the mix of patients. This is the intention-to-treat option, which compares the groups as randomised.

A number of issues arise out of these considerations. While option 1 makes sense from a statistical perspective, does it make sense from a clinical standpoint? Remember that the purpose of this trial is to compare surgery and radiotherapy in operable lung cancer yet we are including 10 patients in the surgery group who did not receive the planned surgery. Well, in fact, option 3 is not comparing surgery with radiotherapy; it is comparing two treatment strategies. Strategy 1 is to give the patient surgery; however, if it is found that the tumour is not operable, then close the patient up and give them radiotherapy, while strategy 2 is to give radiotherapy.

Although you may agree that this provides a comparison of these two treatment strategies, you may say that this is not of interest to you clinically and you are looking for a comparison of pure surgery with pure radiotherapy. On that basis, you may therefore prefer to go for option 1, which seems to provide exactly what you want, as it gives a comparison of pure surgery with pure radiotherapy! This view, however, would be both naive and incorrect. Option 1 does not provide a *valid* comparison of pure surgery and pure radiotherapy because the groups are not alike; it is subject to bias because the radiotherapy group in this comparison is on average a better prognosis group than the surgery *group*.

A question that sometimes arises here is, can't we just remove 10 patients from the radiotherapy group and then compare the 90 who received surgery with the resulting radiotherapy group? No, although this would equalise the numbers in the two groups being compared, it would not necessarily equalise the mix of patients in the two groups. Remember that the 10 patients who did not get surgery are not just any 10 patients; they are a selected group of very poor prognosis patients. Well, as an alternative, could we not remove the 10 patients in the radiotherapy group who turn out to have the worst survival experience? The answer again is no; this would not necessarily make the resulting comparison valid as it is based on a very strong assumption, which could never be verified, that the 10 patients who did not get the intended surgery are indeed the 10 worst patients from that group. Unfortunately, the comparison of pure surgery and pure radiotherapy is not possible in this trial. The only question that can be answered relates to the evaluation of the two treatment strategies as mentioned earlier.

Example 7.2 Clofibrate in the reduction of mortality after myocardial infarction

This is a well-known placebo-controlled trial that evaluated clofibrate in terms of reducing mortality in patients suffering a myocardial infarct that was reported by Coronary Drug Project Research Group (1980).

The groups were compared overall and the five-year death rate among the 1103 patients randomised to clofibrate was 20.0 per cent compared to a five-year death rate among the 2789 placebo patients of 20.9 per cent. These differences were not statistically significant with $p=0.55$.

The trialists then investigated the impact of compliance on these results. Patients were defined as good compliers if they took at least 80 per cent of the prescribed dose during the treatment period. Poor compliers were patients who took less than 80 per cent. In the clofibrate group, the good compliers were seen to have only a 15.0 per cent five-year death rate, while the poor compliers had a 24.6 per cent five-year death rate, a clear difference both clinically and statistically with $p=0.001$. So, in fact, the active medication does work, it is simply a matter of taking the medication. Patients who take the medication do well, while those who fail to take the medication do not.

This same comparison however was then undertaken among the placebo patients. The good compliers on placebo only had a 15.1 per cent five-year death rate, while the poor compliers had a 28.3 per cent five-year death rate with $p=0.0000000000000047$! These placebo tablets are remarkable!

A moment's thought will suffice to realise that the conclusions we are drawing from these analyses are nonsense. The bottom line is that the active medication is having no effect and the initial overall comparison is telling us that. However, compliance is linked to other things that are potentially having an effect, such as giving up smoking, starting to take regular exercise, modifying one's diet to reduce the amount of sugar consumed and so on. The patients who do these things are the ones who do everything that their doctors tell them to do, including taking the medication! So, the taking of the medication is correlated with some other things that are beneficial and causing an apparent *treatment* effect related to compliance.

These two examples should give a clear indication of the dangers of compromising the randomisation at the analysis stage. Even small departures in terms of excluding patients from the analysis could have a major impact on the validity of the conclusions.

The *principle of intention-to-treat* tells us to compare the patients according to the treatments to which they were randomised. Randomisation gives us comparable groups; removing patients at the analysis stage destroys the randomisation and introduces bias. Randomisation also underpins the validity of the statistical comparisons. If we depart from the randomisation scheme, then the statistical properties of our tests are compromised.

The FDA guideline on antimicrobial drugs captures the issues well.

FDA (1998): 'Developing Anti-microbial Drugs – General Considerations for Clinical Trials'

'The intent-to-treat principle suggests that eligible, randomized patients should be evaluated with respect to outcome based on original treatment assignment regardless of modifications to treatment occurring after randomisation. The statistical analysis seeks to establish if the particular assignment received is predictive of outcome, and the study can be interpreted as a strategy trial where the initial assignment is only the beginning of the treatment strategy. However, many researchers seek to glean results from the clinical trial that would have been observed if all patients had been able to remain on their initial assignment. This leads to analysis of subsets that exclude patients with imperfect compliance or follow-up data. However, the validity of these analyses rests on the assumption that the two treatment groups, after excluding such patients, differ only by the treatment received. This assumption could be violated in many subtle ways. For example, differential toxicity related to severity of illness could lead to selection bias. Similarly, the subjects unable to comply with medication may be those most at risk of a negative outcome and their exclusion may bias the treatment comparison.'

7.2 The practice of intention-to-treat

7.2.1 Full analysis set

The previous section clearly indicates the need to conform to the principle of intention-to-treat to ensure that the statistical comparison of the treatment groups remains valid. In practice, compliance with this principle is a little more difficult, and the regulators, recognising these difficulties, allow a compromise. This involves the definition in particular trials of the *full analysis set*, which gets us as close as we possibly can get to the intention-to-treat ideal.

ICH E9 (1998): 'Note for Guidance on Statistical Principles for Clinical Trials'

'The intention-to-treat principle implies that the primary analysis should include all randomised subjects. Compliance with this principle would necessitate complete follow-up of all randomised subjects for study outcomes. In practice this ideal may be difficult to achieve, for reasons to be described. In this document the term "full analysis set" is used to describe the analysis set which is as complete as possible and as close as possible to the intention-to-treat ideal of including all randomised subjects.'

The regulators are telling us therefore, to get as close as possible and they go on in the ICH E9 guideline to outline circumstances where it will usually be acceptable to omit subjects without causing bias.

These potential exclusions are:
- Subjects who violate the inclusion/exclusion criteria
- Subjects who fail to take at least one dose of study medication
- Subjects who do not provide any post-baseline data

These omissions will not cause bias only under some circumstances. In particular, subjects in each of the treatment groups should receive equal scrutiny for protocol violations, and all such violators should be excluded, in relation to the first point. For the second and third points, the fact that patients do not take study medication or do not provide any post-baseline data should be unrelated to the treatments to which such subjects were assigned. Any potential bias arising from these exclusions should be fully investigated.

The term full analysis set was introduced in order to separate the practice of ITT from the principle, but practitioners still frequently use the term *ITT population* when referring to this set. The term *modified ITT population* is also in common use within particular companies and also by regulators in some settings where exclusions from strict ITT are considered. Different therapeutic situations will invariably give rise to different considerations on how best to define the most appropriate analysis sets. Increasingly, we are seeing very specific regulatory guidance in this regard within therapeutic specific guidelines. In the treatment of bacterial infections, for example, the CHMP (2012) guideline recommends defining *clinically evaluable* or *microbiologically evaluable* populations, which are the groups of patients with clinically or microbiologically (respectively) confirmed baseline pathogens as the basis of co-primary analyses together with the *all-treated* population.

In superiority trials, the full analysis set or something akin to that is invariably the basis for the primary analysis. The regulatory preference for this stems in part because the full analysis set also tends to give a conservative view of the treatment difference, as a result of including in the analysis subjects who have not conformed entirely with the protocol. The regulators can be assured that if the analysis based on this set gives a statistically significant result, then the treatment being evaluated is effective. This preference, however, only applies when considering superiority trials. In equivalence and non-inferiority, this analysis set tends to be anti-conservative. This issue will be discussed later, in the chapter on equivalence and non-inferiority testing.

7.2.2 Per-protocol set

The *per-protocol set* is described as follows by the regulators.

ICH E9 (1998): 'Note for Guidance on Statistical Principles for Clinical Trials'

'The "per-protocol" set of subjects, sometimes described as the "valid cases", the "efficacy" sample or the "evaluable subjects" sample, defines a subset of the subjects in the full analysis set who are more compliant with the protocol...'

The definition of a per-protocol set of subjects allows us to get closer to the scientific question by including only those patients who comply with the protocol to a defined extent. The per-protocol set, like the full analysis set, must be pre-specified in the protocol and then defined at the patient level at the blind review, following database lock but before breaking the blind. It must be noted, however, that the per-protocol set is subject to bias and further, tends to over-estimate the treatment effect. For this reason, it is usually used only as a secondary analysis, supportive hopefully of the findings based on the full analysis set.

7.2.3 Sensitivity

It is good statistical practice to evaluate the sensitivity of the conclusions to different choices of the analysis sets.

ICH E9 (1998): 'Note for Guidance on Statistical Principles for Clinical Trials'

'In general, it is advantageous to demonstrate a lack of sensitivity of the principle trial results to alternative choices of the set of subjects analysed. In confirmatory trials it is usually appropriate to plan to conduct both an analysis of the full analysis set and a per-protocol analysis, so that any differences between them can be the subject of explicit discussion and interpretation'.

This regulatory statement is not saying that the analyses based on the full analysis set and the per-protocol set are in any sense co-primary. The full analysis set will provide the primary analysis, and usually this analysis must give $p \le 0.05$ for a positive result. The per-protocol set however, does not need to give $p \le 0.05$, but should provide results that are qualitatively similar in terms of the direction of the treatment effect and with effect size not too dissimilar from that seen for the full analysis set.

***ICH E9 (1998): 'Note for Guidance on Statistical Principles
for Clinical Trials'***

*'When the full analysis set and the per-protocol set lead to essentially the same
conclusions, confidence in the trial results is increased...'*

For further discussion on the definition of analysis sets and additional practical
advice, see Gillings and Koch (1991).

7.3 Missing data

7.3.1 Introduction

The discussion in the previous section regarding the practical application of the
principle of ITT does not, however, give the full picture. While this principle plus
consideration of the per-protocol set may clearly define the sets of subjects to be
analysed, we still have to decide how to deal with the missing data caused by
failure to complete the study entirely in line with the protocol.

***ICH E9 (1998): 'Note for Guidance on Statistical Principles
for Clinical Trials'***

*'Missing values represent a potential source of bias in a clinical trial. Hence, every
effort should be undertaken to fulfill all the requirements of the protocol concerning
the collection and management of data. In reality, however, there will almost always
be some missing data. A trial may be regarded as valid, nonetheless, provided the
methods of dealing with missing values are sensible, and particularly if those
methods are pre-defined in the protocol.'*

It is worth remembering that there is no single, perfect way of handling missing
data. The only truly effective way of dealing with missing data is not to have any
in the first place! In practice, we always need to consider the sensitivity of our
trial results to the methods employed to handle the missing data. This is particularly true if the amount of such data is large.

There are a number of alternative approaches to dealing with missing data in
common practice. Among these are the following:
- Complete cases analysis
- Last observation carried forward (LOCF)
- Success/failure classification
- Worst-case/best-case imputation

Recently, we have seen the development of a collection of more sophisticated
methods that go under the general heading of *Multiple Imputation*. These are
based on certain assumptions about the mechanism that causes the data to be
missing. We will discuss this framework in the final subsection to follow.

7.3.2 Complete cases analysis

One very simplistic way of handling missing data is to remove those patients with missing data from the analysis in a *complete cases analysis* or *completer analysis*. By definition, this will be a per-protocol analysis that will omit all patients who do not provide a measure on the primary endpoint and will of course be subject to bias. Such an analysis may well be acceptable in an exploratory setting where we may be looking to get some idea of the treatment effect if every subject were to follow the protocol perfectly, but it would not be acceptable in a confirmatory setting as a primary analysis.

7.3.3 Last observation carried forward

This analysis takes the final observation for each patient and uses it as that patient's endpoint in the analysis. For example, in a 12-month trial in acute schizophrenia, a patient who withdraws at month 7 due to side effects will have their month 7 value included in the analysis of the data.

In one sense, this approach has clinical appeal. The final value provided by the patient who withdrew at month 7 is a valid measure of how successful we have been in treating this patient with the assigned treatment and so should be part of the overall evaluation of the treatment. In some circumstances, however, this argument breaks down. For example, if there is an underlying worsening trend in disease severity, then patients who withdraw early will tend to provide better outcomes than those who withdraw later on in the treatment period. If one treatment has more early dropouts than the other, say, possibly because of side effects, then there will be bias caused by the use of Last observation carried forward. Multiple sclerosis and Alzheimer's disease are settings where this could apply. The opposite will of course be true in cases where the underlying trend is one of improvement; depression would be one such therapeutic area. These scenarios emphasise the earlier point that there is no universally valid way to deal with missing data.

7.3.4 Success/failure classification

One particularly simple way of dealing with missing data is to use a binary outcome as the endpoint with dropouts being classified as treatment success or failure depending on the outcome at the time of dropping out. For example, in a hypertension trial, success may be defined as diastolic blood pressure below 90 mmHg at the end of the treatment period or at the time of treatment withdrawal with all other outcomes being classified as failures. Reducing the outcome to a dichotomy in this way will, however, lead to a loss of power, and this loss of power needs to be considered when calculating sample size at the planning stage. This kind of analysis is often referred to as a *responder analysis*.

A success/failure approach will be particularly effective if the endpoint is already binary, for example, cured/not cured in a trial of an anti-infective with patients with missing data, perhaps due to withdrawal, treated as failures.

7.3.5 Worst-case/best-case classification

This method gives those subjects who withdraw for positive reasons the best possible outcome value for the endpoint and those who withdraw for negative reasons, the worst value. This may seem a little extreme and a lesser position would be to look at the distribution of the endpoint for the completers and to use, say, the upper quartile (the value that cuts off the best 25 per cent of values) for those subjects withdrawing for positive reasons and the lower quartile (the value that cuts off the worst 25 per cent of values) for those subjects who withdraw for negative reasons.

Alternative applications of these rules would be to use the best-case value for subjects in the control group and the worst-case value for subjects in the test treatment group. Certainly, if the treatment comparison is preserved under such a harsh scheme, then we can be confident of a true benefit for the test treatment!

Example 7.3 Bosentan therapy in pulmonary arterial hypertension

This was a placebo-controlled trial (Rubin *et al.*, 2002) using change from baseline to week 16 in exercise capacity (distance in metres walked in six minutes) as the primary endpoint and change from baseline to week 16 in the Borg dyspnea index and in the WHO functional class as key secondary endpoints. Missing data at week 16 were handled as follows:

'For patients who discontinued the study medication because of clinical worsening, the values recorded at the time of discontinuation were used; patients for whom no value was recorded (including patients who died) were assigned the worst possible value (0 m). For all other patients without a week 16 assessment, the last six-minute walking distance, score on the Borg dyspnea index, and WHO functional class were used as week 16 values.'

So for patients without week 16 values, LOCF was used, unless the patient withdrew because of clinical worsening, in which case either the data at the time of withdrawal was used or a worst-case imputed value (zero metres for the walk test, Borg index = 0 or WHO = IV) if there were no data at withdrawal. This set of rules, which is predefined, is clinically appropriate and should help to minimise bias.

7.3.6 Sensitivity

In all cases, and particularly where the extent of missing data is substantial, several analyses will usually be undertaken to assess the sensitivity of the conclusions to the method used to handle missing data. If the conclusions are fairly consistent across these different analyses, then we are in a good position. If, however, our conclusions are seen to change or to depend heavily on the method used for dealing with missing data, then the validity of those conclusions will be drawn into question.

Our discussion so far regarding sensitivity has focused on using several different approaches to both the definition of the analysis sets and the handling of missing data. One of the main goals of a trial is to estimate the magnitude of the treatment benefit, and these sensitivity evaluations will give a series of estimates. For estimation purposes, and in particular here we are thinking in terms of confidence intervals, we should choose a method of imputation that makes sense clinically rather than go for extremes that, while providing a conservative view of the treatment effect for the purposes of evaluating statistical significance, do not give a sensible, realistic estimate of the clinical benefit.

7.3.7 Avoidance of missing data

The CPMP guideline on missing data (CHMP, 2010) includes several key points on the avoidance of missing data. As we can see from the earlier discussion, missing data causes problems and we should avoid it wherever possible.

CPMP (2010): 'Points to Consider on Missing Data in Confirmatory Clinical Trials'

'Several major difficulties arise as a result of the presence of missing values and these are aggravated as the number of missing values increases. Thus, it is extremely important to avoid the presence of unobserved measurements as much as possible, by favouring designs that minimise this problem, as well as strengthening data collection regardless of the patient's adhesion to the protocol and encouraging the retrieval of data after the patient's drop-out. Continued collection of data after the patient's cessation of study treatment is strongly encouraged, in particular data on clinical outcome. In some circumstances, in particular where this type of "retrieved dropout" information represents the progression of the patient without (or before) impact of further therapeutic intervention, these data give the best approximation to the Full Analysis Set and would generally be seen as a sound basis for the primary analysis.'

Allowing dose reductions or drug *holidays* will possibly keep patients in a trial and avoid them dropping out, in addition to providing a closer model to what will actually happen in practice in real life. Continued follow-up for patients who withdraw from medication should also be considered, and this will give much more flexibility when it comes to analysing the data once the trial is complete. There are of course ethical issues associated with continuing follow-up for patients who wish to withdraw from treatment. In some countries, it is disallowed by law and that of itself may rule out the potential for doing this, or alternatively, we can restrict recruitment to countries where it is feasible. If continued follow-up following withdrawal from treatment is to happen, then the informed consent form will need to be structured taking account of this.

7.3.8 Multiple imputation

Many of the methods we have discussed for dealing with missing data have involved some form of *imputation*. LOCF, success/failure classification and worst-case/best-case classification are all examples where the missing data values have been replaced by certain assumed values. In this section, we will briefly discuss more sophisticated forms of imputation in conjunction with various assumptions regarding the nature of the missing data.

A theoretical framework has been developed that is based on a classification according to the nature of the underlying *missingness* mechanism:

- If the probability that an observation for a patient is missing does not depend on the observed or the unobserved data for that patient, then the observation is said to be *missing completely at random (MCAR)*. This form of missingness occurs, for example, if a patient misses a visit because of some administrative mistake in booking the appointment. Omitting patients with missing data from the analysis under these circumstances will not cause bias.

- If the probability that an observation for a patient is missing depends only on the observed data for that patient, then the observation is said to be *missing at random (MAR)*. This form of missingness occurs if the reason why the data are missing is as a consequence of the deteriorating condition of the patient, but the fact that their condition is deteriorating can be predicted from data for the patient at one or more previous visits. Omitting patients with missing data under these circumstances will cause bias. However, these missing data values can be *predicted* or *imputed* based on other observed data to remove that bias.

- When the observation is neither MCAR nor MAR, then it is said to be *missing not at random (MNAR)*. This kind of missingness will occur, for example, if the reason why data are missing is as a result of the deteriorating condition of the patient but that deterioration cannot be predicted from previous data on the patient. Under these circumstances, omitting patients with missing data will again cause bias; not only that, there is no way to correct for this bias through prediction/modelling as is the case with MCAR and MAR.

Note that in the definitions of MCAR and MAR, when we talk about the *observed data for that patient*, we are thinking in terms of baseline data, observations taken on the variable that is missing at earlier visits as well as data on other variables at the visit where the observation in question is missing. Further details at a technical level on this framework are provided by Carpenter and Kenward (2007), while Sterne *et al.* (2009) give a basic overview.

The difficulty with applying this thinking under most circumstances is that it is not possible to know definitively which situation we are in. Nonetheless, we can make various assumptions about the missingness mechanism and undertake sensitivity analyses of the data based on varying these assumptions.

If the data truly are MCAR, then we can simply undertake an analysis based on those patients with data to get an unbiased view of the treatment differences.

If the data are MAR, then various strategies based on fitting models to the non-missing data and imputing values for the missing data by simulation are available. This is done several times (between 3 and 10 simulations) and the results are averaged. We are beginning to gain more experience in using these methods since the major computer packages have developed routines that implement the approach and the methods seem to have good properties in terms of producing valid estimates for treatment differences and other quantities of interest. There are various options for the choice of the model, and the robustness of the conclusions can be evaluated by varying those options. MNAR is much more difficult to deal with, although some methods are available. See Carpenter and Kenward (2007) for more details.

7.4 Intention-to-treat and time-to-event data

In order to illustrate the kinds of arguments and considerations that are needed in relation to ITT, the discussion in this section will consider a set of applications where problems frequently arise. In Chapter 13, we will cover methods for the analysis of time-to-event or so-called survival data, but for the moment, I would like to focus on endpoints within these areas that do not use the time point at which randomisation occurs as the start point for the time-to-event measure. Examples include the time from rash healing to complete cessation of pain in herpes zoster, the time from six weeks after start of treatment to first seizure in epilepsy and the time from eight weeks to relapse among responders at week 8 in severe depression.

In each of these situations, there are clinical arguments that support the use of the particular endpoint concerned. From a statistical point of view, however, each of these endpoints gives an analysis that is subject to bias in a clear violation of the principle of ITT. We will look at each of the settings in turn.

In the case of a randomised trial in herpes zoster, patients have the potential to cease pain prior to rash healing, and these patients would not enter the analysis of time to cessation of pain from rash healing. Invariably, the likelihood that pain will cease early in this way will depend upon the treatment received. As a consequence, the sets of patients in each of the two treatment groups entering the analysis of time to cessation of pain from rash healing will not necessarily be alike. This selection phenomenon will result in a violation of ITT and the resultant analysis will be biased. See Kay (1995) for further discussion on this point. There have been some attempts (see, e.g. Arani *et al.*, 2001) to justify such an analysis using complex statistical modelling, but this approach has been shown by Kay (2006) to be flawed and the problem of violation of ITT remains. In herpes zoster, the pain that remains following rash healing is known as post-hepatic neuralgia (PHN), and there is strong interest in evaluating the relative effects of treatments on PHN. Looking at time from rash healing to cessation of pain is an attempt to focus on this. Unfortunately, it is not possible, even in a randomised trial, to analyse this endpoint in an unbiased way. The only way to identify the relative effect of the two treatments with regard to PHN is to compare the proportion of all patients in the two treatment groups still with pain at specified points through time.

In newly diagnosed epilepsy, it is common practice to use the time from six weeks (or sometimes three months) following the start of treatment to the first seizure, as the primary or certainly important secondary endpoint. Again, however, we hit problems with selection effects and ITT. Brodie *et al.* (1995) evaluate lamotrigine compared to carbamazepine in a randomised trial in patients with newly diagnosed epilepsy. In a secondary analysis of time (from randomisation) to withdrawal, it is clear that by six weeks, approximately 18 per cent of the patients have withdrawn in the lamotrigine group, while approximately 27 per cent of patients have withdrawn in the carbamazepine group. The analysis of time from six weeks to first seizure excludes these patients. This is a very long way from being a randomised comparison and is potentially subject to substantial bias. Even if the withdrawal rates had been the same, the potential for bias would remain. It is not so much that the numbers of patients withdrawing are different; it is that the comparability in terms of the mix of patients has been compromised, and the differential withdrawal rates just make things worse. From a clinical point of view, excluding the first six weeks of treatment does make sense as it is recognised that it takes some time to stabilise the dose, but again unfortunately, the endpoint that apparently captures this, time from six weeks to first seizure, cannot be evaluated in an unbiased way. An alternative and appropriate approach to look at the effectiveness of treatment following dose stabilisation has been suggested by Brodie and Whitehead (2006). These authors (using three months as the stabilisation period rather than six weeks) consider the following endpoint; time from randomisation to withdrawal, whenever this occurs, or to first seizure from three months onwards.

This endpoint combines both tolerability (withdrawal) and efficacy (first seizure), but does not penalise a treatment in terms of seizures during the stabilisation phase (the first three months) provided that tolerability is not a problem over that period. From a pragmatic perspective, this alternative endpoint makes a lot of sense; from the patients' point of view, the important issue is longer-term stabilisation, free of seizures, and this endpoint captures precisely that.

Finally, in severe depression, many trials are designed to investigate treatment relapse in patients who have responded following treatment. Response could be defined, for example, by a reduction in the score on the 17-point Hamilton Depression Scale (HAMD-17) to below 15 with relapse defined as an increase to 16 or above. Typically, response is assessed following eight weeks of treatment, and the endpoint of interest in evaluating relapse is the time from eight weeks to relapse. Patients who have not responded by week 8 are usually withdrawn for lack of efficacy. These extension studies in responders are not randomised comparisons, and the analysis is based solely on those patients who are responders at eight weeks. Storosum *et al.* (2001) recognise the potential for bias in this analysis. In common with the previous two settings, there is a violation of the principle of ITT. An alternative analysis that looks at time to treatment failure with treatment failure defined as withdrawn from treatment for lack of efficacy up to week 8 or HAMD-17 ≥ 16 beyond week 8 would maintain all patients in the treatment comparison. This comparison takes account of possible differential effects of treatment up to and including week 8 in terms of achieving a response, and beyond week 8 is looking at the proportion of patients whose response is maintained.

As a general rule, time-to-event endpoints that do not use the point of randomisation as the start point should be avoided as there is always the potential for patient selection to take place between the point of randomisation and when the clock starts ticking for the proposed endpoint.

7.5 General questions and considerations

One question that is frequently asked is, what do you do with patients who were given the wrong treatment by mistake? It must be said that this does not happen very frequently, but when it does, it is necessary to dig a little and try to find out why this has happened. If it is an isolated case and is clearly an administrative error, then it seems most reasonable to include that patient in the group according to treatment received. Note that strict ITT would retain this patient in the group to which they were randomised and such an analysis may be imposed by regulators. If, however, it is not an isolated case, maybe there are several such mistakes in the same centre, then this draws into question the validity of what is happening at that centre, and one starts to think in terms of fraud; has the investigator correctly followed the randomisation scheme? In such situations, there may be consideration, ultimately, of removing all of the data from that centre from the analysis.

The considerations so far in this chapter have been on the evaluation of efficacy. For safety, we usually define the *safety set* as the set of subjects who receive at least one dose of study medication. Usually, the safety set will coincide with the full analysis set, but not always. There may well be a patient who started on medication but withdrew immediately because of a side effect. This patient is unlikely to have provided post-baseline efficacy data and so could be excluded from the full analysis set but would still be included in the safety set.

In crossover trials, considerations of analysis sets and missing data are somewhat different. In these trials, each subject provides a response on each of the treatments. The analysis of such data focuses on the treatment difference within each subject. When a subject drops out during the second period and therefore fails to give a response for the treatment given in period 2, then it is not possible to calculate a treatment difference, and so this patient would not be included in the analysis. So, in crossover trials, we are usually forced to exclude the dropouts. Does this compromise the validity of the treatment comparison? In terms of bias, the answer is not usually, since exclusions of this kind will deplete each of the treatment *groups* equally as the same subject is being omitted from both of them, although the potential for bias should always be considered. In terms, however, of extrapolating the conclusions from the trial to the general population, there could be problems. If particular kinds of patients are being omitted from the analysis essentially because they are prone to side effects from one of the two treatments being compared, for example, then the trial population may not be representative of the population defined by the inclusion/exclusion criteria. However, in phase I studies with healthy volunteers, these aspects are unlikely to be an issue, and it is common practice to *replace* dropouts with other subjects in order to achieve the required sample size.

A key aspect of the definition of analysis sets and the way that missing data is to be handled is pre-specification. Usually, these points will be covered in the protocol, if not, in the statistical analysis plan. If methods are not pre-specified, then there will be problems as the way that these issues are dealt with could then be data driven, or at least there may be suspicion of that. This is, of course, not unique to analysis sets and missing data, but is true more generally in relation to the main methods of statistical analysis.

To conclude this discussion, it is worth covering just a few misconceptions:

- Does having equal numbers of subjects in the treatment groups at the statistical analysis stage protect against bias?

  This corresponds to similar dropout rates across the treatment groups. The answer to the question is no! It is the mix of patients that is the basis of a valid comparison, not the numbers of patients. It is almost inevitable that if two treatments are truly different, then different kinds of subjects will drop out from the two groups. For example, in a placebo-controlled trial, those withdrawing from the active treatment group could well be withdrawing for side effects, while the dropouts in the placebo group could be withdrawing because of lack of effect.

- Does basing the sample size calculation on the per-protocol set and then increasing the sample size to allow for dropouts ensure that the per-protocol set will not be subject to bias?

  No! It often makes sense to power for the per-protocol set and then factor upwards to allow for dropouts as this will also ensure that there is enough power for the full analysis set provided that any extra patient-to-patient variation in the full analysis set does not counterbalance the increase in sample size, but the analysis based on the per-protocol set is still subject to bias. See Section 8.5.2 for further discussion on this point.

- Does pre-specifying in the protocol that the analysis based on the per-protocol set will be the primary analysis protect against bias?

  As mentioned elsewhere, it is good scientific practice to pre-specify the main methods of statistical analysis in the protocol, but just because something is specified in the protocol it does not mean that it is correct. So again, the answer is no.

CHAPTER 8

Power and sample size

8.1 Type I and type II errors

The statistical test procedures that we use unfortunately are not perfect, and from time to time, we will be fooled by the data and draw incorrect conclusions. For example, we know that 17 heads and 3 tails can (and will) occur with 20 flips of a fair coin (the probability from Section 3.3.2 is 0.0011); however, that outcome would give a significant p-value, and we would conclude incorrectly that the coin was not fair. Conversely, we could construct a coin that was biased 60 per cent/40 per cent in favour of heads and in 20 flips, see, for example 13 heads and 7 tails. That outcome would lead to a non-significant p-value ($p=0.224$), and we would fail to pick up the bias. These two potential mistakes are termed type I and type II errors.

To explain in a little more detail, consider a parallel-group trial in which we are comparing two treatment means using the unpaired t-test. The null hypothesis $H_0: \mu_1 = \mu_2$ that the treatment means are equal is either true or not true; God knows we don't! We mere mortals have to make do with data, and on the basis of data, we will see either a significant p-value ($p \leq 0.05$) or a non-significant p-value ($p=NS*$). The various possibilities are contained in Table 8.1.

Suppose the truth is that $\mu_1 = \mu_2$, the treatment means are the same. We would hope that the data would give a non-significant p-value and our conclusion would be correct; we are unable to conclude that differences exist. Unfortunately, that does not always occur, and on some occasions we will be hoodwinked by the data and get $p \leq 0.05$. On that basis, we will declare statistical significance and draw the conclusion that the treatment means are different. This mistake is called the *type I error*. It is the *false positive*, sometimes referred to as the *α error*.

Conversely suppose that in reality $\mu_1 \neq \mu_2$, the treatment means are different. In this case we would hope that $p \leq 0.05$, in which case our conclusion will be the correct one, treatment differences. Again this will not always happen, and there will be occasions when, under these circumstances, we get $p=NS*$, a non-significant p-value. On this basis, we will say that we do not have enough

---

$*p$ = NS is shorthand to say that p is not statistically significant at the 5 per cent level. Its use in reporting trial results is not recommended; exact p-values should be used.

Statistical Thinking for Non-Statisticians in Drug Regulation, Second Edition. Richard Kay.
© 2015 John Wiley & Sons, Ltd. Published 2015 by John Wiley & Sons, Ltd.

Table 8.1 Type I and type II errors

	H_0 true, $\mu_1 = \mu_2$	H_0 not true, $\mu_1 \neq \mu_2$
Data gives $p = NS$ (cannot conclude $\mu_1 \neq \mu_2$)	√	x
Data gives $p \leq 0.05$ (conclude $\mu_1 \neq \mu_2$)	x	√

evidence to conclude differences. This second potential mistake is called the *type II error*. This is the *false negative* or the β error, the treatment means really are different, but we have missed it!

There is a well-known theorem in statistics, called the Neyman–Pearson Lemma, which shows that for a given sample size, it is simply not possible to eliminate these two mistakes; we must always trade them off against each another. Usually, the type I error is fixed at 0.05 (5 per cent). This is because we use 5 per cent as the significance level, the cut-off between significance ($p \leq 0.05$) and non-significance ($p > 0.05$). The null distribution tells us precisely what will happen when the null hypothesis is true; we *will* get extreme values in the tails of that distribution, even when $\mu_1 = \mu_2$. However, when we do see a value in the extreme outer 5 per cent, we declare significant differences, and by definition, this will occur 5 per cent of the time when H_0 is true.

The type II error is a little more difficult to pin down. It is related to another quantity called power. If type II error is 10 per cent, then power is 90 per cent; *power* is 100 minus type II error. Type II error is missing a real difference – power is capturing a real difference; if there is a 10 per cent chance of missing the bus, there is a 90 per cent chance of catching the bus, and they are opposites in this sense! We control type II error by controlling power; for example, we may design our trial to have 80 per cent power, in which case the type II error is controlled at 20 per cent.

8.2 Power

As seen in the previous section, power measures our ability to detect treatment differences. A convenient mathematical way of thinking about power is

$$\text{power} = \text{probability} \left(p \leq 0.05 \right)$$

When we say that a trial has 80 per cent power to detect a certain level of effect, for example, 4 mmHg, what we mean is that if we conduct the trial and the true difference really is 4 mmHg, then there is an 80 per cent chance of coming out of the trial with a significant p-value and declaring differences. In other words, if we were to run this same trial 10 times, then on 8 of those occasions, on average, we would get a statistically significant result at the 5 per cent level, and on 2 occasions, on average, we would get a non-significant result.

Table 8.2 Power for various treatment differences, $n = 50$ per group

Treatment difference, $\mu_1 - \mu_2$	Power
0.25	0.206
0.50	0.623
0.75	0.926
1.00	0.995

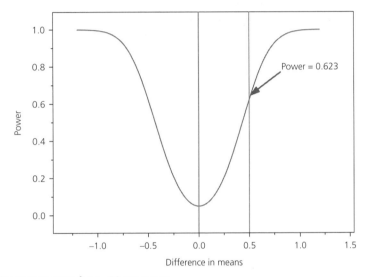

Figure 8.1 Power curve for $n = 50$ per group

We can in fact calculate power in advance of running the trial by speculating about what may happen. Assume in a parallel-group cholesterol lowering study comparing a test treatment with placebo that there are 50 patients per group. The unpaired t-test will be used to compare the mean reduction in cholesterol level between the groups at the conventional two-sided significance level of 0.05. Assume also that the standard deviation for the reduction in cholesterol is 1.1 mmol/l. For various values for the treatment difference, the calculated power is given in Table 8.2.

So, for example, if the true difference between the treatments means was 0.50 mmol/l, then this trial would have a 62.3 per cent chance of coming out with a significant p-value ($p \le 0.05$). Similarly, if the true difference were 0.75 mmol/l, then the chance of getting a significant result would be 92.6 per cent.

Figure 8.1 plots the values for power against the true difference in the treatment means. Certain patterns emerge. Power increases with the magnitude of the treatment difference, large differences give high values for power, and the value for power approaches one as the treatment difference increases in either a negative or a positive direction. The implication here is that large differences are easy to detect and small differences are more difficult to detect. The power curve is symmetric about zero, and this is because our test is a two-sided test; a difference of +1 mmol/l has just the same power as a difference of −1 mmol/l.

Suppose now that the trial in the example were a trial in which a difference of 0.5 mmol/l was viewed as an important difference. Maybe this reflects the clinical relevance of such a difference, or perhaps from a commercial standpoint, it would be a worthwhile difference to have for a new drug in the marketplace. Under these circumstances, only having 62.3 per cent power to detect such a difference would be unacceptable; this corresponds to a 37.7 per cent type II error, an almost 40 per cent chance of failing to declare significant differences. Well, there is only one thing you can do, and that is to increase the sample size. The recalculated values for power are given in Table 8.3 with a doubling of the sample size to 100 patients per group.

The power now to detect a difference of 0.5 mmol/l is 89.5 per cent, a substantial improvement on 62.3 per cent. Figure 8.2 shows the power curve for a

Table 8.3 Power for $n = 100$ per group

Treatment difference, $\mu_1 - \mu_2$	Power
0.25	0.362
0.50	0.895
0.75	0.998
1.00	1.000

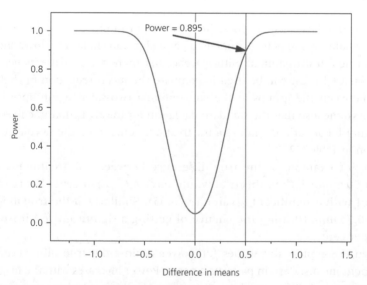

Figure 8.2 Power curve for $n = 100$ per group

sample size of 100 patients per group, and it can be seen that the values for power have increased across all the potential values for the true treatment difference. These arguments form the basis of the sample size calculation; we think in terms of what level of effect it is important to detect, either from a clinical, regulatory or commercial perspective, and choose our sample size to give high power for detecting such an effect. In our example, if we had said that we require 80 per cent power to detect a difference of 0.50 mmol/l, then a sample size of 76 per group would have given us exactly that. For 90 per cent power, we would need 102 patients per group.

Before moving on to discuss sample size calculations in more detail, it is worth noticing that the power curve does not come down to zero at a difference of 0.0 and the curve actually crosses the y-axis at the significance level, 0.05. Recall that power can be thought of as the probability ($p \leq 0.05$). Even when the treatments are identical (difference = 0.0), there is still a 0.05 chance of getting a significant p-value, and this is the type I error and the reason why the power curve cuts at this value. This issue tells as what happens if we want to change the significance level, for example, from 0.05 to 0.01. (We sometimes do this when dealing with multiplicity, and we will look in more detail at this issue in Chapter 10.) Reducing the significance level will pull down the power curve so that it crosses at 0.01, and the effect of this will be to reduce all of the power values. Even when there are true treatment differences, achieving $p \leq 0.01$ is much more difficult than achieving $p \leq 0.05$ and so the power comes down. In practice, of course, we may need to consider increasing the sample size to compensate for this reduction in the significance level to recover the required power.

8.3 Calculating sample size

Once the requirements of a trial have been specified, then calculating sample size is fairly straightforward; formulas exist for all of the commonly occurring situations.

In all cases, we need to specify the required values of the type I error and the power. Usually we set the type I error at 5 per cent, and the recommended minimum value for power is 80 per cent, although for important trials 80 per cent is not enough and 90 per cent at least is recommended.

The remaining quantities that need to be considered when calculating sample size depend upon the particular statistical test to be used:

- For the unpaired t-test, we need to specify the standard deviation, σ, for the primary endpoint and the level of effect, d, we are looking to detect with, say, 90 per cent power.

There is usually an implicit assumption in this calculation that the standard deviations are the same in each of the treatment groups. Generally speaking, this assumption is a reasonable one to make as the effect of treatment will usually be to change the mean with no effect on the variability. We will say a little more about dealing at the analysis stage with situations where this is not the case in a later section. The sample size calculation, however, is also easily modified, if needed, to allow unequal standard deviations.

- For the paired t-test, the standard deviation of the within-patient differences for the primary endpoint needs to be specified, and again, the level of effect to be detected.
- For the χ^2 test, we need to know the success/event rate in the control group and as usual some measure of the treatment difference we are looking to detect.

We commonly refer to the level of effect to be detected as the *clinically relevant difference (crd)*; what level of effect is an important effect from a clinical standpoint. Note also that crd stands for *commercially relevant difference*; it could well be that the decision is based on commercial considerations. Finally, crd stands for *cynically relevant difference*! It does happen from time to time that a statistician is asked to 'do a sample size calculation, oh, and by the way, we want 200 patients!' The issue here of course is budget, and the question really is, what level of effect are we able to detect with a sample size of 200?

The standard deviations referred to earlier often provide the biggest challenge. The information for this will come from previous data; for that same endpoint, from a similar population/sample of patients, treated for the same period of time etc., similar comments apply for the success/event rate in the control group for binary data. We should try and match as closely as possible the conditions of the historical data to those pertaining to the trial being planned.

Example 8.1 Unpaired t-test

In a placebo-controlled hypertension trial, the primary endpoint is the fall in diastolic blood pressure. It is required to detect a clinically relevant difference of 8 mmHg in a 5 per cent level test. Historical data suggests that $\sigma = 10$ mmHg. Table 8.4 provides sample sizes for various levels of power and differences around 8 mmHg; the sample sizes are per group.

So for 90 per cent power, 33 patients per group are required to detect a difference of 8 mmHg. Smaller differences are more difficult to detect, and 59 patients per group are needed to have 90 per cent power to detect a difference of 6 mmHg. Lowering the power from 90 per cent to 80 per cent reduces the sample size requirement by just over 25 per cent.

Table 8.4 Sample sizes per group

crd	Power		
	80%	85%	90%
6 mmHg	44	50	59
8 mmHg	24	29	33
10 mmHg	16	18	22

Example 8.2 χ^2 test

In a parallel-group, placebo-controlled trial in acute stroke, the primary endpoint is success on the Barthel index at month 3. Previous data suggests that the success rate on placebo will be 35 per cent, and it is required to detect an improvement in the active treatment group to 50 per cent. How many patients are needed for 90 per cent power?

For 90 per cent power, 227 patients per group are needed. For 80 per cent power, the sample size reduces to 170 patients per group. If the success rate in the placebo group, however, were to be 40 per cent and not 35 per cent, then the sample size requirements per group would increase to 519 for 90 per cent power and 388 for 80 per cent power to detect an improvement to 50 per cent in the active group.

Machin *et al.* (1997) provide extensive tables in relation to sample size calculations and include in their book, formulas and many examples. In addition, there are several software packages specifically designed to perform power and sample size calculations, namely, nQuery (www.statsol.ie) and PASS (www.ncss. com). The general statistics package S-PLUS (www.insightful.com) also contains some of the simpler calculations, and for those with access to SAS®, O'Brien and Castelloe (2010) give details on the use of that package for calculations.

It is generally true that sample size calculations are undertaken based on simple test procedures, such as the unpaired t-test and the χ^2 test. In dealing with both continuous and binary data, it is likely that the primary analysis will ultimately be based on adjusting for important baseline prognostic factors. Usually, such analyses will give higher power than the simple alternatives. These more complex methods of analysis, however, are not taken into account in the sample size calculation for two reasons. Firstly, it would be very complicated to do so and would involve specifying the precise nature of the dependence of the primary endpoint on the factors to be adjusted for and knowledge regarding how those baseline factors will be distributed within the target population. Secondly, using the simple approach is a conservative approach as generally speaking the more complex methods of analysis that we end up using will lead to an increase in power.

Finally, note that in our considerations we have worked with groups of equal size. It is straightforward to adapt the calculations for unequal randomisation schemes, and the computer packages mentioned earlier can deal with these. Altman (1991) (Section 15.3) provides a simple method for adapting the standard sample size calculation to unequal group sizes as follows. If N is the calculated sample size based on an equal randomisation and k represents the ratio of the number of patients in one group compared to the other group, then the required number of patients for a k to 1 randomisation is

$$N' = N \frac{(1+k)^2}{4k}$$

So, for example, if a 2 to 1 randomisation is required and 200 patients would have been needed for 1 to 1 allocation, then the revised sample size is

$$N' = 200 \times \frac{9}{8} = 225$$

a fairly modest increase. In general, a 2 to 1 randomisation will lead to a 12.5 per cent increase in sample size compared to 1 to 1; a 3 to 1 randomisation would lead to a 33.3 per cent increase.

8.4 Impact of changing the parameters

8.4.1 Standard deviation

It is interesting to see the impact of a change in the standard deviation on the required sample size. Consider the example from the previous section where we were looking to detect a treatment effect of 8 mmHg with a standard deviation of 10 mmHg. For 90 per cent power, the total sample size requirement was 66 patients. If the standard deviation was not 10 mmHg but 20 mmHg, then the required sample size would be 264. A doubling of the standard deviation has led to a fourfold increase in the sample size. The formula for sample size contains not the standard deviation by itself but the variance (=standard deviation squared), and this is what drives this increase. Even a modest increase in the standard deviation, say, from 10 mmHg to 12 mmHg, would require 96 patients in total compared to 66.

There are several implications of this sensitivity of sample size on the standard deviation:

- Good information is needed for the standard deviation; if you get it slightly wrong, you could be severely underpowered. Be realistic, and if anything, conservative.
- Work hard to control the patient-to-patient variability, which not only depends on in-built patient differences but also on extraneous variability caused by an inconsistent measurement technique, data recording and sloppy methodology. Tightening up on these things will over time bring σ down and help to keep sample sizes lower than they would otherwise be.

8.4.2 Event rate in the control group

Again, referring to an example in the previous section where the event was a success on the Barthel index at month 3, we had an event rate in the control group of 35 per cent, and we were looking to detect an improvement of 15 per cent in absolute terms to 50 per cent. A sample size of 227 per group gave 90 per cent power. Figure 8.3 illustrates how this sample size depends upon the success rate in the control group; note we are looking in each case for an absolute 15 per cent improvement.

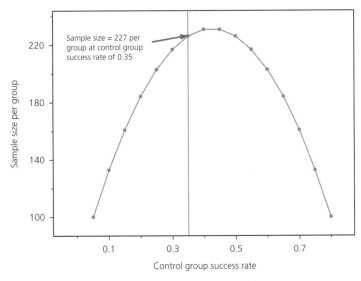

Figure 8.3 Sample size for detecting absolute improvement of 0.15 in success rates

The curve is symmetric around a rate of 0.425 (half-way between 0.35 and 0.50) since we are undertaking two-tailed tests, and changing the labels for success and failure will simply repackage the same calculation. So, for example, comparing 30 per cent to 45 per cent produces the same sample size as comparing 70 per cent to 55 per cent. The sample sizes are much reduced as the success rates move either down towards 0 per cent or up towards 100 per cent. In those regions, of course, the relative changes in either the success rate or the failure rate are large, and it is this that controls the calculation.

One point worth making here is that information on event rates in the control group will inevitably come from studies that took place some time ago. As general patient care is improving in many circumstances over time, these historical rates may not be reflective of what will happen in the future for the trial that is being planned. Moreover, these historical rates, for example, when we are looking at failure rates, could well be overestimates for the current trial. This could lead to the situation where the actual difference in the rates between the control and experimental groups is less than what was assumed in the sample size calculation and a study that is consequently underpowered.

8.4.3 Clinically relevant difference

For continuous data, the sample size is inversely proportional to the square of the clinically relevant difference. So if the crd is reduced by a factor of two, then the sample size is increased by a factor of four; if the crd is increased by a factor of two, then the sample size is reduced by a factor of four. In our earlier example, the sample size requirement to detect a difference of 8 mmHg was 33 patients per group. To detect a difference of 4 mmHg, we require 132 patients per group.

For binary data, this same relationship between the crd, in terms of the absolute difference in success rates, and the sample size is only approximately true. In the example, we were looking to detect an improvement in the success rate from 35 per cent to 50 per cent, an absolute difference of 15 per cent, and we needed a sample size of 227 patients per group. If we were to halve that difference and look for an improvement from 35 per cent to 42.5 per cent, then the sample size requirement would be 885 per group, an increase in the sample size by a factor of 3.9.

8.5 Regulatory aspects

8.5.1 Power >80 per cent

The recommendation for at least 80 per cent power comes from the ICH E9 guideline:

ICH E9 (1998): 'Note for Guidance on Statistical Principles for Clinical Trials'

'The number of subjects in a clinical trial should always be large enough to provide a reliable answer to the questions addressed... The probability of type II error is conventionally set at 10 per cent to 20 per cent; it is in the sponsor's interest to keep this figure as low as feasible especially in the case of trials that are difficult or impossible to repeat'.

The guideline stresses that it is *in the sponsor's interest* to have power as high as possible. Too often, researchers see the power calculation as merely something that has to go into the protocol to satisfy ethics committees and regulators and go for the *minimum* requirement. Also, it is tempting to choose ambitious values for the key parameters, such as the standard deviation of the primary endpoint, or the event rate in the control group, or the crd, to produce a sample size that is comfortable from a budgeting or practical point of view, only to be disappointed once the data appears. Be realistic in the choice of these quantities and recognise that 80 per cent power is 20 per cent type II error, a one in five chance of failing to achieve statistical significance even if everything runs perfectly and in line with assumptions.

8.5.2 Powering on the per-protocol set

Generally speaking, we power based on the per-protocol set and then increase the sample size requirement to give the number of patients for the full analysis set.

So if we need 250 patients for the required power and we expect 10 per cent of patients to be excluded from the full analysis set for the per-protocol analysis, then we need to recruit 278 patients (90 per cent of 278 gives 250). The argument here is that because the full analysis set will be larger than the per-protocol set, then having enough power for the latter will automatically give enough power for both. Generally, this will be true, but sometimes it is not quite so simple.

The variability in the outcome measure across the full analysis set may well be larger than it is in the per-protocol set, and so simply factoring up the sample size to account for the non-evaluable patients may not sufficiently counterbalance the increase in the standard deviation. In a similar way, it may be that the crd seen in the analysis based on the per-protocol set is larger than that seen in the full analysis set, and this anticipated difference may also need to be factored in. It must be noted, however, that even if the sample size calculation gives enough power for the per-protocol analysis, the potential for bias in that analysis still remains.

8.5.3 Sample size adjustment

It will sometimes be the case that there are gaps in our knowledge, and it will not be possible to give values for the standard deviation or for the event rate in the control group with any degree of confidence. In these circumstances, it is possible to revisit the sample size calculation once the trial is underway.

ICH E9 (1998): 'Note for Guidance on Statistical Principles for Clinical Trials'

'In long term trials there will usually be an opportunity to check the assumptions which underlay the original design and sample size calculations. This may be particularly important if the trial specifications have been made on preliminary and/or uncertain information. An interim check conducted on the blinded data may reveal that overall response variances, event rates or survival experience are not as anticipated. A revised sample size may then be calculated using suitably modified assumptions…'.

Note that this calculation must be undertaken on the blinded data, in other words using data on the treatment groups combined. Even evaluating the data with the two groups separated using arbitrary labels A and B (partial unblinding) would not be acceptable. If a comparison based on either partial or complete unblinding were to be made, then there would be a price to pay in terms of the type I error. We will say much more about this in two later sections dealing with interim analysis (Section 8.5.3) and adaptive designs (Section 16.1.2).

Using all of the data as a single group to calculate the standard deviation in the continuous case, however, will give an overestimate of the within-group standard deviation, particularly if the treatment differences are large. It must be accepted therefore that this could lead to some overpowering as a consequence, although in practice experience suggests that this is minor. For binary data, we will end up with a combined event rate, and this must be unpicked to enable a sample size recalculation to be done. For example, if the original calculation is based upon detecting an increase in the success rate from 35 per cent to 50 per cent, then we are expecting an overall success rate of 42.5 per cent. If at the interim check this overall rate turns out to be 45 per cent, then we are looking for an increase from 37.5 per cent to 42.5 per cent if we want to retain the ability of the trial to have enough power to detect an absolute 15 per cent improvement.

8.6 Reporting the sample size calculation

A detailed statement of the basis of the sample size calculation should be included in the protocol and in the final report. This statement should contain the following:

- Significance level to be used. This will usually be 5 per cent and relate to a two-sided test or <5 per cent depending on issues of multiplicity.
- Required power (≥80 per cent).
- The primary endpoint on which the calculation is based together with the statistical test procedure.
- Estimates of the basic quantities needed for the calculation such as the standard deviation or the event rate in the control group and the sources of those estimates.
- The clinically/commercially relevant difference (crd). If the expected difference is larger than this, then it could be worth considering powering for the expected effect and the sample size will be lower.
- The withdrawal rate to enable the trial to be powered based on those patients who do not withdraw, and the resulting recruitment target.

The CONSORT statement (Schulz *et al.*, 2010) sets down standards for the reporting of clinical trials, and their recommendations in relation to the sample size calculation are in line with these points. There may, of course, be cases, especially in the early exploratory phase, where the sample size has been chosen on purely practical or feasibility grounds. This is perfectly acceptable in that context, and the sample size section in the protocol should clearly state that this is the case. The following example is taken from a published clinical trial.

Example 8.3 Xamoterol in severe heart failure

Below is the sample size statement from the Xamoterol in Severe Heart Failure Study Group (1990):

'It was estimated that 228 patients would have to complete the study to give a 90 per cent chance of detecting a 30-second difference in exercise duration between placebo and xamoterol at the 5 per cent level of significance. The aim was therefore to recruit at least 255 patients to allow for withdrawals. A blinded re-evaluation of the variance of the exercise data after the first 63 patients had completed the study, and a higher drop-out rate (15 per cent) than expected (10 per cent) caused the steering committee (in agreement with the safety committee) to revise the recruitment figure to at least 450'.

Consider each of the elements in the calculation and reporting of that calculation in turn:
- The primary endpoint on which the calculation is based is the exercise duration.
- The required power was set at 90 per cent, a type II error of 10 per cent.
- The type I error was set at 5 per cent. Note in general the alternative phrases for the type I error: significance level, α error and false-positive rate.

- Which statistical test was to be used for the comparison of the treatment groups in terms of the primary endpoint do you think? This is a comparison between two independent groups in a parallel-group trial, and the primary endpoint is continuous so the sample size calculation will undoubtedly have been based on the two-sample t-test (although this is not specified).
- The trial appears to have been powered in terms of the per-protocol set. Recruitment was set at 255 patients to allow for dropouts.
- There were two reasons for increasing the sample size: a larger than expected standard deviation (variance) for the primary endpoint and a higher dropout rate (15 per cent compared to 10 per cent).

Most of the elements are contained within the sample size section according to the requirements set down in the CONSORT statement; the only omissions seem to be specification of the statistical test on which the sample size calculation was based, the assumed standard deviation of the primary endpoint and the basis for that assumption.

CHAPTER 9

Statistical significance and clinical importance

9.1 Link between *p*-values and confidence intervals

In Chapter 3, we developed the concepts of both the confidence interval (CI) and the *p*-value. At that stage, these ideas were kept separate. There is in fact a close link between the two, and in this section, we will develop that link.

Consider an application of the unpaired t-test with

$$H_0 : \mu_1 = \mu_2 \quad H_1 : \mu_1 \neq \mu_2$$

Note that the null hypothesis could be rewritten as $H_0 : \mu_1 - \mu_2 = 0$.

The 95 per cent confidence interval (a, b) for the difference in the treatment means, $\mu_1 - \mu_2$, provides a range of plausible values for the true treatment difference. With 95 per cent confidence, we can say that $\mu_1 - \mu_2$ is somewhere within the range from a to b.

Consider the results presented in Table 9.1 for two separate trials. In trial 1, the *p*-value is indicating that the treatment means are different. The confidence interval is also supporting treatment differences, with the magnitude of that difference lying between 2.1 and 5.7 units with 95 per cent confidence. So at least informally in this case, the *p*-value and the confidence interval are telling us similar things; the treatment means are different. In trial 2, the *p*-value is not supporting differences, while the 95 per cent confidence interval tells us that μ_1 could be bigger than μ_2 by as much as 4.6 units but also that μ_2 could be bigger than μ_1 by as much as 1.3 units and everything in between is also possible, so certainly 0 is a plausible value for $\mu_1 - \mu_2$. In this case again, the *p*-value and the confidence interval are saying similar things and neither is able to discount the equality of the treatment means.

In fact, the link between the *p*-value and the confidence interval is not just operating at this informal level; it is much stronger and there is a mathematical connection between the two, which goes as follows:

- If $p < 0.05$, then the 95 per cent confidence interval for $\mu_1 - \mu_2$ will exclude zero (and vice versa).
- If $p = NS$, then the 95 per cent confidence interval for $\mu_1 - \mu_2$ will include zero (and vice versa).

Note that if p is exactly equal to 0.05, then one end of the confidence interval will be equal to zero; this is the boundary between the two conditions above.

Statistical Thinking for Non-Statisticians in Drug Regulation, Second Edition. Richard Kay.
© 2015 John Wiley & Sons, Ltd. Published 2015 by John Wiley & Sons, Ltd.

Table 9.1 p-values and confidence intervals for two trials (hypothetical)

	p-value	95% CI for $\mu_1 - \mu_2$
Trial 1	$p < 0.05$	(2.1 mmHg, 5.7 mmHg)
Trial 2	$p = NS$	(−1.3 mmHg, 4.6 mmHg)

One element that makes the link work is the correspondence between the significance level (5 per cent) and the confidence coefficient (95 per cent). If we were to use 1 per cent as the cut-off for statistical significance, then the same link would apply but now with the 99 per cent Confidence interval.

There is a misunderstanding regarding a similar potential link between the p-value and the Confidence intervals for the individual means. A significant p-value does not necessarily correspond to non-overlapping Confidence intervals for the individual means. See Julious (2004) and Cumming (2009) for further discussion on this issue.

This link applies also to the p-value from the paired t-test and the Confidence interval for μ, the mean difference between the treatments, and in addition extends to adjusted analyses including ANOVA and ANCOVA and similarly for regression. For example, if the test for the slope b of the regression line gives a significant p-value (at the 5 per cent level), then the 95 per cent Confidence interval for the slope will not contain zero, and vice versa.

When dealing with binary data, a similar link applies but now with the Confidence interval for the odds ratio and the p-value for the χ^2 test, with one important difference; it is the value one (and not zero) that is excluded or included from the Confidence interval when p is either significant or non-significant, respectively. Recall that for the odds ratio, it is the value one that corresponds to equal treatments. The link for binary data is not in fact exact in the strict mathematical sense, but in practice, this correspondence can be assumed to apply pretty much all of the time except right on the boundary of 0.05 for the p-value where from time to time one end of the Confidence interval may not quite fall on the appropriate side of one. Similar comments to these apply also to the relative risk.

9.2 Confidence intervals for clinical importance

Example 9.1 presents some hypothetical data from 4 trials in hypertension.
- Trial 1 has given statistical significance and has detected something of clinical importance.
- Trial 2 has also given statistical significance, but the difference detected is clinically unimportant.

In comparing the results from trials 1 and 2, it is clear that the p-value does not tell the whole story. In terms of p-values, they are indistinguishable, but the first trial has demonstrated a clinically important difference, while trial 2 has detected something that is clinically irrelevant.

Example 9.1 A series of trials in hypertension (hypothetical)

In a collection of four placebo-controlled trials in hypertension, a difference of 4 mmHg in terms of mean fall in diastolic bp is to be considered of clinical importance; anything less is unimportant. The results are given in Table 9.2, where μ_1 and μ_2 are the mean reductions in diastolic bp in the active and placebo groups, respectively.

Table 9.2 p-values and confidence intervals for four trials

	p-value	**95% CI for $\mu_1 - \mu_2$**
Trial 1	$p < 0.05$	(3.4 mmHg, 12.8 mmHg)
Trial 2	$p < 0.05$	(1.2 mmHg, 2.9 mmHg)
Trial 3	$p = NS$	(−3.5 mmHg, 3.1 mmHg)
Trial 4	$p = NS$	(−2.6 mmHg, 14.3 mmHg)

Note the mathematical connection again with the first two trials giving significant p-values and the second two trials giving non-significant p-values.

- Trial 3 has given non-significance statistically, and inspecting the confidence interval tells us that there is nothing in terms of clinical importance either; at most with 95 per cent confidence, the benefit of the active treatment is only 3.1 mmHg.
- Trial 4 is different, however. We do not have statistical significance, but the confidence interval suggests that there could still be something of clinical importance with potential differences of 5 mmHg, 10 mmHg and even 14 mmHg. This is classically the trial that is too small with low power to detect even large differences.

Again, the p-value is not giving the whole story. There is clearly nothing of any clinical importance in trial 3, but in trial 4, there could be something worthwhile – it is just that the trial is too small.

It should be clear from the development in this example that statistical significance and clinical importance are somewhat different things. The p-value tells us nothing about clinical importance. Just because we have statistical significance, it does not mean, necessarily, that we have detected a clinically important effect. Vice versa, just because we have a non-significant result does not necessarily indicate the absence of something of clinical importance. The most appropriate way to provide information on clinical benefit is by presenting observed treatment differences together with confidence intervals.

Gardner and Altman (1989) capture the essence of this argument:

'Presenting p-values alone can lead to them being given more merit that they deserve. In particular, there is a tendency to equate statistical significance with medical importance or biological relevance. But small differences of no real interest can be statistically significant with large sample sizes, whereas clinically important effects may be statistically non-significant only because the number of subjects studied was small'.

The regulators are not only interested in statistical significance but also in clinical importance. This allows them, and others, to appropriately balance benefit and risk. It is good practice therefore to present both *p*-values and confidence intervals, and indeed, this is a requirement within a regulatory submission. Most journals nowadays also require results to be presented in the form of confidence intervals in addition to *p*-values.

9.3 Misinterpretation of the *p*-value

9.3.1 Conclusions of similarity

In Section 3.3.1, we defined the *p*-value and briefly mentioned a common incorrect definition. We will return now to discuss why this leads to considerable misinterpretation. In the example of Section 3.3.1, we had observed a treatment difference of 5.4 mmHg with a *p*-value of 0.042 (4.2 per cent), and the proposed incorrect definition was that 'there is a 4.2 per cent probability that $\mu_1 = \mu_2$'.

The problem with this definition is the misinterpretation when the *p*-value is large. As an extreme case, suppose that we ran a trial in hypertension with two patients per group, and also suppose that even though in truth the true treatment means were very different, the patients in the active group had blood pressure reductions of 7 mmHg and 5 mmHg, respectively, while in the placebo group, the reductions were 2 mmHg and 10 mmHg. These data give a mean reduction in the active group of 6 mmHg and a mean reduction in the placebo group of 6 mmHg. In a two-sample t-test, the resulting *p*-value would be one $\left(\text{signal} = \bar{x}_1 - \bar{x}_2 = 0\right)$. A *p*-value of 1 or 100 per cent corresponds to certainty, and taking the aforementioned definition of the *p*-value is telling us on the basis of the observed data that it is certain that the true treatment means are identical! I hope we would all agree that this conclusion based on two patients per group would be entirely inappropriate.

This example, of course, is purely hypothetical, but in practice, we do see large *p*-values, say, of the order of 0.70 or 0.80, that have come from situations where, in truth, the treatments could be very different but we have ended up with a large *p*-value merely as a result of a small sample size or a large amount of patient-to-patient variation (or both), and as a consequence, we have a large amount of noise, a small signal-to-noise (and signal-to-standard error) ratio and a large *p*-value. A *p*-value of this order of magnitude, under this (incorrect) definition, is giving a probability of something close to certainty that the treatment means are identical.

It is all too common to see a conclusion that treatments are the same (or similar) simply on the back of a large *p*-value; this is not necessarily the correct conclusion. Presentation of the 95 per cent confidence interval will provide a statement about the possible magnitude of the treatment difference. This can be inspected and only then can a conclusion of similarity be made if this interval is seen to exclude clinically important differences. We will return to a more formal approach to this in Chapter 12 where we discuss equivalence and non-inferiority.

9.3.2 The problem with 0.05

A further aspect of the p-value that causes some problems of interpretation is the cut-off for significance at 0.05. This issue was briefly raised in Section 3.3.4 where it was pointed out that 0.05 is a completely arbitrary cut-off for statistical significance and that p-values close to 0.05, but sitting on opposite sides of 0.05 should not really lead to different conclusions.

Too often, a p-value <0.05 is seen as definitive proof that the treatments are different, while a p-value above 0.05 is seen as no proof at all. The p-value is a measure of the compatibility of the data with equal treatments, the smaller the p-value the stronger the evidence against the null hypothesis. The p-value is a measure of evidence in relation to the null hypothesis; treating $p \leq 0.05$, $p > 0.05$ in a binary way as proof/no proof is a gross oversimplification, and we must never lose sight of that.

9.4 Single pivotal trial and 0.05

The conventional level for two-sided statistical significance for efficacy is 0.05, but there are some circumstances where a more stringent level is appropriate, in particular where regulatory submission is to be based on a single pivotal trial. A discussion of the two-pivotal-trial rule and under what conditions sponsors may be allowed to deviate from that requirement is included in CPMP (2001) *Points to Consider on Application with 1. Meta-Analysis; 2. One Pivotal Study*.

The repeatability of particular findings gives strong scientific support for the existence of a true treatment effect and is essentially the reason why the regulators in general like to see two pivotal trials that are positive ($p \leq 0.05$ in favour of the experimental treatment) – this clearly then constitutes convincing evidence. In conjunction with this, the two-trial rule provides an opportunity to investigate the treatment effect in different settings, and a demonstration of an effect in both trials adds support to the robustness of that positive finding. The policy of running two separate trials with the same protocol by simply dividing up the centres is not consistent with this thinking and should be avoided.

The two-trial rule, for example, in a placebo-controlled setting, effectively translates into a very stringent requirement for statistical significance. In a single trial, the conventional two-sided type I error rate is 0.05. It follows that in order to obtain a positive result from such a trial, we need the effect to be statistically significant and in favour of the active treatment. The type I error associated with this false-positive result is 0.025 (which is 1 in 40). In two trials, therefore, obtaining two false-positive results carries a combined false-positive rate of $0.025 \times 0.025 = 0.000625$ (which is 1 in 1600). In other words, if the active treatment were to be truly ineffective, then on only 1 in 1600 occasions would we see two positive trials by chance.

In therapeutic settings where there are practical reasons why two trials cannot be easily undertaken or where there is a major unfulfilled public health need, it may be possible for a claim to be based on a single pivotal trial. The regulatory authorities do allow this but only under certain conditions.

CPMP (2001): 'Points to Consider on Application with 1. Meta-Analysis; 2. One Pivotal Study'

'In cases where the confirmatory evidence is provided by one pivotal study only, this study will have to be exceptionally compelling, and in the regulatory evaluation special attention will be paid to:
- *The internal validity. There should be no indications of a potential bias*
- *The external validity. The study population should be suitable for extrapolation to the population to be treated*
- *Clinical relevance. The estimated size of the treatment benefit must be large enough to be clinically valuable*
- *The degree of statistical significance. Statistical evidence considerably stronger than p<0.05 is usually required*
- *Data quality*
- *Internal consistency. Similar effects demonstrated in different pre-specified sub-populations. All important endpoints showing similar findings*
- *Centre effects. None of the study centres should dominate the overall result, neither in terms of number of subjects nor in terms of magnitude of effect*
- *The plausibility of the hypothesis tested'*

Statistical evidence stronger than $p \leq 0.05$ is open to interpretation, but certainly one-sided $p \leq 0.000625$ would be a lower bound on this. In practice, the precise value would depend on the therapeutic setting and likely remain unspecified, although $p \leq 0.01$ would seem a fair compromise in many situations. The only exceptions to this are in orphan indications where the rules tend to be relaxed somewhat. It is difficult to make general statements as things depend so much on the particular situation. With a single pivotal trial in an orphan setting, however, it is unlikely that this requirement for the p-value to be considerable below 0.05 would apply.

It is worth commenting also on the *internal consistency* issue. In general, the regulators are looking for demonstration of a robust treatment effect. Within the context of the intended label there needs to be clear evidence that the treatment is effective in all sub-populations – age groups, disease severity, race, sex (if appropriate) and so on – and this is what is meant by internal consistency. The two-trial rule gives an opportunity to evaluate the treatment across two different settings, for example, different hospital types and different geographies. A single trial will only provide a similar level of assurance if it recruits across the broad range of settings, consistent with the label followed by a thorough demonstration of the homogeneity of the treatment effect across those settings.

CHAPTER 10

Multiple testing

10.1 Inflation of the type I error

10.1.1 False positives

Whenever we undertake a statistical test in a situation where the two treatments being compared are the same (e.g. in terms of equal means), there is a 5 per cent probability of getting a statistically significant result purely by chance; this is the type I error. If we were to conduct several tests in this same setting, then the probability of seeing one or more significant p-values purely by chance will start to mount up. For example, if we were to conduct five tests on independent sets of data, say, on five distinct subgroups, then the probability of getting at least one false-positive result is 22.6 per cent*. For 50 tests, this probability becomes 92.3 per cent, virtual certainty. This should come as no surprise; the 1 in 20 probability of the false positive on each occasion will eventually happen by chance. Certainly with 50 tests under these circumstances, the most surprising thing would be if you did not see the false positive on at least one occasion.

The problem with this so-called multiplicity or multiple testing arises when we make a claim on the basis of a positive result that has been *generated* simply because we have undertaken lots of comparisons and *cherry-picked* the statistically significant differences that are in our favour. Inflation of the type I error rate in this way is of great concern to the regulatory authorities and the clinical community more generally; regulators do not want to be registering, and the clinical community does not want to be adopting, treatments that do not work. It is necessary therefore to control this inflation. The majority of this chapter is concerned with ways in which the potential problem can be controlled, but firstly, we will look to an example to further illustrate the issues.

10.1.2 A simulated trial

Lee *et al.* (1980) report on lessons to be learned in multiple testing by analysing data from a simulated randomised clinical trial. These authors took data from 1073 consecutive, medically treated coronary artery disease patients from the

---

*The probability of no significant results in five tests is $0.95 \times 0.95 \times 0.95 \times 0.95 \times 0.95 = 0.774$, so the probability of one or more significant results is $1 - 0.774 = 0.226$.

Statistical Thinking for Non-Statisticians in Drug Regulation, Second Edition. Richard Kay.
© 2015 John Wiley & Sons, Ltd. Published 2015 by John Wiley & Sons, Ltd.

Duke University data bank and split these patients at random into two groups. They then labelled these groups 1 and 2 and proceeded to analyse these data as if the two groups had in fact received different treatments. These patients had all been treated medically, their data on baseline factors and outcome (survival time) was already complete, and the group 1 and group 2 *treatments* are totally spurious – they do not exist; this is just a random split of a database.

The overall comparison of the two groups in terms of the primary outcome survival time, not surprisingly, gave a non-significant *p*-value ($p > 0.05$). The authors then proceeded to investigate the data in subgroups. The two recognised key prognostic factors are the number of diseased vessels (1, 2 or 3) and left ventricular contraction pattern (LVCP – normal or abnormal). This defines six subgroups, and comparing group 1 with group 2 in each of these subgroups again yielded non-significant *p*-values. The *p*-value in the subgroup of patients with 3 diseased vessels and abnormal LVCP however gave a *p*-value between 0.10 and 0.15 perhaps indicating that there may be something of interest (a *trend*!) in that subgroup. They then analysed the data in this subgroup further by subdividing by a third prognostic factor, history of congestive heart failure (CHF, yes or no). The comparison in the subgroup, the number of diseased vessels = 3, abnormal LVCP and no history of CHF gave a statistically significant difference between group 1 and group 2 ($p < 0.01$). Note that this final comparison comes after 7 previous non-significant results looking at the data overall and in 6 initial subgroups. Even in a setting where the treatments are truly identical a statistically significant result will eventually appear.

Clearly, this difference must be the false positive; the separate group 1 and group 2 *treatments* are totally artificial – they do not exist. Lee *et al.* have used this simulated study to illustrate the false conclusions that potentially can arise through multiple testing. It is not that uncommon unfortunately to see trialists go off on the *fishing trip* in this post hoc way looking for treatment differences and the strategy that they undertook to *discover* this statistically significant *p*-value is maybe not untypical of what could happen in a real situation. This is very dangerous and can easily *uncover* effects that are not real.

10.2 How does multiplicity arise?

There are a number of settings that can result in multiplicity:
• Multiple endpoints
• Multiple pairwise comparisons in multi-arm trials
• Comparing treatments at multiple time points
• Comparing treatments within many subgroups
• Interim analyses
• Using different statistical tests on the same data
• Using different analysis sets or different algorithms for missing data
This list is not exhaustive, but these represent the main areas of concern.

We will explore each of these in turn, but before doing this, it is worth making some preliminary points. Firstly, not all multiple testing is a bad thing. For example, it is good practice to analyse several different analysis sets (the final bullet point) to gauge the robustness of the results to the choice of analysis set. It can also be of value to look at treatment differences in various subgroups in order to assess the homogeneity of the overall finding across the population as a whole. The problem arises when the results of these comparisons are *cherry-picked* with only those analyses that have given significant results being then used to make a confirmatory claim and those giving non-significant results just ignored or pushed to the background. Secondly, if this process of cherry-picking is to be in any sense allowed, then there will be a price to pay in terms of reducing the level at which statistical significance can be declared. We will say more about specific methods for making this reduction later, but basically, the idea is to divide up the 5 per cent allowable false-positive rate across the numerous tests that are going to be the basis of any confirmatory claims. For example, if there are five tests that make up the confirmatory analysis and a claim is going to be made on any of these tests that yield a significant result, then the level at which the statistical significance can be declared will reduce from 5 per cent to 1 per cent; the argument here is that five lots of 1 per cent make up 5 per cent so the overall type I error rate remains controlled at 5 per cent. For 10 tests, the *adjusted significance level* (sometimes denoted by α') would be 0.5 per cent. This is the simplest form of adjustment and is known as the *Bonferroni correction*.

10.3 Regulatory view

The regulatory position with regard to multiplicity is well expressed in ICH E9.

ICH E9 (1998): 'Note for Guidance on Statistical Principles for Clinical Trials'

'When multiplicity is present, the usual frequentist approach to the analysis of clinical trial data may necessitate an adjustment to the type I error. Multiplicity may arise for, example, from multiple primary variables, multiple comparisons of treatments, repeated evaluation over time and/or interim analyses. Methods to avoid or reduce multiplicity are sometimes preferable when available, such as the identification of the key primary variable (multiple variables), the choice of a critical treatment contrast (multiple comparisons), the use of a summary measure such as "area under the curve" (repeated measures). In confirmatory analyses, any aspects of multiplicity which remain after steps of this kind have been taken should be identified in the protocol; adjustment should always be considered and the details of any adjustment procedure or an explanation of why adjustment is not thought to be necessary should be set out in the analysis plan'.

Note that these recommendations relate to confirmatory claims and statements. For post hoc exploratory investigations, there are no restrictions in this multiplicity sense. Any findings arising from such analyses, however, cannot be viewed as confirmatory unless the finding can be (or has been) clearly replicated in an independent setting.

These comments are directed primarily at efficacy and do not tend to be applied to safety, unless a specific safety claim (e.g. drug A reduces the incidence of neutropenia compared to drug B) is to be made. With the routine evaluation of safety, if p-values are being used as a flag for potential concerns, we tend to be conservative and not worry about inflating the type I error. It is missing a real safety concern, the type II error, which troubles us more.

10.4 Multiple primary endpoints

10.4.1 Avoiding adjustment

As mentioned in the previous section, multiplicity can lead to adjustment of the significance level. There are, however, some situations when adjustment is not needed although these situations tend to have restrictions in other ways. We will focus this discussion in relation to multiple primary endpoints and in subsequent sections use similar arguments to deal with other aspects of multiple testing.

As ICH E9 points out, 'There should generally be only one primary variable', and when this is the case, there is clearly no need for adjustment. However, there may well be good scientific and commercial reasons for including more than one primary variable, for example, to cover the different potential effects of the new treatment.

10.4.2 Significance needed on all endpoints

In some therapeutic settings, the regulators require us to demonstrate effects in terms of two or more endpoints. For example, in mild, persistent asthma, we look for effects both in terms of lung function and symptoms.

CPMP (2003): 'Note for Guidance on the Clinical Investigation of Medicinal Products in the Treatment of Asthma'

'For a new controller treatment for mild persistent asthma, equal emphasis should be placed on lung function and the symptom based clinical endpoint. A significant benefit for both primary endpoints, lung function and the symptom based clinical endpoint, should be demonstrated so that no multiplicity adjustment to significance levels is indicated'.

Under such circumstances, no adjustment to the significance level is needed; we have to show significance for both endpoints. Note however that requiring significance on two endpoints will impact on power. If the power attached to each endpoint were 90 per cent, for example, then the combined power (the probability of getting statistical significance on both endpoints) could be as low as 81 per cent (90 per cent × 90 per cent). Increasing the sample size to give power of 95 per cent for each individual endpoint will ensure a combined power of 90 per cent (90.025 per cent = 95 per cent × 95 per cent).

10.4.3 Composite endpoints

Another way of avoiding adjustment is to combine the multiple measurements into a single *composite variable*. Examples would be disease-free survival in oncology, where the variable is the time to disease recurrence or death, whichever occurs first, or a composite of death, non-fatal stroke, myocardial infarction (MI) and heart failure, a binary outcome in a cardiovascular setting. This approach does not require adjustment of the significance level; we are back to having a single primary endpoint. Such endpoints are used extensively in cardiovascular applications where the individual components represent relatively uncommon events; a further issue here is that there is simply not enough power to look at those components individually.

There are some additional requirements, however, when using composite variables. A large positive effect with one of the components could potentially be masking a negative effect in a different component, and this would be unacceptable. Ideally, all component endpoints should be giving differences in the same direction; indeed, it should be expected that treatment will affect all components in a similar way. At the very least, none of the clinically important components should be giving differences in the wrong direction.

In some applications, especially cardiovascular, the separate components or some combination of those components may be secondary endpoints. If specific claims are to be made for any of the components, however, these should be organised within the confirmatory structure of the testing procedures, for example, using hierarchical testing (see Section 10.4.4 and Example 10.1). The CHMP in their guidance on multiplicity talk about these points.

CHMP (2002) 'Points to Consider on Multiplicity Issues in Clinical Trials'

'It is recommended to analyse in addition the single components and clinically relevant groups of components separately, to provide supportive information. There is, however, no need for an adjustment for multiplicity provided significance of the primary endpoint is achieved. If claims are to be based on subgroups of components, this needs to be pre-specified and embedded in a valid confirmatory analysis strategy'.

When they speak here about analysing the separate components, they do not necessarily mean to produce *p*-values but merely to present the individual event rates, for example. There is an acceptance that the power for the individual components may make the *p*-values somewhat irrelevant.

10.4.4 Variables ranked according to clinical importance: Hierarchical testing

It may be possible with several primary endpoints to rank these in terms of their clinical importance and within this structure adopt a testing strategy that avoids having to adjust the significance level. This ranking, which of course should be pre-specified in the protocol, determines the order in which the statistical testing is done. No adjustment to the significance level is required, but claims cannot be made beyond the first non-significant result in the hierarchy. Consider the setting with three primary endpoints, ranked according to their clinical relevance (Table 10.1). In case 1, claims can be made on endpoints 1 and 2. In case 2, a claim can be made on endpoint 1 only, because endpoint 2 is non-significant and we are then not allowed to make a claim for endpoint 3, even though in this case that endpoint may give $p \leq 0.05$. In case 3, no claims can be made. Any p-values ≤ 0.05 lower in the hierarchy than a non-significant endpoint cannot provide the basis for a confirmatory statement/claim; those findings would only be viewed as supportive/exploratory.

The CPMP (2002) *Points to Consider on Multiplicity Issues in Clinical Trials* specifically mentions some examples of the hierarchical strategy:

> *'Typical examples are: (i) acute effects in depressive disorders followed by prevention of progression, (ii) reduction of mortality in acute myocardial infarction followed by prevention of other serious events'.*

Clearly, it is very important that we get the hierarchy correct. Generally, this would be determined by the clinical relevance of the endpoints, although under some circumstances it could be determined, in part, by the likelihood of seeing statistical significance with the easier *hits* towards the top of the hierarchy. These ideas can also be considered as a way of dealing with secondary endpoints, which might be considered for inclusion in a claim. In many cases, secondary endpoints are simply primary endpoints lower down in the hierarchy.

Table 10.1 Hierarchical testing

	Case 1	Case 2	Case 3
Endpoint 1	$p \leq 0.05$	$p \leq 0.05$	$p = NS$
Endpoint 2	$p \leq 0.05$	$p = NS$	
Endpoint 3	$p = NS$		

Example 10.1 Ticagrelor versus clopidogrel in acute coronary syndromes (the PLATO study) (Wallentin *et al.*, 2009)

PLATO was a randomised double-blind trial comparing ticagrelor and clopidogrel in the treatment of patients with acute coronary syndromes for the prevention of cardiovascular events. The primary endpoint was the time to first occurrence of the composite of death from cardiovascular causes, MI or stroke. The principle secondary consideration was in fact the same endpoint but in the subgroup of patients for whom invasive management was planned at randomisation. Additional secondary endpoints (considered for the complete patient population) were organised in a hierarchy below the primary and principle secondary endpoint in the following order:

- The composite of death from any cause, MI or stroke
- The composite of death from vascular causes, MI, stroke, severe recurrent cardiac ischaemia, recurrent cardiac ischaemia, transient ischemic attack or other arterial thrombotic events
- MI alone
- Death from cardiovascular causes alone
- Stroke alone
- Death from any cause

The results for all of these endpoints are given in Figure 10.1. The primary endpoint gave statistical significance with $p < 0.001$. The p-value for the principle secondary endpoint, the primary in a subgroup, gave $p = 0.003$. The next four secondary endpoints in the hierarchy all gave statistical significance at the 5 per cent level. The endpoint stroke however gave a

End point	Ticagrelor group	Clopidogrel group	Hazard ratio for ticagrelor group (95% CI)	p-value†
Primary end point: death from vascular causes, MI or stroke : no./total no. (%)	864/9333 (9.8)	1014/9291 (11.7)	0.84 (0.77–0.92)	<0.001‡
Secondary end points : no./total no. (%)				
Death from any cause, MI, or stroke	901/9333 (10.2)	1065/9291 (12.3)	0.84(0.77–0.92)	<0.001‡
Death from vascular causes, MI stroke, severe recurrent ischaemia, recurrent ischaemia, TIA or other arterial thrombotic event	1290/9333 (14.6)	1456/9291 (16.7)	0.88 (0.81–0.95)	<0.001‡
MI	504/9333 (5.8)	593/9291 (6.9)	0.84 (0.75–0.95)	0.005‡
Death from vascular causes	353/9333 (4.0)	442/9291(5.1)	0.79 (0.69–0.91)	0.001‡
Stroke	125/9333 (1.5)	106/9291 (1.3)	1.17 (0.91–1.52)	0.22
Ischaemic	96/9333 (1.1)	91/9291 (1.1)		0.74
Haemorrhagic	23/9333 (0.2)	13/9291(0.1)		0.10
Unknown	10/9333 (0.1)	2/9291(0.02)		0.04
Other events : no./total no.(%)				
Death from any cause	399/9333 (4.5)	506/9291 (5.9)	0.78 (0.69–0.89)	<0.001
Death from causes other than vascular causes	46/9333 (0.5)	64/9291 (0.8)	0.71 (0.49–1.04)	0.08
Severe recurrent ischaemia	302/9333 (3.5)	345/9291 (4.0)	0.87 (0.74–1.01)	0.08
Recurrent ischaemia	500/9333 (5.8)	536/9291 (6.2)	0.93 (0.82–1.05)	0.22
TIA	18/9333 (0.2)	23/9291 (0.3)	0.78 (0.42–1.44)	0.42
Other arterial thrombotic event	l9/9333 (0.2)	31/9291 (0.4)	0.61 (0.34–1.08)	0.09
Death from vascular causes, MI, stroke : no./total no.(%)				
Invasive treatment planned§	569/6732 (8.9)	668/6676 (10.6)	0.84 (0.75–0.94)	0.003‡
Event rate, days 1–30	443/9333 (4.8)	502/9291 (5.4)	0.88 (0.77–1.00)	0.045
Event rate, days 31–36¶	413/8763 (5.3)	510/8688 (6.6)	0.80 (0.70–0.91)	<0.001
Stent thrombosis : no.of patients who received a stent/ total no. (%)				
Definite	71/5640 (1.3)	106/5649 (1.9)	0.67 (0.50–0.91)	0.009
Probable or definite	118/5640 (2.2)	158/5649 (2.9)	0.75 (0.59–0.95)	0.02
Possible, probable or definite	155/5640 (2.9)	202/5649 (3.8)	0.77 (0.62–0.95)	0.01

* The percentages are Kaplan–Meier estimates of the rate of the end point at 12 months. Patients could have had more than one type of end point. Death from vascular causes included fatal bleeding. Only traumatic fatal bleeding was excluded from the category of death from vascular causes. MI denotes myocardial infarction and TIA transient ischaemic attack.
† p values were calculated by means of Cox regression analysis.
‡ Statistical significance was confirmed in the hierarchical testing sequence applied to the secondary composite efficacy end points.
§ A plan for invasive or non-invasive (medical) management was declared before randomisation.
¶ Patients with any primary event during the first 30 days were excluded.

Figure 10.1 Efficacy endpoints in the PLATO study. Source: Wallentin L, Becker RC, Budaj A, *et al.* (2009) Ticagrelor versus Clopidogrel in Patients with Acute Coronary Syndromes. *NEJM,* **361**, 1045–1057. Reproduced by permission of Massachusetts Medical Society.

non-statistically significant result with $p=0.22$, so a claim cannot be made for that specific endpoint nor for any endpoints, irrespective of their statistical significance, below stroke in the hierarchy. Interestingly, the endpoint below stroke is all-cause mortality with $p<0.001$. In a formal sense, a confirmatory conclusion for all-cause mortality in terms of its statistical significance cannot be made since it violates the strict control of the type I error.

The debate among regulators here would be interesting. All-cause mortality as an endpoint tends to *trump* almost everything else and in that sense stands apart from other considerations. Also in this case, it is not as if the *p*-value has just fallen below 0.05, but it is <0.001. Could this possibly be a false positive given the level of statistical significance and also the results for the other endpoints? This is unlikely, and I think there could be some strong arguments, outside of formal considerations of statistical significance and the control of type I error, that would allow a claim to be made on overall mortality.

There is also the possibility of mixing hierarchical considerations with adjustment. For example, in the case of a single primary endpoint and two secondary endpoints of equal importance to each other, the primary endpoint would be evaluated at $\alpha=0.05$, while each of the secondary endpoints would use $\alpha=0.025$. Claims could only be considered for the secondary endpoints if the primary endpoint gave $p\leq0.05$, but then additional claims could be made on whichever of the secondary endpoints gives $p\leq0.025$. In theory, the use of both a hierarchy and Bonferroni-type adjustments could move beyond a second level; all that is needed is that 0.05 is assigned to each level of the hierarchy. For example, there could be a single endpoint at the first level, two endpoints at the second level (with a Bonferroni adjustment) and finally a single endpoint at the third level. Testing at the second level only occurs if the level 1 endpoint is significant at $\alpha=0.05$, while testing at the third level can take place provided that either of the p-values at the second level is statistically significant at $\alpha=0.025$.

10.5 Methods for adjustment

10.5.1 Bonferroni correction

The Bonferroni method of adjustment has been mentioned earlier in this chapter as a method of preserving the overall 5 per cent type I error rate. In general, if there m confirmatory comparisons with claims to be made on whichever are statistically significant, then the Bonferroni correction requires that each comparison be evaluated at level $\alpha'=\alpha/m$. In a strict statistical sense, this is the correct adjustment only for tests based on independent sets of data. For example, if there are four non-overlapping (independent) subgroups of patients, *males aged under 65, males aged 65 or over, females aged under 65* and *females aged 65 or over*, then an adjustment that uses the 0.0125 level of significance for each of the subgroups will have an overall type I error rate of 5 per cent. In most cases, however, when we use this adjustment, the tests that make up the set of comparisons will not be independent in this sense. With multiple primary endpoints, there will possibly be correlation between those endpoints, and with multiple treatment comparisons of, say, several dose levels with placebo, the placebo group will be common to those comparisons and hence there will be a connection across the tests and so on. Where this is the case, the Bonferroni correction provides a conservative procedure; in other words, the effective overall type I error rate will be <5 per cent. As an extreme example of this conservativeness, suppose that two primary endpoints were perfectly correlated. The Bonferroni adjustment would require each of the endpoints be evaluated at the 2.5 per cent level of significance, but because of the perfect correlation, the overall type I error rate would also be 2.5 per cent, considerably less than the 5 per cent requirement.

The considerations so far are based on the presumption that the type I error rate is divided equally across all of the comparisons. This does not always make sense, and indeed, it is not a requirement that it be done in this way. For example, with two comparisons, there would be nothing to prevent having a 4 per cent type I error rate for one of the comparisons and a 1 per cent type I error rate for the other, provided that this methodology is clearly set down in the protocol. We will see a setting below that of interim analysis, where it is advantageous to divide up the error rate unequally. Outside of the interim analysis, however, it is rare to see anything other than an equal subdivision.

10.5.2 Hochberg correction

The Bonferroni correction is the simplest form of correction but usually not the most efficient. A more efficient, although more complex, correction that protects the overall type I error has been developed by Hochberg and Tamhane (1987). This approach involves ordering the p-values over the endpoints to be considered within the confirmatory structure of the trial and moving through these p-values starting with the largest. If the largest p-value is ≤0.05, then all endpoints can be declared statistically significant (at the 5 per cent level). If however this largest p-value is >0.05, then non-significance is declared for that endpoint and considerations move to the second largest p-value. If the p-value for that endpoint is ≤0.05/2 = 0.025, then all endpoints lower in the order can be declared statistically significant (at the 5 per cent level). If however that endpoint gives a p-value >0.025, then non-significance is declared for endpoint number 2 in the ordering and we move to the endpoint with the third largest p-value. This is then compared to 0.05/3 = 0.017, and the process continues down through the list with the endpoint in position m being compared to 0.05/m. Table 10.2 provides some examples of how this would work in the case of 3 endpoints. In case 1, confirmatory claims can be made on all 3 endpoints since the largest p-value is ≤0.05. In case 2, claims can be made on endpoints 2 and 3, since initially the largest p-value is not ≤0.05 but the second largest p-value is ≤0.025 so all endpoints with p-values below that can also be declared statistically significant. Finally in case 3, it is only the third smallest p-value for which a conclusion of statistical significance can be made; the largest p-value (endpoint 1) was not

Table 10.2 Hochberg correction

	Case 1	Case 2	Case 3
Endpoint 1	$p=0.042$ √	$p=0.17$	$p=0.053$
Endpoint 2	$p=0.029$ √	$p=0.024$ √	$p=0.040$
Endpoint 3	$p=0.019$ √	$p=0.020$ √	$p=0.011$ √

≤ 0.05, the second largest p-value (endpoint 2) was not ≤ 0.025, but the third largest p-value (endpoint 3) was ≤ 0.017. There will be some endpoints within this testing structure that give $p \leq 0.05$ but where a statistically significant difference cannot be declared. Endpoint 2 in case 3 is an example of this. This result would then constitute an exploratory finding.

This process may seem similar to hierarchical testing since they both involve an ordering, but they are fundamentally different. Hierarchical testing defines the order before seeing the data, and this allows the use of 0.05 as the significance level at each step. The Hochberg correction *defines* an ordering once the data have been analysed, and because of that *flexibility* in choosing the order post hoc, there is a price to pay for the significance level as you move through the testing procedure. To reiterate, this method has been shown to preserve the overall type I error at 0.05 in all practical settings. Note that using a pre-planned Bonferroni correction with an adjusted significance level of 0.017 would have led to none of the results in case 1 being declared statistically significant, also none of those in case 2 and only one, the final one, in case 3. As can be seen, Hochberg has performed better than Bonferroni in those first two cases while both methods in case 3 have given the same result.

10.5.3 Interim analyses

Interim analyses arise when we want to look at the data as it accumulates with the possibility of stopping the trial at the interim stage if the data suggests, for example, overwhelming efficacy of the test treatment compared to control. If we were to introduce, say, two interim looks in additional to the final analysis at the end of the trial, then we have an overall testing strategy which consists of three tests and some account of this multiplicity is required. There has been a considerable amount of theory developed in this area, and the resulting procedures not only preserve the 5 per cent type error rate but also do not pay as big a price as Bonferroni. Remember that Bonferroni only strictly applies to independent tests. In the context of interim analysis, the data sets that are being analysed are not independent and are overlapping in a very structured way. With a sample size of 600 and three looks, the first interim analysis after 200 patients provides precisely half of the data on which the second interim analysis, based on 400 patients, is to be undertaken, while these 400 patients provide two-thirds of the data on which the final analysis is to be conducted.

Pocock (1977) developed a procedure that divides the type I error rate of 5 per cent equally across the various analyses. In the example earlier with two interim looks and a final analysis, Bonferroni would suggest using an adjusted significance level of 0.017 (=0.05/3). The Pocock method however gives us the correct adjusted significance level as 0.022, and this exactly preserves the overall 5 per cent type I error rate for the trial as a whole.

While this equal division of the type I error may work for some settings, it is more likely that we would want, firstly, to keep back most of the 5 per cent for the final and most important analysis and, secondly, would only want to stop a trial in the case of overwhelming evidence for efficacy. The methods of O'Brien and Fleming (1979) divide up the type I error rate unequally, with very stringent levels at the early interims, becoming less stringent at subsequent analyses and leaving most of the 5 per cent over for the final analysis. In the case of two interim looks and a final analysis, the adjusted significance levels are 0.00052, 0.014 and 0.045. As can be seen, these adjusted significance levels are very stringent early on with most of the 0.05 left over for the final analysis.

The methods as presented here assume that the analyses are equally spaced in terms of the numbers of patients involved at each stage. It is possible to deviate from this in a planned way using the so-called alpha-spending functions.

It is also possible to stop trials for reasons other than overwhelming efficacy, for example, for futility, where at an interim stage it is clear that if the trial were to continue, it would have little chance of giving a positive result. We will say more about interim analysis in a later chapter and in particular consider the practical application of these methods.

10.6 Multiple comparisons

In the case of multiple treatment groups, it is important to recognise the objectives of the trial. For example, in a three-arm trial with test treatment, active comparator and placebo, the primary objective may well be to demonstrate the effectiveness of the test treatment, and this will be the basis of the claim, while a secondary objective will be to demonstrate the non-inferiority, or perhaps superiority, of the test treatment compared to the active control. This secondary objective may, for example, be driven by market positioning. In this case, we have a hierarchy with the primary objective based on a test undertaken at the 5 per cent level of significance, with the test treatment versus active control comparison relegated to a second level in the hierarchy, and again, this would be conducted with $\alpha = 0.05$. Of course, this second comparison cannot be undertaken if the primary objective is not achieved; this makes sense because it would have little value in this scenario if we were unable to demonstrate that the test treatment works by comparing with placebo.

As a second example, consider a trial with four treatment arms: placebo and low, medium and high doses of drug A. If we wanted to come out of this trial with a confirmatory statement concerning the effectiveness of drug A at a particular dose level, then one strategy would be to undertake three tests, each dose level against placebo, and make a claim based on whichever of these is statistically significant. An adjustment would be required, and Bonferroni would give an adjusted significance level of 0.017. Alternatively, it may be worth considering a hierarchy in the order: high dose versus placebo, medium dose versus placebo and low dose versus placebo, with no adjustment of the 5 per cent significance level. The constraint here, of course, is that you can only make claims down to the first non-significant result. This strategy would get you to the *minimum effective dose* provided that things are well behaved and there is an underlying monotonic dose–response relationship (the higher the dose, the bigger the effect).

10.7 Repeated evaluation over time

It is not uncommon to measure variables of interest at several time points during follow-up. Undertaking statistical testing at each of those time points is inappropriate and leads to inflation of the type I error. By far, the best way to deal with this problem is to reduce the multiple measurements for each subject to a single measure. Several possibilities exist, such as the average of all the measurements, the average of the measurements over the final three months, the achievement of a predefined percentage fall from baseline (a binary outcome) and so on. The ICH E9 guideline as quoted earlier mentions area under the curve (AUC); this is simply a sophisticated form of averaging. The chosen measure should be that measure that provides the clearest clinical interpretation.

There are a set of statistical techniques, which go under the heading of *repeated measures or mixed models ANOVA*, that do not summarise the serial measurements directly for each subject as mentioned earlier, but leave them separated as they are. In the past, these methods have provided *p*-values relating to a comparison of the set of complete profiles for subjects in treatment group A with the set of profiles for subjects in treatment group B. While these methods offered a statistical solution, they were somewhat divorced from methods based on subject level outcomes that offered a clearer clinical interpretation. As a consequence, they were only used to a limited extent in practice, and the approach based upon summary measures was generally preferred by both regulators and practitioners. Matthews *et al.* (1990) gave a general discussion regarding the analysis of repeated measures but in particular, in relation to repeated measures ANOVA and similar approaches, conclude that '*None of these methods provides results that are as easy to understand as the method of summary measures, nor are they as easy to use'.*

More recently, however, developments in the statistical methodology and associated computing routines implemented, for example, in SAS® have enabled more focused clinically interpretable comparisons based around summary measures (termed *contrasts*) to be undertaken within the framework of mixed models. Many situations with multiple measurements per patient are nowadays handled in this way.

10.8 Subgroup testing

Subgroup testing through a post hoc evaluation of treatment effects within those subgroups cannot in general be used to recover a *failed* study. If a claim is to be considered for a specific subgroup, then this would need to form part of the pre-planned confirmatory strategy. As a very simple example, suppose that a trial is to recruit both high-risk and low-risk patients, where a claim is to be considered for either group (or both) depending on the results of significance tests conducted separately within these two subgroups. One possible strategy would then be to use an adjusted significance level of 0.025 (Bonferroni) for each of the subgroups. Alternatively, the Hochberg approach would calculate both *p*-values and base confirmatory conclusions on an ordering of those *p*-values.

Usually, however, evaluation of treatment effects within subgroups is pre-planned and undertaken as part of the assessment of the homogeneity of treatment effect. It is common to display treatment differences within subgroups defined by important prognostic factors, certainly, for example, those that were used as stratification factors, in the form of point estimates of the treatment effect and 95 per cent confidence intervals for the true treatment difference together, possibly, with a *p*-value for an assessment of the treatment-by-covariate interaction (see Sections 5.4 and 6.5.2). In addition, if there were indications that the treatment effect is not homogeneous, then such a display would be of value in explaining the nature of the interaction. In discussing the observed heterogeneity, there should also be comment relating to the clinical plausibility of that heterogeneity.

Recall from Sections 5.4 and 6.5.2 that when assessing interactions, we generally use a significance level of 0.10 rather than 0.05 due to a lack of power. 'Example 10.2 looks at a trial evaluating pravastatin in preventing cardiovascular disease. In Figure 10.2, most of the interactions, except that involving baseline LDL cholesterol, give *p*-values well above 0.10, and so there is no evidence of treatment-by-covariate interactions for most of the baseline factors. This homogeneity of treatment effect can also be seen visually by inspecting the forest plot and observing similar values for the hazard ratios in the various subgroups, for example, males and females, and 95 per cent confidence intervals between those subgroups that are almost completely overlapping. The hazard ratio in all cases is <1, consistent with the overall result. The *p*-value for the treatment-by-LDL cholesterol interaction is, however, almost significant when compared with the 0.10 cut-off, and one might argue some support for a possible differential treatment effect. This only really constitutes an exploratory/interesting finding though, and a confirmatory statement regarding such a differential effect would need to come from another independent study. Note again however that the hazard ratio in both high and low

Example10.2 Pravastatin in preventing cardiovascular disease

Figure 10.2 is taken from Nakamura *et al.* (2006) who reported a large placebo-controlled randomised trial evaluating the effect of pravastatin in preventing cardiovascular disease. The overall treatment effect was positive, with a hazard ratio of 0.67 ($p=0.01$). We will cover hazard ratios and their use in survival analysis in Chapter 13; for the moment, simply note that, like the odds ratio and the relative risk, a value of one corresponds to equal treatments. The homogeneity of the treatment effect was assessed by looking at the p-value for the treatment-by-covariate interaction and also by calculating the hazard ratio separately in various subgroups defined by baseline factors of interest as seen in Figure 10.2.

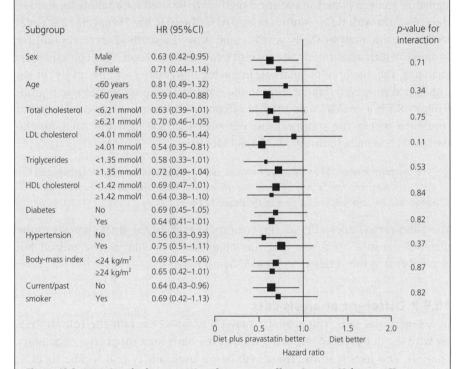

Figure 10.2 Assessing the homogeneity of treatment effect. Source: Nakamura H, Arakawa K, Itakura H, *et al.*, for the MEGA Study Group (2006) 'Primary prevention of cardiovascular disease with pravastatin in Japan (MEGA study): a prospective randomised controlled trial'. *The Lancet*, **368**, 1155–1163. Reproduced by permission of Elsevier.

baseline LDL cholesterol subgroups is below 1 (a quantitative interaction) indicating a benefit of pravastatin, although this benefit is more marginal in those patients presenting with LDL cholesterol <4.01 mmol/l.

The regulators are particularly interested in seeing the homogeneity of treatment effect, and looking in subgroups will be important to give assurance that a positive treatment effect can be assumed across the population as a whole. If there is evidence that this is not the case, especially if the effect in one subgroup is seen to be negative, then specific subgroups could be excluded from the label.

10.9 Other areas for multiplicity

10.9.1 Using different statistical tests

Using several different statistical methods, for example, an unpaired t-test, an analysis adjusted for centre effects, ANCOVA adjusting for centre and including baseline risk as a covariate, etc., and possibly choosing whichever method produces the smallest p-value are other forms of multiplicity and are inappropriate. There is often a temptation to do this: 'torturing the data until it confesses!'.

It is standard practice to pre-specify in the protocol, or certainly in the statistical analysis plan, the statistical method to be used for analysis for each of the endpoints within the confirmatory part of the trial. This avoids the potential for bias at the analysis stage, which could arise if a method were chosen, for example, which maximised the apparent treatment difference. As a consequence, changing the method of analysis following unblinding of the study in an unplanned way, even if there seem sound statistical reasons for doing so, is problematic. Such a switch could only be supported if there was a clear algorithm contained within the statistical analysis plan that specified the rules for the switch. An example of this would be as follows:

> 'The treatment means will be compared using the unpaired t-test. If, however, the group standard deviations are significantly different according to the F-test, then the comparison of the means will be based on Welch's form of the unpaired t-test'.

The blind review does offer an opportunity to make some final changes to the planned statistical methods, and this opportunity should not be missed but remember that this is based on blinded data.

10.9.2 Different analysis sets

In a superiority trial, the primary analysis will be based on the full analysis set with the per-protocol set being used as the basis for a supportive secondary analysis, and in this sense, there will be no multiplicity issues. The form of the analysis, however, depends in addition on the methods to be used to account for missing data, and these should clearly be pre-specified. It is also good practice to explore the robustness of the conclusions to both the choice of the per-protocol set and the methods to be used for missing data. These analyses again will be supportive (or not) of the main conclusions, and no multiplicity aspects arise.

In equivalence and non-inferiority trials (see Chapter 12), the full analysis set and the per-protocol set have equal status and are treated as co-primary. The requirement, therefore, is to show *significance* for each of these analyses. This is another case where statistical significance is needed on all *endpoints* with both analyses being conducted at the usual 5 per cent significance level.

10.9.3 Pre-planning

We have mentioned on several occasions that methods of statistical analysis should be pre-planned. This gives the regulators and others confidence that we are not adapting the methods of analysis or choosing new methods of analysis that somehow maximise the observed treatment benefit. This clearly would be inappropriate. In a sense, not having a pre-planned analysis and having the flexibility to look at several different methods of analysis once the data are in hand constitutes a further form of multiplicity. Any methods that are chosen having seen the data would have little chance of being the basis for confirmatory claims. As is pointed out in ICH E9, *'Only results from analyses envisaged in the protocol (including amendments) can be regarded as confirmatory'*.

In a situation where there is a need to change the statistical methods following finalisation of the protocol and once the trial is underway, it is always advisable to issue a protocol amendment rather than just document this change in the statistical analysis plan. Such a change, for example, could have been motivated by some new knowledge regarding what could be the most efficient method of analysis. Making such of changes however in an unblinded study could lead to concerns if there is suspicion that they were data-driven.

CHAPTER 11

Non-parametric and related methods

11.1 Assumptions underlying the t-tests and their extensions

The t-tests and their extensions ANOVA, ANCOVA and regression all make assumptions about the distribution of the data in the background populations. If these assumptions are not appropriate, then strictly speaking, the p-values coming out of those tests together with the associated confidence intervals are not valid.

The assumptions are essentially of two kinds: *homogeneity of variance* and *normality*. Consider, to begin with, the unpaired t-test. This test assumes that the two population distributions from which the data are drawn firstly have the same standard deviation (homogeneity of variance) and secondly have the normal distribution shape. In contrast, the paired t-test makes only one assumption, and that is that the population distribution of the differences at the patient level (e.g. response on A – response on B) is normal. For the extensions, ANOVA, ANCOVA and regression, there are both homogeneity of variance and normality assumptions underpinning the methods. We will focus primarily on the simple settings in exploring the issues associated with these assumptions and in presenting other methods that are available if these assumptions do not hold.

There is, in fact, one additional assumption that the above procedures make and that is independence; the way a particular patient responds is not linked to the way another patient responds. In a randomised clinical trial, this assumption is unlikely to be violated, and we will not discuss this issue further here.

11.2 Homogeneity of variance

We will focus the development in this section on the unpaired t-test. The constant variance assumption can be assessed by undertaking a test (the so-called F-test) relating to the hypotheses

$$H_0 : \sigma_1 = \sigma_2 \quad H_1 : \sigma_1 \neq \sigma_2$$

Statistical Thinking for Non-Statisticians in Drug Regulation, Second Edition. Richard Kay.
© 2015 John Wiley & Sons, Ltd. Published 2015 by John Wiley & Sons, Ltd.

Here, σ_1 and σ_2 are the true standard deviations within treatment groups 1 and 2, respectively. A significant *p*-value from this test would indicate that constant variance cannot be assumed and therefore that the *p*-value coming out of the unpaired t-test is not correct. Should this happen, then we would need to use an alternative form of the unpaired t-test that allows for non-constant variance. This form of the unpaired t-test is known as *Welch's approximation*. It involves a slightly different formula for the standard error (se) of the difference $\bar{x}_1 - \bar{x}_2$ and a different calculation of the degrees of freedom for the t-distribution on which the *p*-value calculation is based. These details need not concern us here, suffice it to say that the issue of non-constant variance is fairly straightforward to deal with. In addition, our experience in clinical trials tells us that non-constant variance does not seem to occur particularly often in practice and when it does, it tends to be associated additionally with violation of the normality assumption. Conveniently, taking care of the normality assumption by transforming the data (see Section 11.4) often also takes care of the non-constant variance.

11.3 The assumption of normality

While constancy of variance does not seem to be too much of a concern in our clinical trials, it is not uncommon for the assumption of normality to be violated. Many laboratory variables do not usually display the normal distribution shape, while in pharmacokinetics several of the quantities that we routinely calculate, such as AUC and C_{max}, frequently have distributions, which appear as in Figure 11.1. We talk in terms of the data being *positively skewed*. In part, the reason why we often see these positively skewed distributions is that there is a physical boundary at zero; it is not possible to observe a negative value, although it is possible to see larger values for some patients well away from the bulk of the data.

Checking the assumption of normality can be undertaken in one of two ways. Firstly, we have graphical methods, such as a *quantile–quantile plot* (also known as a *normal probability plot*), where normal data displays itself as a straight line. Departures from a straight-line plot are indicative of non-normality. Figure 11.2 is a quantile–quantile plot to assess the normality of 100 observations simulated from the distribution displayed in Figure 11.1, while Figure 11.3 shows the histogram for these same data. The quantile–quantile plot clearly does not conform well to a straight line, and the histogram reflects the positive skewness of these data.

This visual approach based on inspecting the normal probability plot may seem fairly crude. However, most of the test procedures, such as the unpaired t-test, are what we call *robust* against departures from normality. In other words, the *p*-values resulting from these tests remain approximately correct unless we

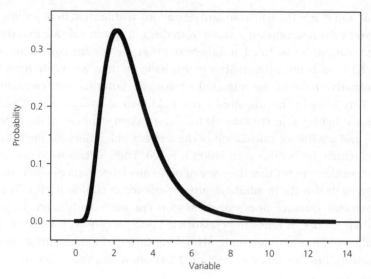

Figure 11.1 Positively skewed (non-normal) distribution

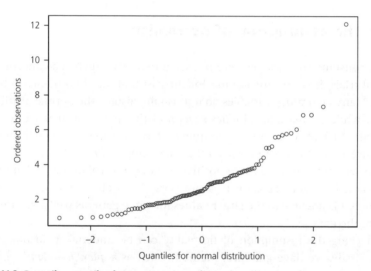

Figure 11.2 Quantile–quantile plot to assess normality

depart substantially from normality, particularly with large sample sizes. The normal probability plot is sensitive enough to detect such substantial departures.

Secondly, we have a statistical test, the *Shapiro–Wilk test*, that gives a *p*-value in the following setting:

H_0 : normal H_1 : non-normal

A significant *p*-value is indicating that the data is not normally distributed and leads to the rejection of H_0; a non-significant *p*-value tells us that there is no evidence for non-normality and in practice it will then be safe to assume that the

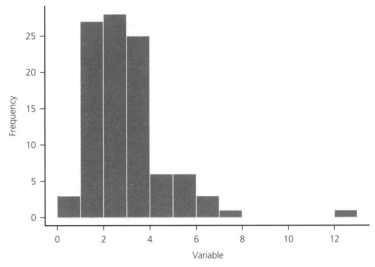

Figure 11.3 Histogram for simulated data

data is at least approximately normally distributed. See Altman (1991) Section 7.5.3 for further details of this test and some examples.

Our discussions here suggest that we look for normality in each of the treatment groups separately. In practice, this is not quite what we do; we look in fact at the two groups combined and evaluate the normality of the so-called residuals. This approach *standardises* the data values in each of the two groups to have mean zero by subtracting the observed mean in group A from the observations in group A and the observed mean in group B from the observations in group B. This standardisation gives the combined group of adjusted observations mean zero and allows all of the data to be considered as a single group for the purpose of evaluating the assumption of normality. In a similar way, this approach is used to deal with ANOVA where there are several *groups* (e.g. A and B observations in each of several centres) and also with more complex structures that form the basis of ANCOVA and regression. For example, in regression, the assumption of normality applies to the vertical differences between each patient's observation y and the value of y on the underlying straight line that describes the relationship between x and y. We therefore look for the normality of the residuals: the vertical differences between each observation and the corresponding value on the fitted line.

11.4 Non-normality and transformations

We will concentrate in this section on the parallel-group case with two treatments where for normally distributed data we would be undertaking the unpaired t-test. If the data are clearly non-normal, then the first approach in analysing the data would be to consider transforming the data to recover normality. As we have

Table 11.1 The log transformation

x	$\log_{10}x$
0	$-\infty$
1	0
10	1
100	2
1000	3

mentioned in the previous section, it is not uncommon to have data that are positively skewed with values that cannot be negative. A transformation that often successfully transforms the data to be normal is the log transformation. It does not matter to which base we take these logs; the usual choices would be to base e (natural logarithms) or to base 10 – either of these is equal to a constant times the other. Table 11.1 shows the effect of taking logs, to base 10, of various values.

The effect of the log transformation on the values 1, 10, 100 and 1000 is to effectively bring them closer together. On the original scale, these numbers are getting progressively further apart, whereas on the log scale, they become equally spaced. Also for values on the original scale between zero and one, the log transformation gives a negative value. The log transformation *brings in* the large positive values and *throws out* the values below one to become negative, and this has the effect of making the positively skewed distribution look more symmetric. If this transformation is successful in recovering normality, then we simply analyse the data on the log scale using the unpaired t-test. The resulting *p*-value provides a valid comparison of the two treatments in terms of the means on the log scale and therefore means on the original scale. Similarly, we can calculate 95 per cent confidence intervals for the difference in the means on the log scale.

While the *p*-value allows us the ability to judge statistical significance, the clinical relevance of the finding is difficult to evaluate from the calculated confidence interval because this is now on the log scale. It is usual to *back-transform* the lower and upper confidence limits, together with the difference in the means on the log scale, to give us something on the original data scale, which is more readily interpretable. The back-transform for the log transformation is the antilog.

Mean values are usually calculated as *arithmetic means*. However, there is another kind of mean value, the *geometric mean*. The arithmetic mean is $(x_1 + x_2 + \ldots + x_n)/n$, while the geometric mean is defined as $\sqrt[n]{x_1 \times x_2 \times \ldots \times x_n}$: the *n*th root of all the data values multiplied together. When the antilog is applied to the difference in the means on the log scale, then the result is numerically equal to the ratio of the geometric means for the original data. This is why in pharmacokinetics, where it is standard practice to log transform C_{max} and AUC prior to analysis, it is the ratio of geometric means together with a confidence interval for that ratio that is quoted. More generally, we often quote geometric means where we are using the log transformation in the analysis of data.

In the paired t-test setting, it is the normality of the differences (response on A – response on B) that is required for the validity of the test. The log transformation on the original data can sometimes be effective in this case in recovering normality for these differences. In other settings, such as ANOVA, ANCOVA and regression, log transforming the outcome variable is always worth trying, where this is a strictly positive quantity, as an initial attempt to recover normality.

Of note finally is that log transforming positively skewed data often kills two pigeons with one pebble, recovering both normality and constant variance. With skewed data, the group with the larger outcome values will tend to have more spread, and the log transformation will then generally bring the spread of the data in each of the groups more into line.

The log transformation is by far the most common transformation, but there are several other transformations that are from time to time used in recovering normality. The *square root transformation*, $\sqrt{x}$, is sometimes used with count data, while the *logit transformation*, $\ell n\{x/(1-x)\}$, can be used where the patient provides a measure that is a proportion, such as the proportion of days symptom-free in a 14-day period. Note that ℓn is the symbol that denotes natural logarithms (log to base e). One slight problem with the logit transformation is that it is not defined when the value of x is either zero or one. To cope with this in practice, we sometimes add $1/2$ (or some other chosen value) to x and $(1-x)$ as a *fudge factor* before taking the log of the ratio.

Figure 11.4 is the quantile–quantile plot for the log-transformed data from Figure 11.3, while Figure 11.5 is the histogram of these same log-transformed data. The quantile–quantile plot is approximately linear indicating that the log transformation has recovered normality for these data and the histogram clearly conforms

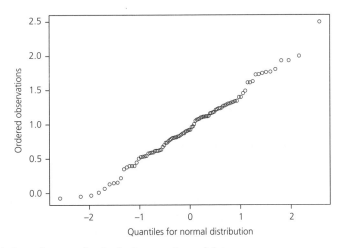

Figure 11.4 Quantile–quantile plot for log-transformed data

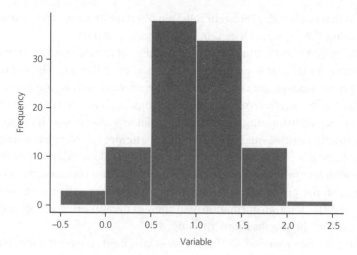

Figure 11.5 Histogram for log-transformed data

more closely to the normal distribution shape. An assumption of normality would now be an entirely reasonable assumption to make on this transformed scale.

If we assume that log of the endpoint follows a normal distribution, then we say that the distribution of the original endpoint is *log-normal*.

There are several other distributions used for certain specialised settings on which statistical tests can be based. The *beta distribution* is often a valid assumption for an endpoint that is recorded as a proportion and is an alternative to using the logit transformation to recover normality. The *gamma distribution* is a distribution that can sometimes be used for *positively skewed data* where the bulk of the data is towards the lower end of the scale and there is a long right tail to the distribution, and statistical tests can be developed for this distribution as an alternative to taking logs and assuming normality. Finally, the *Poisson distribution* is often suited to situations where the endpoint under consideration is a count. These *models* are not non-parametric since they assume a specific distribution for the underlying endpoint but are included here since they move us away from the assumption of normality.

11.5 Non-parametric tests

11.5.1 The Mann–Whitney U-test

The following hypothetical data in Table 11.2 are simulated from two distinct non-normal distributions. The population, from which the observations in group A are taken, has a mean of 3, while the population from which the B group observations were taken has mean equal to 5.

The Mann–Whitney U-test is equivalent to an alternative test called the *Wilcoxon rank sum test*. These tests were developed independently but subsequently

Table 11.2 Hypothetical non-normal data for two groups

Group A (n = 15)	Rank	Group B (n = 16)	Rank
1.45	1	3.54	18
2.55	11	3.04	15
4.35	21	5.33	24
1.93	5	3.16	17
3.95	19	3.10	16
7.90	29	2.69	12
1.78	3	2.95	14
4.60	22	5.89	26
1.84	4	5.17	23
2.54	10	2.13	7
5.47	25	4.30	20
2.29	8	8.48	30
2.91	13	12.88	31
1.46	2	6.43	27
2.30	9	2.01	6
		7.03	28

shown to be mathematically the same. We will develop the test using the Wilcoxon rank sum methodology.

The first step in undertaking this test is to order (or *rank*) the observations in both groups combined, from smallest to largest. This ranking is seen in Table 11.2. There are 31 observations in total, and the average of the numbers 1 through to 31 is 16 (16=(1+31)/2). If there were no differences on average between the two populations, then the average rank in each of the two groups would be close to 16. The *signal* for the Wilcoxon rank sum test is the difference between the observed average rank in the smaller of the two groups (group A in this case) minus the expected average rank (equal to 16) under the assumption that the treatments on average are the same. The average of the ranks attached to the 15 observations in group A is equal to 12.13 (=182/15 since the total of the ranks in this group is 182). This average is below 16 and is an indication that in group A the observations look to be smaller than the observations in group B and the value of the signal is −3.87(=12.13−16). The standard error attached to this signal is given by

$$se = \sqrt{\frac{n_2(n_1 + n_2 + 1)}{12n_1}} = \sqrt{\frac{16 \times (15 + 16 + 1)}{12 \times 15}} = 1.69$$

The signal-to-se ratio for these data is then −2.29. We obtain the *p*-value by comparing the value of this test statistic with what we would expect to see if the treatments were the same. This null distribution is a special form of the normal distribution, called the *standard normal* – the normal distribution with mean zero and standard deviation equal to one. The two-sided *p*-value turns out to be

Example 11.1 Natalizumab in the treatment of relapsing multiple sclerosis

Miller *et al.* (2003) report a trial comparing two dose levels of natalizumab (3 mg/kg and 6 mg/km) with placebo. The primary endpoint was the number of new brain lesions during the six month treatment period. Table 11.3 presents the data.

The distribution of the number of new lesions (count data) is clearly not normal within each of the treatment groups. There is a peak at zero in each of the groups with then fewer patients progressively as the number of lesions increases. A log transformation would not work here because of the presence of the zero values for the endpoint. The authors used the Mann–Whitney U-test to compare each of the natalizumab dose groups with placebo obtaining $p<0.001$ in each case. Each dose level is significantly better than placebo in reducing the number of new enhancing lesions.

Table 11.3 Number of new enhancing lesions

	Placebo (n=71)	Natalizumab (3 mg, n=68)	Natalizumab (6 mg, n=74)
No lesions	23 (32%)	51 (75%)	48 (65%)
1–3 lesions	18 (25%)	14 (21%)	20 (27%)
4–6 lesions	13 (18%)	1 (1%)	5 (7%)
7–9 lesions	0	0	0
10–12 lesions	3 (4%)	1 (1%)	0
>12 lesions	14 (20%)	1 (1%)	1 (1%)

0.022, a statistically significant result indicating treatment differences. Inspecting the data, it is clear that it is group A that, on average, is giving smaller values.

This methodology assumes that all of the observations are distinct so that a unique ranking can be defined. In many cases, however, this will not be true and we will see tied values in the data. In these situations, we assign average ranks to the tied values. For example, had the observations 2.54 and 2.55 both been equal to 2.55, then we would have attached the rank 10.5 (the average of the ranks 10 and 11 corresponding to these two observations) to both values; the ranking then proceeds 8, 9, 10.5, 10.5, 12, 13 and so on. With three values all equal, say, in positions 14, 15 and 16, then the average rank 15 is attached to each of the observations. Provided that the number of tied values is not too large, then the same formulas as earlier can be used to calculate the value of the test statistic. For more frequent ties, then the formula for the se needs to be modified. More details can be found in van Belle *et al.* (2004), Section 8.6.3. Example 11.1 provides an application of the Mann-Whitney U-test in a setting where the data are heavily tied.

11.5.2 The Wilcoxon signed rank test

This test is the non-parametric equivalent of the paired t-test. Recall from Section 11.3 that the paired t-test assumes that the population of differences for each patient follows the normal shape. If this assumption is violated, then the paired t-test does not apply although, as with the unpaired t-test, the paired t-test is fairly robust against modest departures from normality.

The test is again based on a ranking procedure. Under the assumption that the treatments being compared, A and B, are the same, then the number of positive A−B differences should be equal to the number of negative A−B differences.

For example, suppose there are 12 patients; then under the assumption that the treatments are the same, we should see approximately six positive A−B differences and six negative A−B differences. Further, the magnitude of the positive differences and the negative differences should look similar. Having calculated the A−B differences, the first step is to assign ranks to all of the patients according to the magnitude of those differences (ignoring the sign). Secondly, we add up the ranks attached to those differences that were positive. The average rank of the positive differences should be equal to the average rank of the negative differences, and both should be equal to 6.5 (the average of the numbers 1 to 12) under the null hypothesis of no treatment differences. The signal for the test statistic is formed from the observed average rank for the positive differences minus the expected average rank for those positive differences; this latter quantity is 6.5 in the example. The standard error associated with the observed average rank for the positive differences is then calculated, and we compare the signal-to-se ratio with the standard normal distribution to give us the p-value.

Had we chosen to calculate the differences B−A, then the signal would have exactly the same as the signal based on the A−B differences, but with the opposite sign, and the two-sided p-value would be completely unchanged.

11.5.3 General comments

Non-parametric tests, as seen in the two procedures outlined earlier in Section 11.5, are based on some form of ranking of the data. Once the data are ranked, then the test is based entirely on those ranks; the original data play no further part. It is therefore the behaviour of ranks that determines the properties of these tests, and it is this element that gives them their robustness. Whatever the original data looks like, once the rank transformation is performed, then the patterns in the data become predictable.

It may seem strange to see that the normal distribution plays a part in the p-value calculations in Sections 11.5.1 and 11.5.2. The appearance of this distribution is in no sense related to the underlying distribution of the data. For the Mann–Whitney U-test, for example, it relates to the behaviour of the average of the ranks within each of the individual groups under the assumption of equal treatments where the ranks in those groups of sizes n_1 and n_2 are simply a random split of the numbers 1 through to $n_1 + n_2$.

In terms of summary statistics, means are less relevant because of the inevitable skewness of the original data (otherwise, we would not be using non-parametric tests). This skewness frequently produces extremes, which then tend to dominate the calculation of the mean. Medians are usually a better, more stable description of the *average*.

Extending non-parametric tests to more complex settings, such as regression, ANOVA and ANCOVA, is not straightforward although there are some simple extensions, but this is one aspect of these methods that limits their usefulness. The van Elteren test (van Elteren, 1960) is a stratified form of the Mann–Whitney U-test and gives the possibility to undertake simple adjusted analyses.

11.6 Advantages and disadvantages of non-parametric methods

It is fair to say that statisticians tend to disagree somewhat regarding the value of non-parametric methods. Some statisticians view them very favourably, while others are reluctant to use them unless there is no other alternative.

Clearly, the main advantage of a non-parametric method is that it makes essentially no assumptions about the underlying distribution of the data. In contrast, the corresponding parametric methods make specific assumptions, for example, that the data are normally distributed. Does this matter? Well, as mentioned earlier, the t-tests, even though in a strict sense they assume normality, are quite robust against departures from normality. In other words, you have to be some way off normality for the *p*-values and associated confidence intervals to become invalid, especially with the kinds of moderate to large sample sizes that we tend to see in our trials. Most of the time in clinical studies, we are within those boundaries, particularly when we are also able to transform data to conform more closely to normality.

Further, there are a number of disadvantages of non-parametric methods:

*   With parametric methods, confidence intervals can be calculated, which link directly with the *p*-values; recall the discussion in Section 9.1. With non-parametric methods, the *p*-values are based directly on the calculated ranks, and it is not easy to obtain a confidence interval in relation to parameters that have a clinical meaning that links with this. This compromises our ability to provide an assessment of clinical benefit.
*   Non-parametric methods reduce power. Therefore, if the data are normally distributed, either on the original scale or following a transformation, the non-parametric test will be less able to detect differences should they exist.
*   Non-parametric procedures tend to be simple two-group comparisons, although there are some simple extensions to allow stratified analyses. Further, there are some general non-parametric approaches akin to analysis of covariance although they are somewhat complex. The advantages provided by ANCOVA therefore, correcting for baseline imbalances, increasing precision and looking

for treatment-by-covariate interactions, are not readily available within a non-parametric framework.

For these reasons, non-parametric methods are used infrequently within the context of clinical trials, and they tend only to be considered if it is clear that a corresponding parametric approach, either directly or following a data transformation, is unsuitable.

11.7 Outliers

An *outlier* is an unusual data point well away from most of the data. Usually, the outlier in question will not have been anticipated, and the identification of these points and appropriate action should be decided at the *blind review*.

The appropriate method for dealing with an outlier will depend somewhat on the setting, but one or two general points can be made. The first thing that should be done is to check that the value is both possible from a medical perspective and correct. For example, a negative survival time is not possible, and this could well have been as a result of an incorrect date at randomisation being recorded. Hopefully, these problems will have been picked up at the data cleaning stage, but sometimes, things slip through. Clearly, if the data point is incorrect, then it should be corrected before analysis.

An extreme, large positive value may sometimes be a manifestation of an underlying distribution of data that is heavily skewed. Transforming the data to be more symmetric may then be something to consider.

Analysing the data with and without the outliers may ultimately be the appropriate approach, just to ensure that the conclusions are unaffected by their presence. The ICH E9 provides some guidance on this point.

ICH E9 (1998): 'Note for Guidance on Statistical Principles for Clinical Trials'

'If no procedure for dealing with outliers was foreseen in the trial protocol, one analysis with the actual values and at least one other analysis eliminating or reducing the outlier effect should be performed and differences between their results discussed'.

CHAPTER 12
Equivalence and non-inferiority

12.1 Demonstrating similarity

In this chapter, we will move away from superiority trials to look at methods for the evaluation of equivalence and non-inferiority. The setting in all cases here is the comparison of a new treatment to an active control where we are looking to demonstrate similarity (in some defined sense) between the two treatments.

It should be clear from our earlier development, especially the discussion in Sections 9.2 and 9.3, that obtaining a non-significant p-value in a superiority evaluation does not demonstrate that the two treatments are the same or even similar; a non-significant p-value may simply be the result of a small trial, with low power even to detect large differences. ICH E9 makes a clear statement in this regard.

ICH E9 (1998): 'Note for Guidance on Statistical Principles for Clinical Trials'

'Concluding equivalence or non-inferiority based on observing a non-significant test result of the null hypothesis that there is no difference between the investigational product and the active comparator is inappropriate'.

Unfortunately, this issue is not well understood within the clinical trial community, and the misinterpretation of non-significant p-values is all too common. See Jones *et al.* (1996) for further discussion on these points.

Equivalence trials are, of course, routinely used in the evaluation of bioequivalence, and the methodology there is well established; both European and FDA guidelines exist. More recently, we have seen the need to establish therapeutic equivalence, and Ebbutt and Frith (1998) provide a detailed case study in the development of an alternative propellant for the asthma inhaler. More usually, however, in a therapeutic setting, we use a non-inferiority design, where we are looking to establish that our new treatment is *at least as good* or *no worse than* an existing treatment. We will of course need to define what we mean by *at least as good* or *no worse than* in an operational sense for this to be unambiguous.

One question that often arises is, shouldn't such evaluations always be based on non-inferiority rather than equivalence, because surely having a new

Statistical Thinking for Non-Statisticians in Drug Regulation, Second Edition. Richard Kay.
© 2015 John Wiley & Sons, Ltd. Published 2015 by John Wiley & Sons, Ltd.

treatment that is potentially more efficacious than an existing treatment is a positive outcome that we would want to allow? Well, usually this would be the case, but not always. The Ebbutt and Frith (1998) case study is one such situation. The standard metered-dose inhaler has a CFC gas as the propellant, and this causes environmental damage. An alternative propellant was sought to reduce the environmental burden. The primary endpoint for the studies covered by Ebbutt and Frith was peak expiratory flow (PEF) rate, a measure of lung function. The trials developing the alternative propellant were all equivalence trials making comparisons between the two devices, the existing inhaler and the new inhaler with the alternative propellant. It was necessary to show that the new inhaler provided an increase in PEF that was on average the same as that provided by the existing inhaler. The requirement was to match the effectiveness of the two inhalers as eventually the new inhaler would be used as a substitute for the existing inhaler. Should, for example, the new inhaler result in a substantially greater increase in PEF, then this could mean that the new device was delivering a higher dosage, an unsatisfactory situation that could be associated with safety issues. More recently, we have seen guidance from the CHMP (2006) (*Guideline on Similar Biological Medicinal Products Containing Biotechnology-Derived Proteins as Active Substance: Non-Clinical and Clinical Issues*) with regard to establishing similarity for biologics (biosimilars), and equivalence methodology is also required in this case.

As mentioned in Section 1.10, there are essentially two areas where we would want to conduct non-inferiority trials: firstly where inclusion of a placebo for either practical or ethical issues is not possible and we are therefore looking to demonstrate the efficacy of the new treatment indirectly by showing similarity to an established active treatment and secondly where it is necessary to show that there is no important loss of efficacy for a new treatment compared to an existing treatment in a setting where the new treatment offers advantages outside of efficacy. It must also be noted that within the same trial, there may be a mixture of superiority and non-inferiority comparisons. When we talk about a non-inferiority trial, we are usually referring to the fact that the primary comparison is a non-inferiority comparison, but of course, there may be secondary or other comparisons such as safety and tolerability that are evaluating superiority.

Finally, before we move on to look at statistical methods, it is worth mentioning that many people feel uncomfortable with the term non-inferiority. In a strict sense, any reduction in efficacy is saying that the new treatment is not as good as the existing treatment and so is inferior. We are using the term non-inferiority however to denote a non-zero, but clinically irrelevant reduction in efficacy, which we need to define in an appropriate way. Some practitioners use the term *one-sided equivalence* as an alternative to non-inferiority.

A good overview of various aspects of non-inferiority trials is provided by Kaul and Diamond (2006).

12.2 Confidence intervals for equivalence

We will start by looking at equivalence and then move on to consider non-inferiority. The first step in establishing equivalence is to define what we mean by *equivalence*. Following Ebbutt and Frith (1998), suppose we are looking to establish the equivalence of a new asthma inhaler device with an existing inhaler device in a trial setting and further suppose that our clinical definition of equivalence is 15 l/min. In other words, if the treatment difference in the mean increase in PEF following four weeks of treatment is <15 l/min, then we will conclude that the two devices provide a clinically equivalent benefit on average. We may want to argue over whether 15 l/min is the appropriate value, but whatever we do we must choose a value. The ±15 l/min values are termed the *equivalence margins*, and the interval −15 l/min to +15 l/min is also called the *equivalence region* (see Figure 12.1).

The next step is to undertake the trial and calculate the 95 per cent confidence interval for the difference in the means (mean increase in PEF on new inhaler (μ_1) − mean increase in PEF on existing inhaler (μ_2)). As a first example, suppose that this confidence interval is (−7 l/min, 12 l/min). In other words, we can be 95 per cent confident that the true difference, $\mu_1 - \mu_2$, is between 7 l/min in favour of the existing inhaler and 12 l/min in favour of the new inhaler.

As seen in Figure 12.1, this confidence interval is completely contained between the equivalence margins −15 l/min to 15 l/min, and all of the values for the treatment difference supported by the confidence interval are compatible with the definition of clinical equivalence. In this case, we have established equivalence as defined.

In contrast, suppose that the 95 per cent confidence interval had turned out to be (−17 l/min, 12 l/min). This interval is not entirely within the equivalence margins, and the data are supporting potential treatment differences below the lower equivalence margin. In this case, we have not established equivalence.

Note that there are no conventional *p*-values here. Such *p*-values have no role in the evaluation of equivalence; establishing equivalence is based entirely on the use of confidence intervals.

ICH E9 (1998): 'Note for Guidance on Statistical Principles for Clinical Trials'

'Statistical analysis is generally based on the use of confidence intervals. For equivalence trials, two-sided confidence intervals should be used. Equivalence is inferred when the entire confidence interval falls within the equivalence margins'.

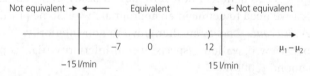

Figure 12.1 Establishing equivalence

The confidence intervals we have used to date are all two-sided. We will talk later about one-sided confidence intervals.

12.3 Confidence intervals for non-inferiority

For non-inferiority, the first step involves defining a non-inferiority margin. Suppose that we are developing a new treatment for hypertension and potentially the reason why the new treatment is better is that it has fewer side effects, although we are not anticipating any improvement in terms of efficacy. Indeed, suppose that we are prepared to pay a small price in terms of efficacy for a reduction in the side effects profile, say, up to 2 mmHg in the mean reduction in diastolic blood pressure.

In Figure 12.2, μ_1 and μ_2 are the mean reductions in diastolic blood pressure in the test treatment and active control groups, respectively. If the difference in the means is above zero, then the test treatment is superior to the active control; if the difference is zero, then they are identical. If the difference falls below zero, the test treatment is not as good as the active control. This, however, is a price we are prepared to pay, but only up to a mean reduction in efficacy of 2 mmHg; beyond that, the price is too great. The non-inferiority margin is therefore set at −2 mmHg.

Step 2 is then to run the trial and compute the 95 per cent confidence interval for the difference, $\mu_1 - \mu_2$, in the mean reductions in diastolic blood pressure. In the aforementioned example, suppose that this 95 per cent confidence interval turns out to be (−1.5 mmHg, 1.8 mmHg). As seen in Figure 12.2, all of the values within this interval are compatible with our definition of non-inferiority. In this case, the non-inferiority of the test treatment has been established. In contrast, had the 95 per cent confidence interval been, say, (−2.3 mmHg, 1.8 mmHg), then non-inferiority would not have been established since the lower end of that confidence interval falls below −2 mmHg. Note again that there is no mention of conventional *p*-values; they have no part to play in non-inferiority.

In order to demonstrate non-inferiority, it is only one end of the confidence interval that matters; in our example it is simply the lower end that needs to be above −2 mmHg. It is therefore not really necessary to calculate the upper end of the interval, and sometimes we leave this unspecified. The resulting confidence interval with just the lower end is called a *one-sided 97.5 per cent confidence interval*; the two-sided 95 per cent confidence interval cuts off 2.5 per cent at each of the lower and upper ends, and having the upper end undefined leaves just 2.5 per cent cut off at the lower end. The whole of this confidence interval must be entirely to the right of the non-inferiority margin for non-inferiority to be

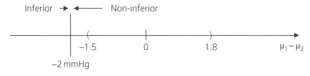

Figure 12.2 Establishing non-inferiority

established. Note that the conclusions we draw are unchanged when we use a one-sided 97.5% confidence interval in place of a two-sided 95% confidence interval as the lower end of the interval is unaffected.

ICH E9 (1998): 'Note for Guidance on Statistical Principles for Clinical Trials'

'For non-inferiority a one-sided confidence interval should be used'.

Example 12.1 provides an application that we will return to later in this chapter.

Example 12.1 Fluconazole compared to amphotericin B in preventing relapse in cryptococcal meningitis

The aim of this study reported by Powderly *et al.* (1992) was to establish the non-inferiority of a test treatment, fluconazole, compared to an established treatment, amphotericin B, in preventing the relapse of cryptococcal meningitis in HIV-infected patients. It was thought that fluconazole would be less effective than amphotericin B but would offer other advantages in terms of reduced toxicity and ease of administration; fluconazole was an oral treatment, while amphotericin B was given intravenously. The non-inferiority margin was set at −15 per cent in terms of relapse rates:

Let θ_F = relapse rate on fluconazole

Let θ_A = relapse rate on amphotericin B

In Figure 12.3, a positive difference for $\theta_A - \theta_F$ is indicating that fluconazole is a better treatment, while a negative difference is indicating that amphotericin B is better.

The non-inferiority margin has been set at −15 per cent. Figure 12.4 displays the non-inferiority region, and we need the (two-sided) 95 per cent confidence interval, or the one-sided 97.5 per cent confidence interval, to be entirely within this non-inferiority region for non-inferiority to be established, that is, to the right of −15 per cent.

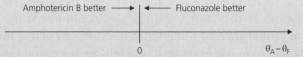

Figure 12.3 Difference in relapse rates

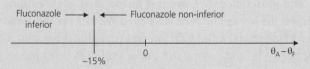

Figure 12.4 Definition of non-inferiority

12.4 A *p*-value approach

Although conventional *p*-values have no role to play in equivalence or non-inferiority trials, there is a *p*-value counterpart to the confidence interval approach. The confidence interval methodology was developed by Westlake (1981) in the context of bioequivalence, and Schuirmann (1987) developed a *p*-value approach that was mathematically connected to these confidence intervals, although much more difficult to understand! It nonetheless provides a useful way of thinking, particularly when we come later to consider type I and type II errors in this context and also the sample size calculation. We will start by looking at equivalence and use $\pm \Delta$ to denote the equivalence margins.

Within the framework of hypothesis testing, the null and alternative hypotheses of interest for equivalence when dealing with means are as follows:

$$H_0 : \mu_1 - \mu_2 \leq -\Delta \text{ or } \mu_1 - \mu_2 \geq \Delta$$
$$H_1 : -\Delta < \mu_1 - \mu_2 < \Delta$$

In this case, the alternative hypothesis states that the two treatments are equivalent; the null hypothesis is saying that the two treatments are not equivalent. Note that the alternative encapsulates the *objective*; we are trying to disprove the null in order to establish equivalence.

The hypotheses stated earlier can be expressed as two separate sets of hypotheses corresponding to the lower and upper ends of the equivalence range:

$$H_{01} : \mu_1 - \mu_2 \leq -\Delta \quad H_{11} : \mu_1 - \mu_2 > -\Delta$$
$$H_{02} : \mu_1 - \mu_2 \geq \Delta \quad H_{12} : \mu_1 - \mu_2 < \Delta$$

Undertaking two tests each at the 2.5 per cent level, one for H_{01} versus H_{11} and one for H_{02} versus H_{12}, can be shown to be mathematically connected to the confidence interval approach developed earlier. In particular, if each of these tests gives significant *p*-values at the 2.5 per cent significance level, then the 95 per cent confidence interval for the difference in the means will be entirely contained within the equivalence margins $\pm \Delta$. Conversely, if the 95 per cent confidence interval is contained within the equivalence margins, then each of the aforementioned sets of tests will give *p*-values significant at the 2.5 per cent level. These two sets of hypotheses are both one-sided comparisons; the first set is looking to see whether the treatment difference, $\mu_1 - \mu_2$, is either $\leq$ or $> -\Delta$, while the second set is looking to see if $\mu_1 - \mu_2$ is either $\geq$ or $< \Delta$. The approach using *p*-values is therefore known as the *two one-sided tests approach*. Following on from the earlier quote specifying the role of confidence intervals, ICH E9 states:

ICH E9 (1998): 'Note for Guidance on Statistical Principles for Clinical Trials'

'Operationally, this is equivalent to the method of using two simultaneous one-sided tests to test the (composite) null hypothesis that the treatment difference is outside the equivalence margins versus the (composite) alternative hypothesis that the treatment difference is within the margins'.

With the *p*-value methodology, we are rejecting the null hypothesis H_0 in favour of the alternative hypothesis H_1, provided the two (one-sided) *p*-values are

≤2.5 per cent. We have then established equivalence, and we can talk in terms of the treatments being *significantly equivalent*. The terminology sounds almost contradictory, but is a correct statement. If either of the two *p*-values is above 2.5 per cent, then the treatments are *not significantly equivalent*.

For non-inferiority, the one-sided comparison

$$\text{H}_0 : \mu_1 - \mu_2 \leq -\Delta \quad \text{H}_1 : \mu_1 - \mu_2 > -\Delta$$

yields a *p*-value that links with the one-sided 97.5 per cent confidence interval for establishing non-inferiority. If the *p*-value from this test is significant at the 2.5 per cent level, then the one-sided 97.5 per cent confidence interval will be entirely to the right of the non-inferiority margin – Δ, and vice versa. If we see this outcome, then we can talk in terms of the new treatment being *significantly non-inferior* to the active control. Alternatively, if we get a non-significant *p*-value, then the new treatment is *not significantly non-inferior*.

Using a 2.5 per cent significance level for non-inferiority in this way may initially appear to be out of line with the conventional 5 per cent significance level for superiority. A moment's thought should suffice, however, to realise that in a test for superiority we would never make a claim for a new treatment if that treatment was significantly worse than control, and we would only ever make a claim if the new treatment was significantly better than control, so effectively for superiority, we are conducting a one-sided test at the 2.5 per cent level to lead us to a positive conclusion for the new treatment.

In practice, I would always recommend using confidence intervals for evaluating equivalence and non-inferiority rather than these associated *p*-values. This is because the associated *p*-values tend to get mixed up with conventional *p*-values for detecting differences. The two are not the same and are looking at quite different things. The confidence interval approach avoids this confusion and provides a technique that is easy to present and interpret.

12.5 Assay sensitivity

One concern with equivalence and non-inferiority trials is that a positive conclusion of equivalence/non-inferiority could result from an insensitive trial by default. If, for example, equivalence is established, then this could mean either that the two treatments are equally effective or indeed equally ineffective. If the chosen endpoints are insensitive, dosages of the drugs too low, patients recruited who are not really ill and the trial conducted in a sloppy fashion with lots of protocol deviators and dropouts, then the treatments will inevitably look very similar! Clearly, we must ensure that a conclusion of equivalence/non-inferiority from a trial is a reflection of the true properties of the treatments. Regulatory guidelines (see in particular ICH E10) talk in terms of *assay sensitivity* as a requirement of a clinical trial that ensures this.

ICH E10 (2001): 'Note for Guidance on Choice of Control Group in Clinical Trials'

'Assay sensitivity is a property of a clinical trial defined as the ability to distinguish an effective treatment from an ineffective treatment'.

Of course, assay sensitivity applies in the same way to trials that evaluate superiority, but in those cases, things take care of themselves. A conclusion of superiority by definition tells us that the trial is a sensitive instrument; otherwise, superiority would not have been detected.

Ensuring assay sensitivity is best achieved through good design and trial conduct to a high standard. From a design perspective, the current design should be in line with trials historically that have shown the active control to be effective. The following aspects need to be carefully considered:

- Entry criteria: the patients should preferably be at the moderate to severe end of the disease scale.
- Dose and regimen of the active control: in line with standard practice.
- Endpoint definition and assessment: use established endpoints.
- Run-in/washout period to exclude ineligible patients: avoids diluting the patient population.

Further, the trial conduct should protect against any compromise of assay sensitivity, and the following in particular should be avoided:

- Poor compliance
- Use of concomitant medication that could interfere with response to the new and active treatments
- Poor application of diagnostic criteria
- Unblinding
- Unnecessary dropouts
- Lack of objectivity and consistency in the evaluation of endpoints

It is also possible at the analysis stage to use the trial data to support assay sensitivity. Ebbutt and Frith (1998) investigate the mean change from baseline in both test treatment and active control groups and observe that the magnitude of these changes is in line with what one would expect historically in terms of the effect of the active control over placebo. In a trial where the primary endpoint is a binary outcome, seeing a response rate in the active control group similar to response rates seen historically in placebo-controlled trials that demonstrated the active control to be an effective treatment supports assay sensitivity. In contrast, if the response rate in the current trial is higher or lower than expected, then assay sensitivity could be drawn into question. A higher rate may indicate a population that is less severe than that used previously, while a lower rate could indicate dosages that are too low, for example.

Finally, one sure way to investigate assay sensitivity is to include a placebo group as a third arm in the trial. This allows direct assessment of assay sensitivity by comparing the active control with placebo where statistically significant differences would need to be seen. However, including a placebo arm will only be possible where it is ethically and practically reasonable to do so, and in many equivalence/non-inferiority settings, this will not be the case. A related point is that there are some therapeutic settings that are unsuitable for equivalence/non-inferiority trials unless a placebo arm is included, for example, depression, anxiety, allergic rhinitis and Alzheimer's disease and other dementias, where established effective drugs do not consistently demonstrate effects over placebo. The inclusion of a placebo arm would allow direct evaluation of assay sensitivity. Many therapeutic specific regulatory guidelines in these areas actively discourage the use of non-inferiority trials in the absence of a placebo group.

CHMP (2008): Guideline on Medicinal Products for the Treatment of Alzheimer's Disease and Other Dementias

'Active control parallel group trials comparing the new treatment to an already approved treatment are needed in order to give the comparative benefit/risk ratio of the new treatment, at least in those treatments intended for symptomatic improvement. However, due to concerns over assay sensitivity, the use of a non-inferiority design versus active control only, will not be accepted as proof of efficacy'. Therefore three-arm studies with placebo, test product and active control or a superiority trial are the preferred design options.

The CHMP (2012) addendum to the note for guidance on bacterial infections states that for certain infections, for example, acute bacterial sinusitis and superficial skin infections, *'An approval based solely on non-inferiority studies is not currently acceptable'*.

A related concept that is used in this area is *historical evidence of sensitivity to drug effects*. This idea, introduced initially in ICH E10, refers to the ability of effective treatments to consistently show an advantage over placebo in appropriately designed and conducted clinical trials. As mentioned in the previous paragraph, there are certain therapeutic settings where this is not the case.

12.6 Analysis sets

In superiority trials, the full analysis set is the basis for the primary analysis. As discussed in Section 7.2, the regulators prefer this approach, in part, because it gives a conservative view of the new treatment. In equivalence/non-inferiority trials, however, the full analysis set is not conservative and may result in the treatments looking more similar than, in reality, they are. This is because the full analysis set will include the patients who have not complied with the medication schedules and who have not followed the study procedures and the inclusion of such patients will tend if anything to weaken treatment differences.

For equivalence and non-inferiority trials, therefore, the regulators like to see analyses undertaken on both the full analysis set and the per-protocol set with positive conclusions being drawn from both. In this sense, these two analyses are considered co-primary. There is a common misconception here that for equivalence/non-inferiority trials, the per-protocol set is primary. This is not the case. The per-protocol set is still potentially subject to bias because of the exclusion of randomised patients and so cannot supply the complete answer; both analysis sets need to be supporting equivalence/non-inferiority in order to have a robust conclusion.

CPMP (2000): 'Points to Consider on Switching Between Superiority and Non-inferiority'

'In a non-inferiority trial, the full analysis set and the per-protocol analysis set have equal importance and their use should lead to similar conclusions for a robust interpretation'.

Similar comments apply to therapeutic equivalence trials also.

12.7 The choice of Δ

One of the most difficult aspects of the design of equivalence and non-inferiority trials, with the exception of bioequivalence, is the choice of the margin(s).

12.7.1 Bioequivalence

The equivalence margins for bioequivalence specified by both the FDA (2001) *Statistical Approaches to Establishing Bioequivalence* and the CPMP (2001) *Note for Guidance on the Investigation of Bioavailability and Bioequivalence* require that the ratios of the geometric means, μ_1^{GM}/μ_2^{GM}, for the two treatments lie between 0.80 and 1.25. This requirement applies to both AUC and C_{max}. A deviation from the rules for therapeutic equivalence is that 90 per cent confidence intervals are used rather than 95 per cent leading to a more relaxed requirement.

The reason why ratios of geometric means are used in this context follows on from what was discussed in Section 11.4; the distributions of AUC and C_{max} tend to be positively skewed, and the log transformation is applied to recover normality.

By taking logs, the condition, $0.8 < \left(\mu_1^{GM}/\mu_2^{GM}\right) < 1.25$, can be translated into the following requirement for $\mu_1^* - \mu_2^*$ where μ_1^* for example is the mean AUC on the log scale for the test treatment and μ_2^* for example is the mean AUC on the log scale for the active control:

$$ln(0.80) < \mu_1^* - \mu_2^* < ln(1.25)$$
or equivalently $-0.22 < \mu_1^* - \mu_2^* < 0.22$

12.7.2 Therapeutic equivalence

The rules for therapeutic equivalence are different from those for bioequivalence. The choice of margin will be a mixture of statistical and clinical reasoning. Strict equivalence is appropriate when we want to consider essential similarity or where the test treatment is to be used as an exact replacement for the new treatment. In these cases, Δ should be chosen to be a completely irrelevant difference from a clinical point of view. Ebbutt and Frith (1998) based their choice of $\Delta = 15\,l/min$ on several considerations:

- Previous trials with the beta-agonist salmeterol had given an average difference from placebo in PEF of $37\,l/min$, while the effect of inhaled steroids was of the order of $25\,l/min$, and Δ was chosen as a proportion of those effects.
- Typically, a mean improvement of $70\,l/min$ would be seen following treatment with a short-acting beta-agonist, and Δ was chosen to be about 20 per cent of this.
- Discussion with practitioners suggested that $15\,l/min$ was clinically irrelevant.

In the next section, we will discuss the non-inferiority setting, and many of the considerations there also apply to the situation of therapeutic equivalence.

12.7.3 Non-inferiority

In the context of using a non-inferiority trial to demonstrate that a test treatment is efficacious, the following provides a statistical approach for the choice of Δ. Consider, in the setting of hypertension, the trials that historically compared the active control with placebo. In a meta-analysis (see Chapter 18), suppose that the 95 per cent confidence interval for the active control treatment effect in terms of the fall in diastolic blood pressure was $(4.5\,mmHg, 10.3\,mmHg)$. Clearly, Δ would need to be chosen to be considerably less than $4.5\,mmHg$. The confidence interval is telling us that the active control may only be $4.5\,mmHg$ better than placebo. If we allow a margin equal to $4.5\,mmHg$ in the non-inferiority trial comparing the new treatment to the active control, then we are postulating that the new treatment is just as good as the active control if it gets within $4.5\,mmHg$, and under these circumstances, we could find ourselves simply developing another placebo! Defining Δ to be one-half $(=2.25\,mmHg)$ or one-third $(=1.50\,mmHg)$ of the lower bound of this confidence interval would give us statistical confidence coming out of our non-inferiority trial with a positive result, that the test treatment is at worst either $2.25\,mmHg$ or $1.50\,mmHg$ less efficacious than the active control and that the test treatment therefore still maintains a clear advantage over placebo. This value for Δ would then need to be additionally justified on clinical grounds, that is, as an irrelevant difference clinically. Example 12.2 provides an application of this way of thinking.

In situations where we are trying to show no important loss of efficacy of a test treatment to an active control, it is not possible to be entirely prescriptive

---

Example 12.2 Prevention of venous thromboembolism after total hip replacement

The RE-NOVATE trial (Eriksson *et al.*, 2007) compared dabigatran etexilate at two doses (150 mg and 220 mg) with enoxaparin 40 mg once daily (active control) in a randomised, double-blind non-inferiority trial. The primary efficacy outcome was a composite of total venous thromboembolic events and all-cause mortality during the four- to five-week treatment period. In the absence of placebo-controlled trials using enoxaparin for four to five weeks, the authors undertook a meta-analysis of placebo-controlled trials that used enoxaparin for one to two weeks. The 95 per cent confidence interval for the difference in event rates was (23.2 per cent, 42.6 per cent), showing that with 95 per cent confidence, enoxaparin shows a reduction in the rate of venous thromboembolic events and all-cause mortality at least as big as 23.2 per cent. From this, a conservative non-inferiority margin of 7.7 per cent was chosen equal to one-third of the lower end of the 95 per cent confidence interval. A positive result in favour of non-inferiority would therefore support the conclusion that the experimental treatment was no more than 7.7 per cent worse than enoxaparin still keeping it well away from placebo.

The 95 per cent confidence intervals for the difference between the event rates for the two doses of dabigatran etexilate and enoxaparin were (−0.6 per cent, 4.4 per cent) for the 150 mg dose and (−2.9 per cent, 1.6 per cent) for the 220 mg dose, in both cases leading to a conclusion of non-inferiority since the upper ends of these confidence intervals are below 7.7 per cent, the pre-specified margin. It is perfectly acceptable and appropriate to claim, with 95 per cent confidence, that the 150 mg and 220 mg doses have event rates at most 4.4 per cent and 1.6 per cent higher than the rate for enoxaparin.

---

about methods for the choice of Δ. For example, if a new treatment provides an advantage over the existing treatment in terms of safety, the price we are prepared to pay for this in terms of efficacy will clearly depend on the extent of the safety advantage. In these cases, it is not appropriate to think in terms of preserving a proportion of the effect of the active control over placebo.

Further, if the active control effect over placebo is large, then preserving only a proportion does not fit with the objectives of the non-inferiority evaluation if we are looking to conclude *similarity*.

CHMP (2005): 'Guideline on the Choice of Non-Inferiority Margin'

'Alternatively the aim may be to provide data to show that there is no important loss of efficacy if the test product is used instead of the reference. This is probably the most common aim of non-inferiority trials. The choice of delta for such an objective cannot be obtained by looking only at past trials of the comparator against placebo. Ideas such as choosing delta to be a percentage of the expected difference between active and placebo have been advocated, but this is not considered an acceptable justification for the choice. To adequately choose delta an informed decision must be taken, supported by evidence of what is considered an unimportant difference in the particular disease area'.

As the regulators point out, the choice when we are looking to demonstrate no important loss of efficacy needs to be based on clinical reasoning.

Finally, the importance of justifying the choice for Δ cannot be overstated, and there is a clear recommendation from the CHMP regarding its justification.

CHMP (2005): 'Guideline on the Choice of Non-Inferiority Margin'

'The choice of non-inferiority margin should be justified in the study protocol'.

12.7.4 The 10 per cent rule for cure rates

It has been relatively common practice, historically, to use a Δ of 10 per cent for cure rates when dealing, for example, with anti-infectives and vaccines.

CPMP (1999): 'Note for Guidance on Clinical Evaluation of New Vaccines'

'In individual trials, Δ can often be set to about 10 per cent, but will need to be smaller for very high protection rates'.

CPMP (2003): 'Note for Guidance on Evaluation of Medicinal Products Indicated for Treatments of Bacterial Infections'

'In most studies with antibacterial agents in common indications this (Δ) should likely be 10 per cent, but may be smaller when very high cure rates are anticipated'.

The message here appears consistent; 10 per cent is likely to be acceptable except when rates are high, say, >90 per cent, and although these regulatory guidelines are from Europe, the FDA position has been similar. In more recent times, however, the regulators have been happy to deviate from this 10 per cent, in both directions! In a rare disease in which only one or a small number of treatments currently exist, the regulators may be willing to relax the 10 per cent to 12.5 per cent or even 15 per cent. In contrast, for common diseases, the regulators may suggest a tighter Δ, arguing that in the interests of public health, the new treatment will only be acceptable if its performance is very close to the active control.

There are one or two other specific therapeutic settings where there is more guidance on the choice of Δ. For example:

CPMP (2003): 'Points to Consider on the Clinical Development of Fibrinolytic Medicinal Products in the Treatment of Patients with ST Segment Evaluation Acute Myocardial Infarction (STEMI)'

'In the recent past differences of 14 per cent relative or 1 per cent absolute (whichever proves smallest) have been accepted. These margins were based on "all cause mortality" rates at day 30 close to 6.5–7 per cent'.

One final point on the choice of delta that is relevant in all therapeutic settings, and certainly in relation to cure rates, is that the regulators could very well change their minds about what is and what is not acceptable for Δ if the performance of the active control in the trial deviates from what was expected. For example, suppose that a Δ = 10 per cent was chosen with an expected cure rate of 85 per cent for the active control. If in the trial the cure rate on the active control turns out to be 93 per cent, then the regulators may view 10 per cent as too large a value and may suggest a reduction to, say, 5 per cent for this particular trial.

12.7.5 The synthesis method

The method detailed in Section 12.7.3 for determining Δ is called the *fixed margin approach*. In this approach the value for Δ is determined from historical data together with clinical considerations and the data from the current active controlled trial used to establish (or not) non-inferiority based on this margin.

There is an alternative approach, the *synthesis approach*, which does not require a margin to be pre-specified. This method combines the estimated treatment effect from the active control trial with the estimated effect of the active control compared to placebo from the historical data to provide an indirect estimate of the treatment effect of the experimental treatment compared to placebo.

In the example introduced at the beginning of Section 12.7.3, we were considering a hypothetical example where the primary endpoint was the fall in diastolic blood pressure and historical data on the reference product suggested that it was on average 7.4 mmHg better than placebo. So if $\bar{x}_R^* - \bar{x}_P^* = 7.4$ mmHg represents the treatment difference between the reference (active control) mean and the placebo mean in the meta-analysis while $\bar{x}_T - \bar{x}_R = -0.6$ mmHg equals the observed difference in the test and reference treatments in the non-inferiority trial, then assuming that the conditions of the trials are similar (termed constancy – see Section 12.7.6) so that we can assume that $\bar{x}_R \approx \bar{x}_R^*$, an estimated difference between test treatment and placebo means, is, by adding these two effects together, equal to 6.8 mmHg. The standard error (*se*) attached to each of these differences, say, se_1 and se_2, can be combined to give a standard error (*se*) for $\bar{x}_T - \bar{x}_P^*$ using the formula $se = \sqrt{se_1^2 + se_2^2}$. The 95 per cent confidence interval for the true test treatment effect (vs. placebo) is then given approximately by $\bar{x}_T - \bar{x}_P^* \pm 2 * se$.

This synthesis method treats the data from the current trial and the data from the historical data as if they came from the same randomised trial to indicate what treatment difference would have been seen had placebo been included as an additional arm in the current trial. Clearly, there are some very strong assumptions that are being made here, and these are largely unverifiable. For this reason, this method is less popular with regulators who like to see a fixed pre-specified value for Δ, justified based on statistical and clinical arguments, independently from the active control trial currently being conducted.

12.8 Biocreep and constancy

One valid concern that regulators have is the issue of so-called *biocreep*. Demonstrating that a second-generation active treatment is non-inferior to the active control may well mean that the new treatment is slightly less efficacious than the active control. Evaluating a third-generation active treatment to the now established second-generation active treatment may lead to a further erosion of efficacy and so on, until at some stage a new active treatment, while satisfying the *local* conditions for non-inferiority, is, in reality, indistinguishable from placebo. The FDA discussed this issue many years ago specifically in relation to anti-infectives (FDA (1992) *Points to Consider on Clinical Development and Labeling of Anti-Infective Drug Products*).

The issue of *constancy* concerns the conditions under which the current active control trial is being conducted compared to the conditions under which the active control was established historically. Things may well have changed. For example, the nature of the underlying disease or the effectiveness of ancillary care may be such that the active control performs rather differently now than it did when the original placebo-controlled trials were undertaken. This may well be true, for example, for antibiotics where populations of patients will have developed resistance to certain treatments. If this were the case, then the current non-inferiority trial could lead to a misleading conclusion of effectiveness for the new active when in the context of the current trial the comparator treatment is ineffective.

Both of these elements cause nervousness among regulators. So much so that for example, the FDA Anti-Infective Drugs Advisory Committee (AIDAC) recommended that the non-inferiority design should no longer be used in trials for acute bacterial sinusitis (CDER Meeting Documents; Anti-Infective Drugs Advisory Committee (29 October 2003), www.fda.gov).

12.9 Sample size calculations

We will focus our attention to the situation of non-inferiority. Within the testing framework, the type I error in this case is, as before, the false positive (rejecting the null hypothesis when it is true), which now translates into concluding non-inferiority when the new treatment is in fact inferior. The type II error is the false negative (failing to reject the null hypothesis when it is false), and this translates into failing to conclude non-inferiority when the new treatment truly is non-inferior. The sample size calculations below relate to the evaluation of non-inferiority when using either the confidence interval method or the alternative *p*-value approach detailed in Section 12.4; recall these are mathematically the same.

The sample size calculation requires pre-specification of the following quantities:
- Type I error; for non-inferiority, this is one-sided and will usually be set at 2.5 per cent.
- Power = 1 − type II error, which would usually be at least 80 per cent.
- Δ, the non-inferiority margin.

The remaining quantities would depend on the primary endpoint and the design. Assume we are dealing with the parallel group case.

For a continuous endpoint, we would need:
- The standard deviation of the endpoint
- The anticipated true difference in the two mean values

For a binary endpoint, we would need:
- The response rate in the active control group
- The anticipated true difference in the response rates

Usually, we conduct these calculations assuming there is no difference between the treatments in terms of means (or rates), but this is not always a realistic assumption. It is good practice to at least look at the sensitivity of the calculation to departures from this assumption.

Example 12.3 Evaluating non-inferiority for cure rates

In an anti-infective non-inferiority study, it is expected that the true cure rates for both the test treatment and the active control will be 75 per cent. Δ has been chosen to be equal to 15 per cent. Using the usual approach with a one-sided 97.5 per cent confidence interval for the difference in cure rates a total of 176 patients per group will give 90 per cent power to demonstrate non-inferiority. Table 12.1 gives values for the sample size per group for 90 per cent power and for various departures from the assumptions.

When the cure rates are equal, the sample size decreases as the common cure rate increases. When the test treatment cure rate is above the active control cure rate, then the test treatment is actually better than the active control, and it is much easier to demonstrate non-inferiority. When the reverse happens, however, where the true cure rate under the test treatment falls below that of the active control, then the sample size requirement goes up; it is much more difficult under these circumstances to demonstrate non-inferiority. It is also worth noting that when the test treatment is truly 15 per cent (the value for Δ in this example,) below the rate in the active control, planning a trial to demonstrate non-inferiority is simply not possible.

Table 12.1 Sample sizes per group

| | | Cure rate (test treatment) | | | |
		65%	70%	75%	80%
	65%	213	115	70	46
Cure rate (active control)	70%	460	197	105	63
	75%	1745	418	176	91
	80%	∞	1556	366	150

As with sample size in superiority trials, we generally power on the basis of the per-protocol set and increase the sample size to account for the non-evaluable patients. This is particularly important in non-inferiority trials where the full analysis set and the per-protocol set are co-primary analyses. Note also, as is the case in superiority trials, that further factoring up may be needed if there are randomised patients who are being systematically excluded from the full analysis set, as could be the case for example, in anti-infective trials where we tend to deal with the clinically or microbiologically evaluable patients (see Section 7.2.1).

There is a perception that non-inferiority trials are inevitably larger than their superiority counterparts. Under some circumstances, this is true, but is by no means always the case. One crucial quantity in the sample size calculation for a non-inferiority trial is Δ, which plays a role similar to the clinically relevant difference (crd) in a superiority sample size calculation. The sample size (this is also true for equivalence) is inversely proportional to the square of Δ. If Δ is small, then the sample size will be large, and the constraints placed upon us by regulators together with the clinical interpretation of *irrelevant differences* tend to make Δ small in such trials. In a superiority trial, the choice of the crd to detect is an internal, clinical, sometimes commercial decision that is under the control of the trialists, and we are at liberty to power a trial on the basis of a large value. The net effect of these considerations is that non-inferiority trials tend to be larger than trials designed to demonstrate superiority. However, and in contrast to this, if we truly feel that the test treatment is in reality, somewhat better than the active control, then assuming such a positive advantage can have the effect of considerably reducing the sample size, as seen in Example 12.3.

12.10 Switching between non-inferiority and superiority

In a clinical trial with the objective of demonstrating non-inferiority, suppose that the data are somewhat stronger than this and the 95 per cent confidence interval is not only entirely to the right of $-\Delta$ but also completely to the right of zero as in Figure 12.5; there is evidence that the new treatment is in fact superior.

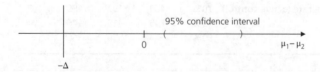

Figure 12.5 Concluding superiority in a non-inferiority trial

What conclusions can we draw in this situation? Can we conclude superiority even though this was not the original objective? Well, generally the answer is yes, superiority can be claimed.

CPMP (2000): 'Points to Consider on Switching Between Superiority and Non-Inferiority'

'If the 95 per cent confidence interval for the treatment effect not only lies entirely above − Δ but also above zero, then there is evidence of superiority in terms of statistical significance at the 5 per cent level (p<0.05). In this case, it is acceptable to calculate the exact probability associated with a test of superiority and to evaluate whether this is sufficiently small to reject convincingly the hypothesis of no difference... Usually this demonstration of a benefit is sufficient for licensing on its own, provided the safety profiles of the new agent and the comparator are similar'.

There are no multiplicity arguments that impact on this switch. Essentially, we can think of the two tests, a test of non-inferiority followed by a test of superiority, as a hierarchy, and we will only be considering the second provided the first one gives a significant result, and as pointed out by the FDA there are no multiplicity issues in these considerations.

FDA Guidance for Industry: Non-Inferiority Clinical Trials (2010)

'In some cases, a study planned as an NI study may show superiority to the active control. ICH E-9 and FDA policy has been that such a superiority finding arising in an NI study can be interpreted without adjustment for multiplicity'.

Perhaps the safest thing to do in this setting though is to pre-specify a hierarchy in the protocol with a test for non-inferiority followed by a test for superiority; there can then be no dispute about such a switch in the eyes of regulators. Following calculation of the exact *p*-value for superiority, the 95 per cent confidence interval allows the clinical relevance of the finding to be evaluated. Presumably, however, any level of benefit would be of value given that at the outset we were looking only to demonstrate non-inferiority and that in this regard the new treatment is likely to have other benefits outside of efficacy.

For superiority, the full analysis set is usually the basis for the primary analysis, so the emphasis in the superiority claim would then need to be based around this. We will now return to Example 12.1 and see a situation where switching from non-inferiority to superiority was possible.

Moving in the opposite direction and concluding non-inferiority in a superiority trial is much more difficult, as this would generally require pre-specification of a non-inferiority margin. Such pre-specification would usually not have been considered in a trial designed to demonstrate superiority. However, if a conclusion of non-inferiority would be a useful outcome, then it could be appropriate to consider such pre-specification.

Example 12.1 (Revisited) Fluconazole compared to amphotericin B in preventing relapse in cryptococcal meningitis

This example has been presented earlier in this chapter. The initial objective was to demonstrate the non-inferiority of fluconazole compared to amphotericin B in the prevention of cryptococcal meningitis in patients with AIDS. The non-inferiority margin was set at −15 per cent for the difference in the relapse rates.

The 95 per cent confidence interval for $\theta_A - \theta_F$ was in fact (7 per cent, 31 per cent), and this is entirely to the right, not only of −15 per cent but also of zero. In this case, a claim for the superiority of fluconazole is supported by the data. The authors concluded that non-inferiority had been established, but additionally, there was evidence that fluconazole was more effective than amphotericin B:

'These data allow us to conclude that fluconazole was at least as effective as weekly amphotericin B... Indeed, the 19 per cent difference in the probability of relapse at one year... suggests that fluconazole was more effective than amphotericin B in preventing a relapse of crytococcal disease in this population of patients'.

FDA (2010): 'Non-Inferiority Clinical Trials'

'Seeking an NI conclusion in the event of a failed superiority test would almost never be acceptable. It would be very difficult to make a persuasive case for an NI margin based on data analyzed with study results in hand'.

Switching from superiority to non-inferiority also presents additional problems. Assay sensitivity may well be one reason why the trial, initially designed to detect superiority, has not done so. The design would need to be very robust and the data compelling if assay sensitivity were to be supported.

Given the various possibilities regarding switching, there may well be a strong argument in any active control comparison to always go for non-inferiority. If the data then turn out to be stronger and support superiority, then this additional conclusion can be made. There are some drawbacks, however, with this way of thinking:

- Non-inferiority trials are more difficult to design; assay sensitivity and the choice of non-inferiority margin are just two of the issues that would additionally need to be considered.
- Non-inferiority trials can often require large sample sizes.
- Designing the trial as a non-inferiority evaluation may give a negative perception external to the company and the clinical trial team.

Nonetheless, this may be a strategy worth considering under some circumstances.

CHAPTER 13

The analysis of survival data

13.1 Time-to-event data and censoring

In many cases, an endpoint directly measures time from the point of randomisation to some well-defined event, for example, time to death (survival time) in oncology or time to rash healing in herpes zoster. The data from such an endpoint invariably has a special feature, known as censoring. For example, suppose the times to death for a group of patients in a 24-month oncology study are as follows:

14 7 24* 15 3 18 9* 10 24* 9...

Here, the first patient died after 14 months from the time of randomisation, and the second patient after 7 months. The third patient however is still alive at the end of the study, while patients 4, 5 and 6 died after 15, 3 and 18 months, respectively. Patient 7 was lost to follow-up at 9 months, and patient 8 died after 10 months. Patient 9 is also still alive at the end of the trial, while patient 10 died after 9 months. As can be seen, the primary endpoint, survival time, is not available for all of the patients. It is not that we have no information on patients 3, 7 and 9, but we do not have complete information – we know only that their survival times are at least 24, 9 and 24 months, respectively. These patients provide what we call *censored observations*. Unfortunately, we cannot even do some simple things. For example, it is not possible to calculate the mean survival time. You might say, well, can't we just ignore the fact that these observations are censored and calculate the average of the numerical values? Well, you could, but clearly this would give an underestimate of the true mean survival time since eventually the actual survival times for patients 3, 7 and 9 will be greater than the numerical values in the list. Can't we just ignore the censored values and calculate the mean of those that remain? Again, this calculation would give an underestimate of the true mean, the censored values tend to come from the patients who survive a long time, and ignoring then would systematically remove the patients that do well and give a biased value for the mean.

It is this specific feature that has led to the development of special methods to deal with data of this kind. If censoring were not present, then we would probably just takes logs of the patient survival times and undertake the unpaired

---

Statistical Thinking for Non-Statisticians in Drug Regulation, Second Edition. Richard Kay.
© 2015 John Wiley & Sons, Ltd. Published 2015 by John Wiley & Sons, Ltd.

t-test or its extension analysis of covariance (ANCOVA) to compare our treatments. Note that survival time, by definition, is always positive while frequently the distribution is positively skewed and taking logs will often be successful in recovering normality.

The special methods we are going to discuss were first developed primarily in the 1970s and applied in the context of analysing time to death, and this is why we generally refer to the topic as *survival analysis*. As time has gone by, however, we have applied these same techniques to a wide range of time-to-event type endpoints. The list below gives some examples:

- Time to rash healing in herpes zoster
- Time to complete cessation of pain in herpes zoster
- Disease-free survival in oncology
- Time to first seizure in epilepsy
- Time to alleviation of symptoms in flu
- Time to cure for an infectious disease

Throughout this section, we will adopt the conventions of the area and refer to survival analysis and survival curves, accepting that the methods are applied more widely to events other than death.

Censoring in clinical trials usually occurs because the patient is still alive at the end of the period of follow-up. In the earlier example, if this were the only cause of censoring, then all of the censored observations would be equal to 24 months. There are, however, other ways in which censoring can occur, such as loss to follow-up or withdrawal. These can sometimes raise difficulties, and we will return to discuss the issues in a later section. Also, at an interim analysis, the period of follow-up for the patients still alive in the trial will be variable, and this will produce a whole range of censored event times; our methodology needs to be able to cope with having censored survival times that are distributed over the period of follow-up.

In the next section, we will discuss Kaplan–Meier (KM) curves, which are used both to display the data and also for the calculation of summary statistics. We will then cover the logrank and Gehan–Wilcoxon tests, which are simple two-group comparisons for censored survival data (akin to the unpaired t-test), and then extend these ideas to incorporate baseline covariates and centre effects.

13.2 Kaplan-Meier curves

13.2.1 Plotting Kaplan-Meier curves

Kaplan and Meier (1958) introduced a methodology for estimating, from censored survival data, the probability of being event-free as a function of time. If the event is death, then we are estimating the probability of surviving, and the resultant plots of the estimated probability of surviving as a function of time are called either *Kaplan-Meier curves* or *survival curves*.

Example 13.1 Carvedilol in severe heart failure

A placebo-controlled randomised trial reported by Packer *et al.* (2001) investigated the effect of carvedilol on survival time in severe heart failure. Figure 13.1 shows the survival curve for each of the two treatment groups following the early termination of the trial at a planned interim analysis.

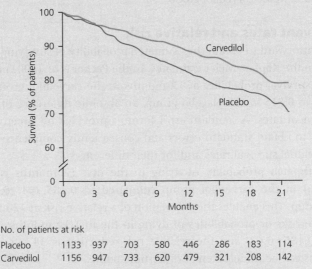

No. of patients at risk								
Placebo	1133	937	703	580	446	286	183	114
Carvedilol	1156	947	733	620	479	321	208	142

Figure 13.1 Kaplan–Meier survival curves in placebo and carvedilol groups. Source: Packer M, Coats AJS, Fowler MB, *et al.* for the Carvedilol Prospective Randomised Cumulative Survival Study Group (2001). Effect of carvedilol on survival in severe chronic heart failure. *NEJM* **344**, 1651–1658. Reproduced by permission of Massachusetts Medical Society.

The Kaplan-Meier method looks at the patterns of deaths over time to estimate the probability of surviving. The censored values make a contribution to this estimation process; if a patient is censored at 12 months, then that patient is involved in estimating the probability of surviving beyond any time up to and including 12 months, but not beyond those times. The form of the estimated survival curves is a so-called step function, with steps down occurring at those time points where there are deaths. As patients die or are censored, the number of patients remaining alive in the trial in each of the treatment groups is diminishing. The probabilities of surviving are, as a consequence, estimated from fewer and fewer patients as time goes on, and once these groups of patients become small, the estimated curves become less stable. That is why generally you will see greater instability in the curves at the longer follow-up times. To give information in relation to this, it is common practice to record the *number of patients at risk* through time; these are the numbers of patients alive and in the trial at particular time points. In the Packer *et al.* (2001) study, there were 1133 patients randomised to placebo and 1156 patients randomised to carvedilol;

at 12 months following randomisation, there were 446 patients at risk in the placebo group compared to 479 in the carvedilol group. This means that there were 687 (=1133−446) patients in the placebo group who either died before month 12 or gave censored observations that were less than 12 months. Similarly, there were 677 (=1156−479) patients in the carvedilol group who either died or were censored prior to month 12. By 21 months, the risk sets comprised 114 patients in the placebo group and 142 in the carvedilol group.

13.2.2 Event rates and relative risk

It is straightforward to obtain the estimated probability of surviving for key time points from the Kaplan-Meier estimates. In the Packer *et al.* (2001) example, the estimated survival probability at 12 months in the carvedilol group was 0.886 compared to 0.815 in the placebo group, an absolute difference of 7.1 per cent in the survival rates. A standard error formula provided by Greenwood (1926) enables us to obtain standard errors and consequently confidence intervals for these individual survival rates and for their differences.

The estimated probability of dying in the first 12 months is then 0.114 (=1−0.886) in the carvedilol group compared to 0.185 (=1−0.815) in the placebo group. This enables the calculation of a relative risk at 12 months as the ratio of the risks or probabilities of dying in the first 12 months. This is given by 0.114/0.185=0.62, and the relative risk reduction is 38 per cent. Similar calculations can be undertaken at other time points.

13.2.3 Median event times

We have mentioned earlier in this chapter that it is not possible to calculate the mean survival time. It is, however, often possible to obtain median survival times from the Kaplan-Meier curves. The median survival time for a particular group corresponds to the time on the *x*-axis when the survival probability on the curve takes the value 0.5. In order for this statistic to be obtained, the survival curves must fall below the 0.5 value on the *y*-axis. In Example 13.1, this has not happened. In such cases, we use the survival rates at various time points as summary descriptions of the survival experience in the groups. We will see an example later where the curves do fall below the 0.5 point. When the median times are available, it is also possible to obtain associated standard errors and confidence intervals.

It is usual to estimate and plot the probability of being event-free, but there will be occasions, in particular when the event rates are low, where interpretation is clearer when the opposite of this, cumulative incidence (or cumulative probability of experiencing the event by that time), is plotted. This is simply obtained as 1−probability of being event-free. Pocock, Clayton and Altman (2002) discuss issues associated with the interpretation of these plots. Figure 13.2 provides some examples of these kinds of plots in a trial looking at several cardiovascular events in the primary prevention of cardiovascular disease with pravastatin (Nakamura *et al.*, 2006). When the event rates are low, it is common in the conventional type of plot to put a break in the *y*-axis. As Pocock *et al.* point

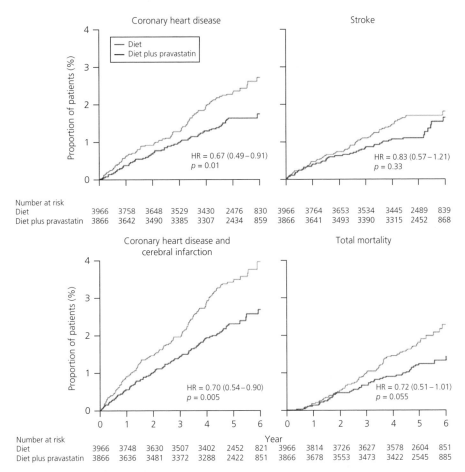

Figure 13.2 Inverted Kaplan–Meier curves for the primary and secondary endpoints.
Source: Nakamura H, Arakawa K, Itakura H, *et al.*, for the MEGA Study Group (2006) 'Primary prevention of cardiovascular disease with pravastatin in Japan (MEGA study): a prospective randomised controlled trial'. *The Lancet*, **368**, 1155–1163. Reproduced by permission of Elsevier.

out, this can sometimes visually exaggerate the treatment difference, so take care with interpretation in this case!

13.3 Treatment comparisons

The Kaplan-Meier curves do not of themselves provide a formal, *p*-value, comparison of the treatments. This comparison of the survival curves is undertaken using either the logrank test or the Gehan–Wilcoxon test. We will look at these two test procedures in turn.

The *logrank test* was developed by Peto and Peto (1972). The *p*-value resulting from this test is not a comparison of the survival curves at a particular time point (although such a test could be constructed) but a test comparing the two complete

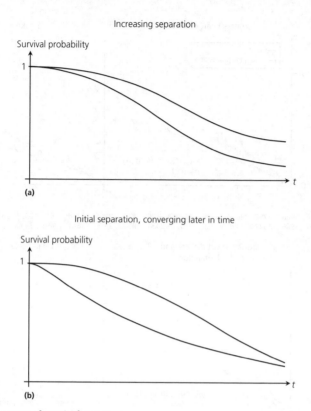

Figure 13.3 Patterns of survival curves

curves. A statistically significant *p*-value indicates that the survival experience in the two groups is different. The *Gehan–Wilcoxon test* (Gehan, 1969) (sometimes referred to as the *generalised Wilcoxon test*) is an alternative procedure for producing a *p*-value comparison of two survival curves. Why do we need two different tests? Well, the reasons relate to the basic shape of the curves that we are comparing. Both tests provide valid *p*-values, but these two tests are designed in different ways to pick up different patterns of treatment difference.

Figure 13.3 provides two sets of hypothetical population survival curves. In part a), the curves are seen to separate out gradually over the period of follow-up. In contrast, the curves in part b) separate out fairly rapidly but then start to converge later on in time.

The curves in part a) represent, over the period of follow-up, a *permanent* treatment effect. There is a long-term advantage in survival for one group compared to the other group. The interpretation of the curves in part b), however, is different. Here, we see a short-term benefit of one treatment group over the other, but as time goes on, this relative benefit diminishes, leaving little long-term effect. This pattern of differences represents a delay in the occurrence of the event in one group compared to the other group.

The two tests mentioned earlier are designed to look for these different patterns. The logrank test is best able to pick up the longer-term differences as seen in Figure 13.3a, while the Gehan–Wilcoxon test focuses on short-term effects or a delay as seen in Figure 13.3b. The appropriate test to use depends upon what kind of differences you are expecting to see.

In the Packer *et al.* (2001) trial in Figure 13.1, we see longer-term differences displayed over the 21-month follow-up period, and the logrank test is entirely appropriate here. The *p*-value from the logrank test was 0.00013, a highly significant result.

Generally, it is these kinds of patterns we see in long-term cardiovascular and oncology trials. In other applications, however, such long-term effects are not anticipated and indeed do not fit with the objectives of the study. For example, in flu trials, where the primary endpoint is the time to alleviation of symptoms, we are looking for rapid resolution of symptoms in the active group compared to placebo. Treatment effects are seen in the first two or so days with many more patients symptom-free in the active group compared to placebo. By the time we get out to seven days, however, most of the patients in each of the two groups have only minor symptoms remaining, so the probability of being event-free (still having symptoms) is the same in the two groups. In this case, it is the Gehan–Wilcoxon test that is best suited to picking up differences. Similar comments often apply to progression-free survival in advanced cancer trials where the best we can hope for is that the test treatment delays the event (death or progression). It is unfortunately the case that the logrank test dominates this area of statistics and there are many applications that have failed to detect important short-term differences between survival curves as a result of using a test that is insensitive to the detection of those differences. One of many examples is Okwera *et al.* (1994) who compared two treatments (thiacetazone and rifampicin) for pulmonary tuberculosis in HIV-infected patients. The survival curves at 300 days following randomisation were separated by more than 10 per cent (77 per cent surviving in one group compared to around 66 per cent in the second group). In other words, 10 per cent more patients, at least, were alive at 300 days in the rifampicin arm compared to the thiacetazone arm, a clear and important benefit of one treatment over the other. At 600 days, however, the survival curves had come together showing no long-term benefit. The quoted *p*-value from the logrank test was >0.50. Now, one could argue whether a short-term benefit is clinically important, but the issue here is that the test used was not sensitive in terms of picking up differences between the curves. The Gehan–Wilcoxon test would have stood a much better chance of yielding statistical significance and at least generated some interest in discussing the implication of those short-term differences.

One question that often arises is, which test should I use as I don't know what kind of effect I am going to see? My short answer to this question is that in a confirmatory setting you should know! By the time you reach that stage in the drug development programme, your knowledge of the disease area and the treatment, in combination with the endpoint, should enable accurate prediction of what is likely to happen. Of course, earlier on in the programme, you may not know, and in this exploratory non-confirmatory phase, it is perfectly valid to undertake both tests to explore the nature of the effects.

13.4 The hazard ratio

13.4.1 The hazard rate

In order to be able to understand what a hazard ratio is, you first need to know what a hazard rate is. The *hazard rate (hazard function)* is formally defined as the conditional death (or event) rate calculated through time. What we mean by this is as follows. Suppose in a group of 1000 patients 7 die in month 1; the hazard rate for month 1 is 7/1000. Now suppose that 12 die in month 2; the hazard rate for month 2 is 12/993. If now 15 die in month 3, then the hazard rate for month 3 is 15/981 and so on. So the hazard rate is the death (event) rate for that time period among those patients still alive at the start of the period.

There are several things to note about the hazard rate. Firstly, it is unlikely that the hazard rate will be constant over time. Secondly, even though we have introduced the concept of the hazard rate as taking values for monthly periods of time, we can think in terms of small time periods with the hazard rate essentially being a continuous function through time.

The hazard rate can be estimated from data by looking at the patterns of deaths (events) over time. This estimation process takes account of the censored values in ways similar to the way such observations were used in the Kaplan-Meier curves.

Figure 13.4 shows a schematic plot of two hazard rates corresponding to two treatment groups in a randomised trial. As can be seen from this plot, the hazard rates in each of the two treatment groups start off just after randomisation ($t=0$) at a fairly modest level and then increase to a peak after a certain period of time, say, one year, and then begin to decrease. This is telling us that at one year the

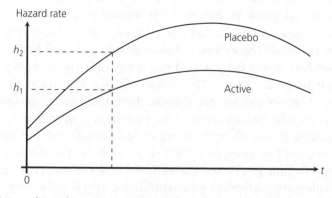

Figure 13.4 Hazard rates for two groups of patients

death rates in each of the groups are at their maximum; prior to that, they have been steadily increasing, and following one year, the death rates are tending to tail off. It is also clear from the plot that the hazard rate in the placebo group is always higher than the hazard rate in the active group, at every time point.

13.4.2 Constant hazard ratio

Even though the individual hazard rates seen in Figure 13.4 are not constant, it would be reasonable to assume, wherever we look in time, that the ratio of the hazard rates is approximately constant. In fact, these hazard rates have been specifically constructed to behave in this way. When this is the case, the ratio of the hazard rates will be a single value, which we call the *hazard ratio*. We will denote this ratio by λ so that $\lambda = h_1/h_2$ where h_1 and h_2 are as displayed in the plot; this ratio would take the same value at each and every point in time.

It is convention for the hazard rate for the test treatment group to appear as the numerator and the hazard rate for the control group to be the denominator in the definition of the hazard ratio.

A hazard ratio of one corresponds to exactly equal treatments; the hazard rate in the active group is exactly equal to the hazard rate in the placebo group. If we adopt the aforementioned convention and the event is death (or any other undesirable outcome), then a hazard ratio less than one is telling us that the active treatment is a better treatment. This is the situation we see in Figure 13.4. A hazard ratio greater than one is telling us that the active treatment is the poorer treatment.

Even if the hazard ratio is not precisely a constant value as we move through time, the hazard ratio can still provide a valid summary provided the hazard rate for one of the treatment groups is consistently above the hazard rate for the other group. In this case, the value we get for the hazard ratio from the data represents an average of that ratio over time.

Confidence intervals for the hazard ratio are straightforward to calculate. Like the odds ratio (see Section 4.5.5), this confidence interval is firstly calculated on the log scale and then converted back to the hazard ratio scale by taking antilogs of the ends of that confidence interval.

13.4.3 Non-constant hazard ratio

However, it is not always the case, by any means, that we see a constant or approximately constant hazard ratio. There will be situations, as seen in Figure 13.5, when the hazard rate for one group starts off lower than the hazard rate for a second group and then as we move through time they initially move closer together, but then a switch occurs. The hazard rate for the first group then overtakes that for the second group, and they continue to move further apart from that point on.

In this case, it clearly makes no sense to assign a single value to the hazard ratio. When this happens the hazard ratio will start off below one, increase towards one as we move through time, but then flip over and start to increase above and away from one. The hazard ratio still exists, but it is not constant and varies over time. See Kay (2004) for further discussion on these points.

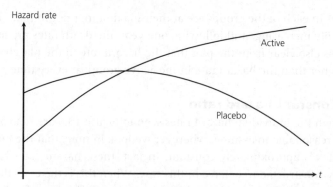

Figure 13.5 Hazard rates for two groups of patients where the hazard ratio is not constant

13.4.4 Link to survival curves

In an earlier section, we saw two different patterns for two sets of survival curves. In Figure 13.3a, the survival curves move further and further apart with increasing time. This pattern is consistent with one of the hazard rates (think in terms of death rates) being consistently above the other hazard rate. This in turn corresponds to a fairly constant hazard ratio, the situation we discussed in Section 13.4.2. So a constant hazard ratio manifests itself as a continuing separation in the two survival curves as in Figure 13.3a. Note that the higher hazard rate (more deaths) gives the lower of the two survival curves.

In Figure 13.3b, the survival curves move apart very early on in time and then start to converge later. This pattern is consistent with one of the hazard rates being above the other initially; this corresponds to the survival curve that decreases most rapidly due to the high death rate early on. In order for the survival curves to begin to converge, however, a reversal of the death rates in the two groups needs to take place, so that the death rate in the group that did well initially now starts to increase and overtakes the death rate in the other group. This is the only way that the catchup can take place to ensure that the probability of surviving beyond the end of the observation period is approximately equal in the two groups. In turn, this pattern is consistent with a hazard ratio that is not constant. Here, the hazard ratio starts off well below one, increases to one and then moves above one through time as the death rates in the two groups reverse.

For the pattern of survival curves in Figure 13.3b, the hazard ratio, because it is not constant, does not take a single value. A better way to summarise the relative performance in the two groups in this case would be to use median survival times or relative risk at particular time points of interest. We mentioned in Section 13.3 that the logrank test is specifically designed to provide a p-value for a pattern of survival curves as in Figure 13.3a. As we have now seen, this pattern corresponds to a constant hazard ratio; indeed, the logrank test is essentially a test of the hypothesis H_0: $\lambda = 1$ against the alternative H_1: $\lambda \neq 1$ where λ is the hazard ratio.

13.4.5 Calculating Kaplan-Meier curves

It is worth revisiting the calculation of the Kaplan-Meier curve following on from the discussion of the hazard rate, in order to see, firstly, how censoring is accounted for and, secondly, how the two are linked in terms of the calculation.

As in Section 13.4.1, consider a group of 1000 patients at the point of randomisation. Again, suppose that in month 1, 7 die – then the hazard rate for month 1, as before, is 7/1000. Now assume that in addition 10 are censored at the end of month 1, while among the 983 ($=1000-7$ (deaths)-10 (censorings)) remaining in the study at the beginning of month 2, 15 die in that month. The hazard rate for month 2 is 15/983. Next, assume that 8 patients are censored at the end of month 2, so that 960 patients are in the study at the beginning of month 3, and of these, 12 die in that month; the hazard rate for month 3 is 12/960 and so on. The calculation of the hazard rate through time takes account not only of the number of patients dying but also of the censoring patterns. Patients with censored observations contribute to the denominator of the hazard rate calculation in the months prior to the time at which they are censored but not after that.

Now to the calculation of the Kaplan-Meier survival probabilities, using this example, the estimated probability of surviving beyond month 1 is $1-(7/1000)=0.9993$. The probability of surviving beyond month 2 is the probability of surviving beyond month 1 × the probability of surviving beyond month 2 among those alive at the start of month 2, and from the data, this is estimated to be $0.9993 \times (1-(15/983))=0.984$. Continuing this process, the probability of surviving beyond month 3 is the probability of surviving beyond month 2 × the probability of surviving beyond month 3 among those alive at the start of month 3; this is estimated to be $0.984 \times (1-(12/960))=0.972$. In general, if h_t is the hazard rate for month t, then the estimated probability of surviving beyond month t is equal to

$$(1-h_1) \times (1-h_2) \times \ldots \times (1-h_t)$$

Note also here that the numbers 1000, 983 and 960 are the numbers of patients alive in the trial, in that group at the start of months 1, 2 and 3, respectively, that is, the number at risk.

This calculation in relation to both the hazard rate and the survival probabilities has been undertaken at intervals of one month. In practice, we use intervals that correspond to the unit of measurement for the endpoint itself, usually days, in order to use the total amount of information available.

13.5 Adjusted analyses

In Chapter 6, we covered methods for adjusted analyses and analysis of covariance in relation to continuous (ANOVA and ANCOVA) and binary and ordinal data (CMH tests and logistic regression). Similar methods exist for survival data. As with these earlier methods, particularly in relation to binary and ordinal data, there are numerous advantages in accounting for such factors in the analysis. If the randomisation has been stratified, then such factors should be incorporated into the analysis in order to preserve the properties of the resultant p-values.

13.5.1 Stratified methods

Both the logrank and Gehan–Wilcoxon tests can be extended to incorporate stratification and other factors, for example, baseline covariates and centres. These methods provide p-value comparisons of treatments, allowing for the main effects of baseline covariates and centre to be accounted for. Although possible, extensions of these procedures to evaluate the homogeneity of the treatment effect, that is, the investigation of treatment-by-covariate or treatment-by-centre interactions, are not so straightforward. Consequently, we tend to build the covariates into the modelling through methods that will be covered in the next two sections.

13.5.2 Proportional hazards regression

The most popular method for covariate adjustment is the *proportional hazards model*. This model, originally developed by Cox (1972), is now used extensively in the analysis of survival data to incorporate and adjust for both covariate effects and centres.

The method provides a model for the hazard function. As in Section 6.6, let z be an indicator variable for treatment taking the value one for patients in the active group and zero for patients in the control group and let x_1, x_2, etc. denote the covariates and possibly centre indicators. If we let $\lambda(t)$ denote the hazard rate as a function of t (time), the main effects model takes the form

$$\ell n(\lambda(t)) = a + cz + b_1 x_1 + b_2 x_2 + \ldots$$

As before, the coefficient c measures the effect of treatment on the hazard rate. If $c < 0$, then the log hazard rate, and therefore the hazard rate itself, in the active group is lower than the hazard rate in the control group. If $c > 0$, then the reverse is true, and the active treatment is giving a higher hazard rate, and if $c = 0$, then there is no treatment difference. An analysis using this model then largely revolves around testing the hypothesis H_0: $c = 0$ and subsequently presenting an estimate for the treatment effect. The structure of the model is such that c is the log of the hazard ratio and the antilog, e^c, is the (adjusted) hazard ratio. This, together with a confidence interval for the hazard ratio, gives us a measure of the treatment effect, adjusting for baseline factors.

Treatment-by-covariate and treatment-by-centre interactions can be investigated by including cross-product terms in the model as with binary data and logistic regression, although it is more usual to evaluate these potential interactions visually (see Example 13.1 (revisited)). All of the remarks made previously in Section 6.7 regarding regulatory aspects of the inclusion of covariates apply equally well to the survival data setting and the proportional hazards model.

Example 13.1 (Revisited) Carvedilol in severe heart failure

The proportional hazards model was fitted to the survival data overall and additionally within subgroups defined according to key baseline prognostic factors in order to calculate hazard ratios and evaluate the homogeneity of the treatment effect. Figure 13.6 shows these hazard ratios together with 95 per cent confidence intervals. Such plots were discussed earlier in Section 10.8 in relation to subgroup testing. The data in Figure 13.6 indicate that there is a consistency of treatment effect across the various subgroups investigated.

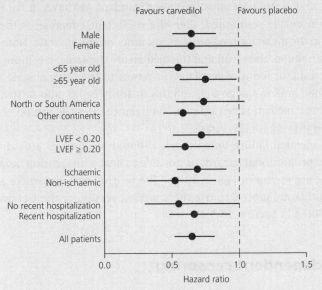

Figure 13.6 Hazard ratios (and 95 per cent confidence intervals) for death in subgroups defined by baseline characteristics. Source: Packer M, Coats AJS, Fowler MB, *et al.* for the Carvedilol Prospective Randomised Cumulative Survival Study Group (2001). Effect of carvedilol on survival in severe chronic heart failure. *NEJM*, **344**, 1651–1658. Reproduced by permission of Massachusetts Medical Society.

The proportional hazards model, as the name suggests, assumes that the hazard ratio is a constant. As such, it provides a direct extension of the logrank test, which is a simple two treatment group comparison. Indeed, if the proportional hazards model is fitted to data without the inclusion of baseline factors, then the p-value for the test $H_0: c=0$ will be very similar to the p-value arising out of the logrank test. Any differences are due to the subtleties of the slightly different formulas for constructing the test statistic.

13.5.3 Accelerated failure time model

As we have already seen, there will be settings where the pattern of differences between treatment groups does not conform to proportional hazards, where the hazard ratio is not a constant, single value. Such situations are best handled by using an alternative model to incorporate baseline factors. The *accelerated failure time model* is an analysis of variance technique that models the survival time itself but on the log scale:

$$\ell n T = a + cz + b_1 x_1 + b_2 x_2 + \ldots$$

We mentioned earlier, in Section 13.1, that if we did not have censoring, then an analysis would likely proceed by taking the log of survival time and undertaking the unpaired t-test. This model simply develops that idea by now incorporating covariates, and centre indicators through a standard ANCOVA. If we assume that $\ell n T$ is also normally distributed, then the coefficient c represents the (adjusted) difference in the mean (or median) survival times on the log scale. Note that for the normal distribution, the mean and the median are the same; it is more convenient though to think in terms of medians. To return to the original scale for survival time, we then antilog c to give e^c, and this quantity is the ratio (active divided by control) of the median survival times. Confidence intervals can be obtained in a straightforward way for this ratio.

The accelerated failure time model, although it provides a model that does not assume proportional hazards, is not able to deal with crossing hazards, which is what we are seeing in Figure 13.5b. The best way to undertake an adjusted analysis in this situation is to use the stratified version of the Gehan–Wilcoxon test as outlined in Section 13.5.1.

13.6 Independent censoring

One important assumption that we have made in the analyses presented so far is that the censoring process is independent of the process associated with the event that we are looking at. This is the assumption of *independent censoring*. If, for example, patients were being withdrawn from the trial and therefore giving censored survival times at the time of withdrawal because their health was deteriorating, then this assumption would be violated. Doing this would completely fool us as to the true hazard rate. In the extreme, if this happened with every patient, we would never see any deaths!

Usually, censoring occurs at the end of the predefined observation/follow-up period, and in these cases, the issue of independent censoring is not a problem; the censoring process is clearly unconnected with the underlying process for the events. Similarly there are no problems if in an interim analysis, censoring occurs only because for many patients follow-up is not yet complete but they are still alive. When patients are lost to follow-up or withdrawn, however, there is the potential for bias. Unfortunately, there is no easy way to deal with this. The recommended approach is to analyse the data as it is collected and presented but then undertake one or more sensitivity analyses. For example, for patients who withdraw for negative reasons (deteriorating health, suffering a stroke), assume that the censoring is in fact a death; for patients who withdraw for positive reasons (disease-free for six months), assign the maximum length of follow-up to those patients and censor them at that time. This is the worst-case scenario for the withdrawals for negative reasons and the best-case scenario for the withdrawals for positive reasons. If the conclusions are essentially unchanged when these assumptions are made, then you can be assured that this conclusion is fairly robust to any violation of the assumption of independent censoring. An alternative, and certainly this is possible with a hard endpoint such as death, is to continue follow-up, even though the patient has withdrawn from treatment, to obtain the required information on the time to death.

Example 13.1 (Revisited) Carvedilol in severe heart failure

A total of 12 patients (six in each of the two treatment groups) underwent cardiac transplantation during the study. One issue was how to deal with these patients in the analysis as receiving a transplant will impact on the survival prospects for that patient. In the primary analysis, these patients were censored at the time of transplantation. As a sensitivity analysis, the eventual time to death (or censoring at the end of follow-up if they were still alive) was included in the analysis. Parker *et al.* (2001) reported that the conclusions were essentially unchanged.

13.7 Sample size calculations

The power of a study where the primary endpoint is time to event depends not so much on the total patient numbers, but on the number of events. So a trial with 1000 patients with 100 deaths has the same power as a trial with only 200 patients but also with 100 deaths. The sample size calculation for survival data is therefore done in two stages. Firstly, the required number of patients suffering events is calculated in the two groups as a whole, and secondly, this is factored upwards by an assumed proportion of patients who are expected to suffer events, again in the two groups as a whole, to give the required number of patients for the trial.

Example 13.2 Sample size calculation for survival data

Suppose that on a standard treatment it is expected that the five-year survival rate will be 35 per cent. It is desired to detect an increase in this rate to 55 per cent with 90 per cent power in a 5 per cent level test. The required number of deaths to give this level of power is 133. The overall survival rate at five years is expected to be 45 per cent (the average of 35 per cent and 55 per cent), and therefore, we expect to see 45 per cent of patients dying. It follows that 133/0.45 = 296 patients need to be recruited overall or 148 patients per group. We would then expect to see 81 deaths in the first group and 52 in the second group. Adding these two together gives the required number of events needed overall for 90 per cent power.

There is of course no guarantee that things will turn out as expected, and even though we require 133 events in our example, 296 patients may not give us that. An alternative way of designing the trial would be to continue follow-up until the required number of events is observed. Having an *event-driven study* is frequently a safer option to ensure that the required power is achieved although it does add another element of uncertainty and that is the duration of the study. Careful management of the whole trial process is then needed.

Example 13.1 (Revisited) Carvedilol in severe heart failure

This trial adopted a design that continued follow-up until the required number of events was observed:

'The sample size was estimated on the basis of the following assumptions: the one-year mortality in the placebo group would be 28 per cent; the risk of death would be altered by 20 per cent as a result of treatment with carvedilol; the study would have 90 per cent power (two-sided $\alpha = 0.05$) to detect a significant difference between the treatment groups. Since it was recognised that the estimate of the rate of events might be too high, the trial was designed to continue until 900 deaths had occurred'. *(Packer et al., 2001)*

This sample size methodology depends upon the assumption of proportional hazards and is based around the logrank test as the method of analysis. If this assumption is not appropriate and we do not expect proportional hazards, then the accelerated failure time model may provide an alternative framework for the analysis of data. In this case, it is no longer strictly true that the power of the study depends only on the number of events (and not directly on the number of patients). However, this still gives a solution that is approximately correct, so we first of all undertake a sample size calculation based on the unpaired t-test for the difference in the medians (means) on the log scale and then factor up by the expected number of patients dying to give the total number of patients needed. Alternatively, the trial follow-up continues until the specified numbers of deaths have been seen. The resulting power in each case will be slightly higher than the required power.

CHAPTER 14

Interim analysis and data monitoring committees

14.1 Stopping rules for interim analysis

In Chapter 10, we spoke extensively about the dangers of multiple testing and the associated inflation of the type I error. Methods were developed to control that inflation and account for multiplicity in an appropriate way.

One area that we briefly mentioned was interim analysis, where we are looking at the data in the trial as it accumulates. The method by Pocock (1977) was discussed to control the type I error rate across the series of interim looks. The Pocock methodology divides up the 5 per cent type I error rate equally across the analyses. So, for example, for two interim looks and a final analysis, the significance level at each analysis is 0.022. For the O'Brien and Fleming (1979) method, most of the 5 per cent is left over for the final analysis, while the first analysis is at a very stringent level and the adjusted significance levels are 0.00052, 0.014 and 0.045.

These two methods are the most common approaches seen in pharmaceutical applications. A third method, which we see used from time to time, is by Haybittle (1971) and Peto *et al.* (1976). Here, a significance level of 0.001 is used for each of the interims, again leaving most of the 5 per cent for the final analysis. For two interims and a final analysis, the adjusted significance level for the final analysis is in fact 0.05 to two decimal places; for three interims, we have 0.049 left over. Clearly, this method has little effect on the final evaluation, but associated with that, there is also little chance of stopping at an interim stage.

Each of these methods assumes that the analyses take place at equally spaced intervals. So for example, if the total sample size is 600 and we are planning two interims and a final analysis, then the interims should take place after 200 and 400 patients have been observed for the primary endpoint, in order for these adjusted significance levels to apply. Small deviations from this make little difference; conducting analyses after, say, 206 and 397 patients, for example, would essentially work fine under the same scheme. More major deviations, however, would have an impact. Also, we may for practical reasons, not want the analyses to be equally spaced and we will see an example of this later in this chapter. In both these cases, we would need to use a more general methodology,

Statistical Thinking for Non-Statisticians in Drug Regulation, Second Edition. Richard Kay.
© 2015 John Wiley & Sons, Ltd. Published 2015 by John Wiley & Sons, Ltd.

α-spending functions. The application of these methods requires some fairly sophisticated computer software. There are several packages available for these calculations including ADDPLAN (www.addplan.com), EasT (www.cytel.com) and S-Plus (www.insightful.com).

On a final point, for survival data information is carried through the numbers of patients with events and not directly the number of patients in the trial. So for example, if the trial is continuing until we have seen 900 deaths, then the equally spaced interim analyses would be conducted after, respectively, 300 and 600 deaths have been observed.

14.2 Stopping for efficacy and futility

There are several potential reasons why we would want to stop a trial on the basis of the data collected up to that point:

- Overwhelming evidence of efficacy (or harm) of the test treatment.
- Futility: the data are such that there is little chance of achieving a positive result if the trial were continued to completion.
- Safety: collective evidence that there are serious safety problems with the test treatment.

We will deal with safety and this final point separately in Section 14.3.

14.2.1 Efficacy

Each of the schemes outlined in Section 14.1 for dividing up the 5 per cent type I error can be applied for the evaluation of efficacy in theory. In practice, however, we would only want to be stopping for efficacy if the evidence was absolutely overwhelming. For this reason, the O'Brien and Fleming scheme appears to be the most useful in that it has a sliding scale of adjusted significance levels starting from very stringent through less stringent to something close to 5 per cent for the final analysis. The Pocock scheme pays too big a price for the early looks, and at the final analysis the adjusted significance level is well below 5 per cent; it would be very unfortunate indeed if, with two interims and a final analysis, the final analysis gave $p = 0.03$. Statistical significance could not be claimed because the p-value has not fallen below the required 0.022. The Haybittle and Peto *et al.* scheme is also a possibility but giving only a small chance for stopping early.

Note that the schemes we are discussing here are based upon the calculation of standard two-sided p-values. Clearly, we would only be claiming overwhelming efficacy if the direction of the observed treatment effect were in favour of the test treatment. If the direction of the treatment effect were in the opposite direction then we would still be stopping the trial, but now concluding differences in the negative direction and for certain endpoints, for example, survival time, this would constitute harm. It could also be appropriate in such cases to consider stopping for harm on the basis of somewhat weaker evidence and using an overall one-sided significance level of 0.025 for efficacy and an overall one-sided significance level of say 0.10 for harm. It is straightforward to construct such asymmetric schemes by undertaking two calculations: one with a one-sided significance level of 0.025 (for efficacy) and the other with a one-sided significance level of 0.10 (for harm) and in each case dividing the corresponding adjusted two-sided significance levels by two. A further generalisation would allow the use of separate schemes for efficacy and harm, say, O'Brien and Fleming for efficacy and Pocock for harm. Such a structure would sensibly be more cautious early on for harm and prepared to stop on modest evidence rather than imposing a much more stringent adjusted significance level using an O'Brien and Fleming scheme.

Example 14.1 Separate one-sided schemes

With two interims and a final analysis looking at both overwhelming efficacy and harm, the adjusted one-sided O'Brien–Fleming significance levels for efficacy of 0.0003, 0.0071 and 0.0225 would give an overall one-sided significance level of 0.025. A Pocock scheme for harm with an overall conservative one-sided significance level of 0.10 would use the adjusted significance levels of 0.0494 at each of the interims and the final analysis.

14.2.2 Futility and conditional power

In addition to looking for overwhelming efficacy, there is also the possibility of stopping the trial for futility at an interim stage. It may be for example, that the analysis of the interim data is not especially favourable for the test treatment and were the trial to continue to the end, there would simply be no real possibility of obtaining a positive (statistically significant) result. For commercial reasons, it may be better to abandon the trial to save on additional costs and resources.

There are several approaches to evaluating futility but the most common method is based on *conditional power*. At the design stage, we may have based the sample size calculation on a power of say, 90 per cent to detect a certain level of effect, the clinically relevant difference, d, arguing that a difference less than d was of little or no clinical importance. It is possible at an interim stage to recalculate the power of the trial to detect a difference d given that we already have a proportion of the data on which the final analysis will be based in hand. Suppose that this so-called conditional power was equal to 20 per cent. In other words, were we to continue this trial (and the treatment difference that we have observed to date reflected the true treatment difference), then there would only be a 20 per cent probability of seeing a significant p-value at the end. Under these circumstances it may not be worth continuing. In contrast, if the conditional power turns out to be 50 per cent, then it may be worth carrying on with the trial. The cut-off that is chosen, which, ideally to avoid ambiguity, should be pre-specified is based on commercial risk/benefit considerations but generally speaking is around 20–30 per cent.

This method of calculating the conditional power assumes that the observed difference between the treatments at the interim stage is the true difference, termed the conditional power *under the current trend*. It is also possible to calculate conditional power under other assumptions, for example, that the true treatment difference in the remaining part of the trial following the interim analysis will be equal to d. This is a much more optimistic assumption and will lead to a larger value for the conditional power. What we are saying is that even though in the first part of the trial the treatment difference is less than the difference d that we assumed at the start, we still believe that d is the true treatment difference. These calculations under different assumptions about how the future data will behave will provide a broad basis on which to make judgements about terminating the trial for futility.

14.2.3 Some practical issues

In general, it is not a requirement for a trial to have an interim analysis, either for efficacy or for futility. In most long-term trials, however, where there is the opportunity for an interim evaluation, then it may be something worth putting in place. The interim can involve only efficacy, only futility, or both and may indeed involve some other things as well, such as a re-evaluation of sample size (see Section 8.5.3). One thing that must be borne in mind however is that stopping a trial early for overwhelming evidence of efficacy based on the primary endpoint may compromises the ability to gain good information on important secondary endpoints, detailed efficacy information in subgroups and also safety. If this is a possibility, then introducing interim analyses with associated stopping rules may not be the sensible thing to do. See Example 14.2 for a situation that related to these points.

For practical reasons, the number of interims should be small. Undertaking interims adds cost to the trial and they also need to be very carefully managed. In particular, the results of each interims must be made available in a timely way in order for go/no-go decisions to be made in good time. Remember that the trial does not stop to allow the interims to take place; recruitment and follow-up continue. So do not overburden the clinical trial with lots of interim analyses; two at most is my recommendation. In some situations, trial recruitment may be complete once the results on the interim analysis are known. Is this of any value? Well commercially it could be, in that it could enable a regulatory submission to be made earlier than would have been the case had the trial run its full course.

The results of interim analyses are not formally binding, but it would be a very brave decision to continue a trial when the decision coming out of the interim was to stop. If the trial data at the interim has given a statistically significant result, then there would clearly be ethical problems in continuing randomising patients or even continuing treating patients with a treatment that was known to be inferior. The investigators would likely not be willing to continue with the study in its current form. For futility, this is less of an issue; there are no real ethical problems with continuing the trial with two treatments that evidence suggests are somewhat similar. There are, however, technical problems when a trial is designed with pre-planned stopping boundaries for futility and then the boundaries are ignored. The type I error of 5 per cent, which has been carefully preserved with the interim analysis plan, is slightly inflated. This is a technical point a little beyond the scope of this text and expert statistical advice should be sought to avoid the problem.

It is almost self-evident that all analyses of the kind we are discussing here must be pre-planned in a detailed way. The regulators, in particular, are very unhappy with unplanned interims or interims that are ill defined. Such situations would give rise to major problems at the time of submission.

Example 14.2 Lapatinib plus capecitabine for HER2-positive advanced breast cancer

This was a phase III trial in HER2-positive breast cancer comparing lapatinib plus capecitabine versus capecitabine monotherapy (Geyer *et al.*, 2006). The planned sample size was 528 with a final analysis of time to progression scheduled to take place after 266 progression events. A single interim analysis was prospectively included for this endpoint after approximately 133 progression events using an adjusted one-sided significance level according to an O'Brien–Fleming scheme. The interim analysis actually took place following 146 events and at that time, 324 patients had been recruited. The O'Brien–Fleming adjusted significance level to preserve an overall one-sided significance level of 0.025, calculated using an alpha-spending function, was 0.0014. The observed p-value for this interim analysis for time to progression was 0.00016 well below the required cut-off for statistical significance, and the independent DMC recommended stopping the trial based on this evidence for overwhelming efficacy. Recruitment was stopped and patients in the control arm were offered treatment with lapatinib.

While the data for time to progression were convincing, there was concern expressed among regulators however that this early stopping effectively prevented the collection of long-term survival data. The results for overall survival at the time of the interim gave a non-significant two-sided p-value of 0.72; there were 36 deaths in the lapatinib group compared to 35 in the control arm. These data nonetheless led to the successful filing for lapatinib in this indication.

14.2.4 Analyses following completion of recruitment

Analyses of data are sometimes undertaken by the sponsor following completion of recruitment but before follow-up of all patients according to the study schedule for a variety of reasons. The two most common situations are:

- The sponsor is looking for preliminary information to allow for strategic planning.
- To accelerate regulatory approval. The data may be sufficiently compelling for a regulatory submission to be made.

These analyses are not interims in the usual sense, in that generally there is no associated *stopping rule* and the trial will continue to completion irrespective of what the results look like. Great care needs to be taken with regard to these analyses however, and in particular, the question needs to be asked: is this analysis going to compromise the integrity of the study as a whole? If the answer to this question is potentially yes, then the analysis is ill advised. Given that there is no stopping rule, it is very difficult to know what kind of price to pay in terms of α. If this analysis is to be considered as an analysis where confirmatory conclusions are to be drawn if the data are compelling, then it should be considered in the same way as a standard interim analysis with a pre-planned α adjustment. If however it is to be considered as an analysis that will simply provide preliminary data, then it can be considered as a so-called *administrative* analysis with an adjusted α of 0.001 leaving the final (primary analysis) unaffected, or little affected, with an α close to 0.05. A further potential for bias to be introduced is associated with dissemination of the results. Will the investigators and others who are made aware of the interim results behave in a way that could compromise the ability of the trial to reach valid conclusions? This aspect of dissemination will be a common theme throughout the remainder of this chapter and needs to be carefully controlled.

14.3 Monitoring safety

In addition to considerations of efficacy and futility, it will usually be appropriate in most long-term trials to consider safety in an ongoing way. This is not new and we have always, for example, looked at accumulating data on individual serious adverse events (SAEs) and considered stopping (or modifying) trials if these are indicative of problems with the trial or with the treatments.

As time has gone by we have increasingly done this in a very structured way. Data Monitoring Committees (DMCs) have a major role here and we will consider various aspects of their structure and conduct later. For the moment, we will just focus on associated statistical methodologies. Usually, this ongoing safety monitoring is done by looking at various aspects of safety: adverse events (serious and non-serious), vital signs, key laboratory parameters, physical examination, ECGs, etc., both in individual cases and overall across the treatment groups or the study as a whole. I hesitate to say that this is done in an informal way, because it is taken very seriously, but what I mean is that there is usually little formal statistical structure wrapped around the process. Yes, we may put p-values on the adverse events, suitably grouped, but these are simply used as flags for potential problems. A discussion ensues and decisions are taken by members of the DMC. Producing p-values in this way is not necessarily a bad thing; it fits with a broad requirement to look at many different aspects of safety across the trial as a whole although as a result of the multiplicity involved in this process, we should be careful not to jump every time we see a statistically significant p-value. Conversely there may be safety issues of concern even though formal statistical significance has not been achieved.

If, at the design stage and based on the nature of the disease and the treatment, specific potential safety issues can be identified, then more formal rules can be set up. These rules are unlike those considered earlier for overwhelming efficacy. For safety, it would not usually be appropriate to look just at one or two interim stages; we must look more frequently than that.

There is further discussion on these points in Section 19.3.

14.4 Data monitoring committees

14.4.1 Introduction and responsibilities

In this section, we will cover several aspects, particularly in relation to statistical issues, associated with DMCs. This is not meant to be a comprehensive discussion of the area and the reader is referred to the book by Ellenberg, Fleming and DeMets (2003) for an excellent and exhaustive coverage that in addition contains a plethora of case studies. There are two guidelines, one from the FDA (2006), *Establishment and Operation of Clinical Trial Data Monitoring Committees*, and one from the CHMP (2005), *Guideline on Data Monitoring Committees*, which outline the roles and responsibilities of DMCs in the regulatory environment. DMCs are also referred to as Data Monitoring Boards (DMBs) and Data and Safety Monitoring Committees/Boards (DSMCs/DSMBs).

It is clearly important that the trial sponsor remain blind to the accumulating data within the separate treatment groups and an important reason for having a DMC is to enable trial data to be looked at without compromising that blinding. The main responsibilities of a DMC will vary depending on the particular circumstances. The main responsibility, however, will always be to protect the safety of the trial participants and to ensure that the trial is being conducted in an ethical way. There may also be additional responsibilities associated with interim analyses if these are to be incorporated in the trial. The DMC may or may not have access to evolving efficacy data, as the committee may only be looking at safety. This can cause problems. It is difficult for DMCs to make recommendations based on safety in isolation in that the absence of efficacy makes it impossible to make a risk/benefit judgement. There should therefore be provision for the committee to access efficacy data should they request it.

CHMP (2005): 'Guideline on Data Monitoring Committees'

'In most cases, safety monitoring will be the major task for a DMC. Even if the safety parameters monitored are not directly related to efficacy, a DMC might need access to unblinded efficacy information to perform a risk/benefit assessment in order to weigh possible safety disadvantages against a possible gain in efficacy'.

The DMC will also have responsibilities in relation to protecting the scientific integrity of the trial, and in particular the DMC must ensure that all interim analyses and safety monitoring activities are conducted in an appropriate way to protect blinding and the type I error to avoid problems with multiplicity. There is also the responsibility to oversee the overall conduct of the trial to make sure that it will fulfil its objectives.

FDA (2006): 'Establishment and Operation of Clinical Trial Data Monitoring Committees'

'A DMC will generally review data related to the conduct of the study (that is, the quality of the study and its ultimate ability to address the scientific questions of interest), in addition to data on effectiveness and safety outcomes. These data may include, among other items:
- Rates of recruitment, ineligibility, non-compliance, protocol violations and drop-outs, overall and by study site;
- Completeness and timeliness of data;
- Degree of concordance between site evaluation of events and centralized review;
- Balance between study arms on important prognostic variables;
- Accrual within important subsets'.

It is important that interaction between the sponsor and the DMC is kept to an absolute minimum to avoid any inadvertent communication of unblinded information. Sponsor exposure to unblinded interim results, except in terms of the communication of go/no-go decisions associated with interim analyses, can seriously compromise the scientific validity of the study. The sponsor is in the position of being able to influence the future conduct of the trial, and exposure to interim results could influence aspects of that, leading to bias. There can also be pressure from the sponsor to provide interim results for planning purposes: taking decisions about future production facilities, agreeing budgets for further trial activity and so on. Such pressure should be resisted as it can lead to the integrity of the trial being seriously undermined. Where this need is compelling, then communication should be managed in a very tight way. Further discussion of this point is provided in the FDA (2006) guideline in Section 6.5.

A DMC is usually needed in long-term trials in life-threatening diseases and sometimes in non-life-threatening diseases where there are potential safety concerns. It may also be necessary to have DMCs in studies in specific and vulnerable or fragile populations such as children, pregnant women or the very elderly, but DMCs are not usually necessary in phase I and early phase II trials or in short-term studies where the goal is relief of symptoms.

14.4.2 Structure and process

The independence of the committee from the sponsor is important, and there should also be no conflicts of interest among the participants, for example, holding equity in the sponsor's company or a direct competitor's company.

The members of the committee should also not otherwise be involved in the study, for example, as investigators, or, in the case of the statistician the final analysis of the data. The DMC consists of at least three participants, one of which will be a statistician; the remaining participants will be clinicians with expertise in relevant clinical disciplines associated with the disease under study or with the potential side effects. If the trial is an international study, then it is advisable to have members of the committee from the spread of geographical regions in which the trial is to be conducted. It is often this final point that determines the ultimate size of the DMC.

There will also be at least one other statistician involved closely with the activities of the DMC, and this is the statistician who supplies data tables to the committee for their deliberations. This statistician should also not be otherwise involved in the trial as they will potentially be supplying unblinded information to the DMC and attending their meetings. In the way that these things tend to be organised, this individual may be part of a CRO that is providing this service (and potentially other services) to the sponsor. See Pocock (2004) and the FDA (2006) guideline for further discussion on this and related points. In some cases, the DMC will also receive details of individual patient SAEs, usually in the form of narratives, and these will often be supplied directly from the sponsor, provided that this is not too burdensome. An alternative to this is to provide summary tables for these SAEs periodically, for example, monthly. These patients can be unblinded by the independent statistician if this has not already been done by the sponsors pharmacovigilance group.

Data tables produced for the DMC should contain separate summaries by treatment group, with the treatment groups labelled A and B (partially blinded). A separate sealed envelope or a password-protected electronic file should be provided to the members with decodes for A and B to enable the DMC members to be completely unblinded. This may seem an elaborate process, but it protects against inadvertent unblinding.

FDA (2006): 'Establishment and Operation of Clinical Trial Data Monitoring Committees'

'A common approach is presentation of results in printed copy tables using codes (for example, Group A and Group B) to protect against inadvertent unblinding should a report be misplaced, with separate access to the actual study arm assignments provided to DMC members by the statistical group responsible for preparing DMC reports'.

The activities of the DMC should be covered by a charter, prepared in advance of running the trial. The charter should detail the participants, their responsibilities, the format and conduct of meetings, communication pathways with the sponsor, decision making, confidentiality, indemnity and conflict of interest issues together with details regarding the format of the data supplied to the DMC by the independent statistician and the supply of other data, details of SAEs. It is advisable to involve the DMC members as early as possible in the review and possibly the construction of this document in order to gain clear buy-in to their role in the successful conduct of the trial.

14.4.3 Meetings and recommendations

The DMC should meet at a set of predefined time points during the course of the trial, typically following completion of a proportion of the patients. For example, four meetings could be organised, following completion of 25 per cent, 50 per cent and 75 per cent of the patients and finally at trial completion. If the trial is to involve interim analyses, then some of the meetings will revolve around those. Summary tables should be supplied in conjunction with all meetings. Meetings of the committee will usually be organised in open and closed sessions. The open sessions, which will also involve, for example, members of the sponsor company and the steering committee, will cover general issues such as recruitment rates, timelines and the presentation of summary demographic and baseline data tables. Details can also be given during these open sessions on the progress and results from other trials within the drug development programme. The closed sessions will involve only the members of the DMC plus the independent statistician supplying data to the DMC, if required. Minutes of both closed and open sessions of these meetings should be kept, and the closed minutes should be stored securely and confidentially by the chair of the DMC until trial completion. Electronic copies of the data sets on which interim analyses are based should also be retained as these may be requested by regulators.

Outside of the regular planned meetings, details of all SAEs can be supplied to the DMC in real time or at regular intervals, and the DMC members should arrange to discuss these, by email or teleconference, as and when they feel necessary.

Recommendations to the sponsor coming out of the regular DMC meetings will be one of the following:

- Trial to continue unchanged;
- Modification of the protocol to protect the safety of the trial participants;
- Termination of the trial.

Clearly, if the recommendation is anything other than *continue unchanged*, then additional information would need to be supplied to the sponsor to support these recommendations. The recommendations are not binding on the sponsor, although as mentioned earlier it would be very unusual to see these recommendations being ignored.

CHAPTER 15

Bayesian statistics

15.1 Introduction

The methods for statistical inference that we have discussed so far in this book fall under the heading of *classical* or *frequentist* methods. These methods are those that are most usually applied in analysis of clinical trial data. They are however not the only methods and Bayesian methodology provides an alternative way of thinking about statistical inference. In this section, we will outline the Bayesian approach and contrast this with the frequentist way of thinking. We will then set down how Bayesian methods can be applied in the analysis of data and also discuss implications for trial design. Finally, we will look at an application of these methods within a regulatory context.

Frequentist methods centre on making treatment comparisons using *p*-values and confidence intervals in relation to the value of an unknown parameter. In the comparison of two treatments means μ_1 and μ_2, for example, frequentist statisticians view these means as fixed unknown numerical values. They are the mean values you would see if you were able to treat the complete population of patients with drug A (μ_1) or with drug B (μ_2). Bayesian statisticians however view these means differently, as variables about which we can make probability statements. As we will see in the next section, it is possible within this framework to develop methods akin to *p*-values and confidence intervals that have different and, many people would say, more straightforward interpretations.

The Bayesian approach also allows the incorporation of *beliefs* (called prior beliefs) about parameters based on knowledge (and opinions) and information from outside of the particular clinical trial under consideration. It is this aspect that causes the biggest concern from regulators and we will address this point in subsequent sections.

15.2 Prior and posterior distributions

15.2.1 Prior beliefs

In order to develop the methodology underpinning the Bayesian approach, consider the following simple example. Suppose we are planning to run a single-arm phase II study to gain information about the cure rate of a particular new antibiotic and

Statistical Thinking for Non-Statisticians in Drug Regulation, Second Edition. Richard Kay.
© 2015 John Wiley & Sons, Ltd. Published 2015 by John Wiley & Sons, Ltd.

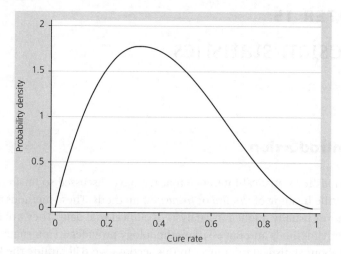

Figure 15.1 Prior distribution for cure rate

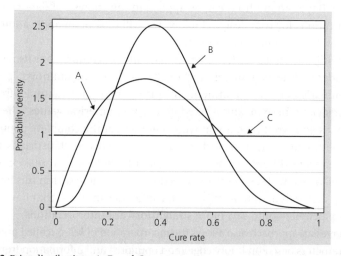

Figure 15.2 Prior distributions A, B and C

suppose that based on our knowledge of the disease setting, the population under study, the preclinical performance of this agent and its therapeutic class, we feel that the cure rate will be around 40 per cent. Assume that the probability distribution in Figure 15.1 captures our *prior beliefs* with regard to the likely values for the cure rate. This distribution (distribution A) is just one possibility; we will discuss other possibilities later. This prior distribution is centred on 0.4 (the mean of this distribution = 0.4) but we are not ruling out that the cure rate, for example, could be as low as 0.1 or as high as 0.8 although we are saying that these values are less likely based upon our knowledge before we run the study.

Figure 15.2 presents alternative prior distributions. Distribution B which also has a mean of 0.4, is less spread out compared to distribution A. Distribution C,

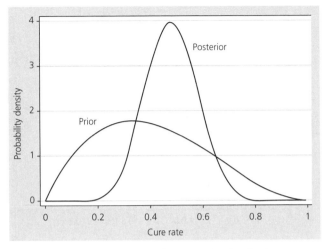

Figure 15.3 Prior distribution A and corresponding posterior distribution

which is a so-called uniform distribution (known as a *vague* prior distribution), gives equal prior probability to any value between 0 and 1.

15.2.2 Prior to posterior

Now, let's suppose that our study recruits 20 patients and at the day 21 test of cure visit, 10 of those patients are cured. The observed cure rate is 50 per cent, which is a little bit higher than what we were expecting based on our prior beliefs. The Bayesian analysis combines the observed data with the prior beliefs to produce *posterior beliefs* in the form of a second probability distribution, the *posterior distribution*. We will discuss later in this section how this combination is done.

Figure 15.3 shows the posterior distribution for these data together with our original *prior* distribution A. Note that our posterior beliefs are now centred at a value between 0.4 and 0.5; the observed data have influenced our prior beliefs and moved them in the direction of 0.5.

Figure 15.4 shows the posterior distributions A, B and C for the alternative prior distributions A, B and C, respectively. It can be seen that the data have strongly influenced our beliefs (as they should) about the cure rate. Indeed, the posterior beliefs have very much come together, and this is generally what happens; it is the data, especially with larger sample sizes, that ultimately dominates our views. The influence of our prior beliefs would have been greater had the sample size been smaller.

15.2.3 Bayes theorem

The term Bayesian statistics derives from the mathematical theorem, known as *Bayes theorem*, which uses data to convert prior beliefs into posterior beliefs.

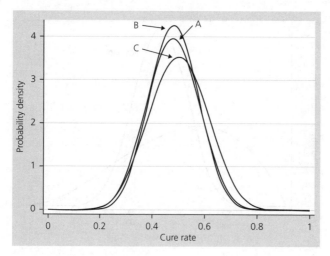

Figure 15.4 Posterior distributions A, B and C

The simple form of Bayes theorem (called the *Bayes rule*) is as follows. If E_1 and E_2 denote any two events, then

$$p(E_1|E_2) = \frac{p(E_2|E_1) \times p(E_1)}{p(E_2)}$$

Here, $p(E_1)$, for example, denotes the probability of event E_1, while $p(E_1|E_2)$ denotes the probability of event E_1 given that we know that event E_2 has occurred, called the *conditional probability of E_1 given E_2*.

To take a simple example, consider throwing two perfectly balanced 6-sided dice and suppose that event E_1 is getting a 6 on the first throw and E_2 is getting a total score of at least 9. The outcomes that give a total score of at least 9 (event E_2) are 3 6, 4 5, 4 6, 5 4, 5 5, 5 6, 6 3, 6 4, 6 5 and 6 6, and each of these is equally likely to occur when throwing two fair dice. Of these 10 outcomes, 4 involve getting a 6 on the first throw so that if you have a total of 9, the probability that you got a 6 on the first throw is $p(E_1|E_2) = \frac{4}{10}$. Let us now evaluate the right side of the Bayes rule and see if this gives the same answer. The probability of getting a total of at least 9 given that the first throw gives a 6 is $p(E_2|E_1) = \frac{4}{6}$ since 4 of the 6 outcomes (6 1, 6 2, 6 3, 6 4, 6 5 and 6 6) that involve a 6 on the first throw result in a total of 9 or above. Further, the probability of a 6 on the first throw is $p(E_1) = \frac{1}{6}$ and the probability of a total of at least 9 on the two throws is $p(E_2) = \frac{10}{36}$. The right-hand side of the Bayes rule is then

$$\frac{p(E_2|E_1) \times p(E_1)}{p(E_2)} = \frac{4/6 \times 1/6}{10/36} = \frac{4}{10}$$

So the equation works!

Further mathematical detail is beyond the scope of this book, but simply speaking, if $p(\theta)$ denotes the equation for the prior distribution and $p(\theta|y)$ denotes the equation for the posterior distribution where y are the data (10 patients cured in the example in Section 15.2.2), then the Bayes rule tells us that

$$p(\theta|y=10) = \frac{p(y=10|\theta) \times p(\theta)}{p(y=10)}$$

This equation allows us then to calculate the posterior distribution $p(\theta|y=10)$ based on the prior distribution $p(\theta)$ and probabilities associated with the observed data $y=10$.

15.3 Bayesian inference

15.3.1 Frequentist methods

The statistical methods we have used to make inferences within the frequentist framework are p-values and confidence intervals. Let us just recap on the way that these quantities are defined in the context of comparing two treatments in a superiority study.

The p-value is the probability associated with observed difference (or a larger difference) when the null hypothesis is true. The precise nature of this p-value was introduced in Chapter 3 and discussed in detail in Section 3.3.1. For many who work in the field of clinical research, this definition is not easy to grasp, and the p-value is often misinterpreted as the probability that the null hypothesis is true. In the next section, we will see how the Bayesian equivalent to the p-value can be interpreted in this way.

A 95 per cent confidence interval for the difference in the treatment means will contain the true difference on 95 per cent of occasions when the trial is repeated. So on any single occasion, we can be 95 per cent confident that the true difference is within the range given by the confidence interval. See Section 3.1.1 for further discussion. The corresponding quantity coming out of the Bayesian framework is a 95 per cent *credible interval*, which has a much simpler and, some would say, more useful interpretation.

15.3.2 Posterior probabilities

Bayesian methods allow us to calculate probabilities, based on the posterior distribution, that are of interest to us. For example, when evaluating an experimental treatment for blood pressure lowering in a placebo-controlled trial, there may be interest in calculating the probability that the mean reduction in blood pressure in the active group is less than or equal to the mean reduction in the placebo group in other words that the active drug is ineffective. If μ_1 and μ_2 denote the mean reductions in the active and placebo groups, respectively, then we are looking to obtain

$$p(\mu_1 \leq \mu_2) = p(\mu_1 - \mu_2 \leq 0)$$

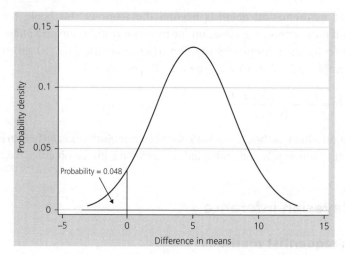

Figure 15.5 Posterior distribution for difference in means and probability that the drug is ineffective

Figure 15.5 presents a typical posterior distribution $(\mu_1 - \mu_2)$ in this setting and the marked area is this probability.

This probability (0.048 in the example) is akin to a (one-sided) p-value within the frequentist framework, and if this is small, then we are thinking in terms of rejecting the null hypothesis that the active treatment is ineffective. We could of course calculate this the opposite way around, the probability that the new treatment does work, $p(\mu_1 - \mu_2 > 0) = 1 - 0.048 = 0.952$. We could also obtain other probabilities of interest from this posterior distribution. Let's suppose that 4 mmHg is viewed as being a difference in the means that is of clinical importance. We can calculate $p(\mu_1 - \mu_2 \geq 4)$ to address this issue, the probability that the new treatment has efficacy that is of clinical relevance. For this example, this probability is 0.63 (or 63 per cent).

15.3.3 Credible intervals

Credible intervals are the Bayesian equivalent of the confidence interval and can be produced directly from the posterior distribution. For example, if we want a 95 per cent *credible interval*, we calculate the lower end of that interval as the value c_1 on the x-axis that cuts off the lowest 2.5 per cent probability. Figure 15.6 shows this graphically. Similarly, the upper end of this interval is the value c_2 on the x-axis that cuts off the upper 2.5 per cent probability. The 95 per cent credible interval is then $(c_1, c_2) = (-0.9, 10.9)$. The interpretation of this 95 per cent credible interval is very straightforward, and we can say there is 95 per cent probability that the difference in the means $\mu_1 - \mu_2$ lies between −0.9 and +10.9.

It is straightforward to extend this to other coverage probabilities, for example, 99 per cent where we would cut off the lower and upper 0.5 per cent probabilities.

Wijeysundera *et al.* (2008) provide an extended discussion of the interplay between frequentist and Bayesian methodologies.

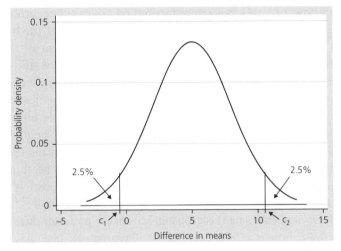

Figure 15.6 Posterior distribution for difference in means and 95 per cent credible interval (c_1, c_2)

15.4 Case study

In this section, we will consider a specific example and contrast the frequentist and Bayesian approaches to the analysis of data and the associated interpretations. Wijeysundera *et al.* (2008) report a clinical study evaluating the effectiveness of paclitaxel in addition to platinum-based chemotherapy as second-line treatment in women with ovarian cancer originally reported by The ICON and AGO Collaborators (2003). The trial was designed to detect an improvement in overall survival in the paclitaxel group with a hazard ratio of 0.71.

In the classical analysis reported in the trial publication, the hazard ratio was 0.82 with a 95 per cent confidence interval of (0.69, 0.97) and a statistically significant one-sided *p*-value of 0.012. Note that the authors actually reported a two-sided *p*-value, but for the purposes of this comparison between classical and Bayesian methods, I have converted this to be one-sided. The confidence interval tells us that the true hazard ratio is, with 95 per cent confidence, somewhere in the range 0.69 to 0.97. The one-sided *p*-value tells us that the probability of seeing a hazard ratio (in favour of paclitaxel) at least as low as 0.82 is only 1.2 per cent and of course it is on this basis that we declare statistically significant differences.

Wijeysundera *et al.* (2008) reanalysed these data from a Bayesian point of view. They assumed a normal distribution prior for the hazard ratio on the log scale with a mean of zero and a standard deviation equal to 0.21. This prior assumes that the most likely value for the hazard ratio is 1 (no treatment benefit) with only a 5 per cent a priori probability of there being a treatment benefit given by a hazard ratio of 0.71 or better. This therefore represents a very conservative prior distribution; we would call this a *sceptical prior*. The posterior distribution, again on the log hazard ratio scale, given the data, also turns out to be normal but with a mean of −0.17 and a standard deviation of 0.081.

We can now use this posterior distribution to calculate probabilities of interest. In particular, the probability that the hazard ratio is ≥1 (no benefit from paclitaxel) is equal to 0.019. This is the Bayesian equivalent of the classical p-value. Its interpretation however is much more straightforward; we can say that the probability of no benefit is 1.9 per cent. Conversely, we can conclude that there is a 98.1 per cent probability that paclitaxel treatment is beneficial in terms of improving overall survival. The 95 per cent credible interval for the hazard ratio based on the posterior distribution is calculated to be (0.72, 0.99) so we can say with 95 per cent probability that the true hazard ratio is within this range. Further probabilities can also be calculated. It may be that clinicians would only view this treatment as being beneficial clinically, possibly because of associated risks, if the hazard ratio were 0.90 or lower, for example. The Bayesian analysis allows us to calculate this probability from the posterior distribution and its value is 0.78; there is a 78 per cent probability that paclitaxel has a clinically relevant beneficial effect in terms of overall survival.

Note that in one sense the Bayesian and classical analyses are not too dissimilar. The classical p-value is 0.019, and the Bayesian posterior probability of no effect is 0.021. The 95 per cent confidence interval for the hazard ratio is (0.69, 0.97). The 95 per cent Bayesian credible interval is (0.72, 0.99). In part, it is the assumption of a sceptical prior that has given marginally less impressive results for the Bayesian analysis compared to the classical analysis. But that is not the point really. The main distinction between the two approaches is in the interpretation. The Bayesian approach has given quantities that are much easier to interpret; we are able to present and discuss probabilities of interest to us. This kind of interpretation is simply not available to us under the classical approach.

15.5 History and regulatory acceptance

It was Thomas Bayes (1702–1761) who first set down the basis for what we now know as Bayes theorem, but it was Pierre-Simon Laplace (1749–1827) who developed the ideas and applied them to problems in medical statistics. So these methods have been around for an awful long time! The widespread application of the methods however has until very recently been constrained by the practicalities of actually doing the calculations. Until maybe around 15 years ago, strict mathematical assumptions regarding the prior distribution were needed before problems could be solved. In recent years, however, the development of the so-called Markov Chain Monte Carlo (MCMC) methods and computer algorithms that apply these methods has enabled tremendous flexibility in the range of problems that can now be addressed within the Bayesian framework; mathematical constraints are no longer an issue. WinBUGS (http://www.mrc-bsu.cam.ac.uk/bugs/welcome.shtml) is a well-established computer package that applies the Bayesian methodology to the design and analysis of clinical trials.

How do regulators view Bayesian methods?

ICH E9 (1998): 'Note for Guidance on Statistical Principles for Clinical Trials'

'Because the predominant approaches to the design and analysis of clinical trials have been based on frequentist statistical methods, the guidance largely refers to the use of frequentist methods when discussing hypothesis testing and/or confidence intervals. This should not be taken to imply that other approaches are not appropriate: the use of Bayesian and other approaches may be considered when the reasons for their use are clear and when the resulting conclusions are sufficiently robust'.

There are two issues here. Firstly, the *'reasons for their use are clear'*. The prior distribution is by definition based on prior beliefs, and it is this that is the basis of the concern over the use of the Bayesian methods; those beliefs potentially have an element of subjectivity. The basis for a reasoned choice for the prior distribution should be set down and, in line with general regulatory thinking, must be pre-specified before the experiment. Secondly, *'the resulting conclusions are sufficiently robust'*. My take on this is that sensitivity analyses based on other choices for the prior distribution should essentially lead to the same result and conclusions.

In some cases, prior distributions are based entirely on data, perhaps from a previous trial or from some other alternative source, external to the trial. When the prior distribution is obtained in this way and does not involve any elements of subjectivity, then we talk in terms of *empirical Bayes methods*. This overcomes to a certain extent the issues associated with subjectivity although the choice of the data on which to base the calculation of the prior is still subjective in a sense. Nonetheless, following the empirical Bayes pathway can alleviate some concerns.

Bayesian methods are potentially of great concern to regulators however when applied to the sequential (interim) analysis of data. The Bayesian approach in this setting takes a prior distribution at the start of the study and updates this to produce a posterior distribution based on the prior and the data up to that first interim. This posterior distribution then becomes the prior distribution at this point in time, which is itself updated at the second interim analysis using the new data to that point to produce a second posterior distribution. This again then becomes the prior at that point in time and so on until the end of the study. This general approach pays no price for many looks at the data; there are no type I errors in Bayesian statistics. There are however hybrid approaches in this setting, which while using Bayesian methods also pay a price for the multiple looks associated with the interim analyses. The interested reader is referred to Spiegelhalter, Abrams and Myles (2004), Section 6.6.5, for discussion of this issue.

There is one area however where the Bayesian methods generally have gained greater acceptance and that is in the area of medical devices. The FDA has produced a guideline (FDA, 2006) entitled *Guideline on the Use of Bayesian Statistics in Medical Device Clinical Trials*. The document points out that Bayesian statistics are generally more acceptable in these kinds of trials.

FDA (2006): 'Guideline on the use of Bayesian Statistics in Medical Device Clinical Trials'

'Good prior information is often available for a medical device; for example from earlier studies on previous generations of the device or from studies overseas. These studies can often be used as prior information because the mechanism of action of medical devices is typically physical, making the effects local and not systemic. Local effects are often predictable from prior information when modifications to a device are minor'.

15.6 Discussion

There has been some resistance in the past to the use of Bayesian methods. This has been linked firstly to concerns about the incorporation of prior beliefs into the inferential process, especially when the methodology was constrained by the mathematical limitations of undertaking calculations of posterior probabilities and credible intervals. Secondly, regulators and others have concerns about the Bayesian treatment of multiple testing where the pure Bayesian view does not incorporate the idea of a false positive. The false positive is essentially a frequentist concept built around the frequency of drawing an incorrect conclusion based on repeated looks at the data. In Bayesian statistics, the focus is on expressing information in terms of posterior distributions rather than on control of false-positive rates.

The development of specialist statistical software has essentially eliminated the first of these concerns in that realistic priors can be specified and the robustness of conclusions can be easily evaluated by choosing a range of different priors. The second concern can be addressed by using hybrid solutions that on the one hand do calculate Bayesian posterior probabilities and credible intervals but on the other hand incorporate multiplicity considerations.

In some circumstances as we have mentioned, it is possible to base prior beliefs entirely on data, for example from other trials that have already been conducted. Using such *empirical* priors can alleviate some of the regulatory concern regarding the basis for prior beliefs.

Two major benefits of the Bayesian methods relate to the way that results can be expressed and interpreted. It is certainly true that many practitioners misinterpret *p*-values, no matter how hard we as statisticians try to explain. Similar comments apply to confidence intervals. Maybe frequentist statisticians should accept defeat, climb over the fence and move to using posterior probabilities and credible intervals that avail themselves to a much more straightforward interpretation.

CHAPTER 16
Adaptive designs

16.1 What are adaptive designs?

16.1.1 Advantages and drawbacks

There has been a tremendous amount of recent interest, both from statisticians and non-statisticians, in so-called adaptive or flexible designs where certain aspects of the clinical trial design can be changed based on accumulating data from within the trial. These designs have the potential, at least in theory, to improve the efficiency of decision making, by reducing sample size, reducing costs, avoiding waste and reducing timelines. In practice, however, things are not quite so simple and very careful thought should be given to the use of such designs. In particular, the validity and integrity of the trial in terms of maintaining control of the type I error and avoiding bias in the eventual treatment comparison, must be maintained. These aspects cannot be compromised; if they are, then this can completely destroy the trial in the eyes of the regulators and the scientific community in general. This is rather a negative statement to start out with, but such cautionary words are justified. There has been a tendency to view adaptive designs as the Holy Grail with an ability to recover failing trials or to avoid careful planning at the design stage. The CHMP is clear on this point in their guidance on adaptive designs:

CHMP (2007): 'Reflection Paper on Methodological Issues in Confirmatory Clinical Trials Planned with an Adaptive Design'

'… adaptive designs should not be seen as a means to alleviate the burden of rigorous planning of clinical trials'.

Regulators make a clear distinction between exploratory and confirmatory trials, and adaptations in a confirmatory trial may destroy the ability of that trial to make confirmatory statements and claims.

CHMP (2007): 'Reflection Paper on Methodological Issues in Confirmatory Clinical Trials Planned with an Adaptive Design'

'Adaptations to confirmatory trials introduced without proper planning will render the trials to be considered exploratory'.

Statistical Thinking for Non-Statisticians in Drug Regulation, Second Edition. Richard Kay.
© 2015 John Wiley & Sons, Ltd. Published 2015 by John Wiley & Sons, Ltd.

The FDA talks of the *'learn versus confirm' paradigm* (Wang, Hung and O'Neill, 2011); the exploratory phase II trial is used for proof of concept, for gaining information about the statistical aspects of endpoints of interest, for the identification of appropriate inclusion/exclusion criteria and to choose a single dose (or a limited number of doses) for phase III. Having gained this information, we then finalise our plans for the subsequent phase III studies, and in that confirmatory phase, we establish the efficacy of the drug and evaluate its risks. Allowing uncontrolled design adaptations within a phase III clinical trial clearly conflicts with the confirmatory nature of that trial.

Nonetheless, there are certain adaptations that, if carefully planned do not undermine the ability of the trial to provide confirmatory conclusions, and it is these adaptations that we will explore in this chapter.

Throughout the remainder of this chapter, we will focus our attention primarily on evaluating treatments in terms of continuous or score data where we are comparing mean values. Extensions to other data types are straightforward; this restriction simply allows us to be economical with the language that we use.

16.1.2 Restricted adaptations

We have in fact already considered adaptations to the design of a phase III trial of two kinds. Firstly, in Section 8.5.3, we spoke about the reassessment of sample size based on a blinded evaluation of the variance of the primary endpoint or the overall event rate. Such adaptations are allowed by regulators and have no effect on the type I error provided that blinding is maintained. The FDA in their guidance makes these issues clear:

FDA (2010): 'Guidance for Industry. Adaptive Design Clinical Trials for Drugs and Biologics'

'There is a critical distinction between adaptations based on an interim analysis of unblinded results of the controlled trial (generally involving comparative analyses of study endpoints or outcomes potentially correlated with these endpoints) and adaptations based on interim noncomparative analyses of blinded data (including study endpoint data but also including data such as discontinuation rates and baseline characteristics). ... Protocol revisions intended to occur after unblinded analysis should be prospectively defined and carefully implemented to avoid risking irresolvable uncertainty in the interpretation of study results. In contrast, revisions based on blinded interim evaluations of data (e.g. aggregate event rates, variance, discontinuation rates, baseline characteristics) do not introduce statistical bias to the study or into subsequent study revisions made by the same personnel'.

Secondly, in Section 14.2, we considered group sequential designs and stopping for both futility and for overwhelming efficacy. Various schemes were considered, using strict rules about the preservation of the type I error rate. Again, if these rules are followed, then there should be no regulatory concerns.

We will refer to adaptations of these kinds as *restricted adaptations*. They are restricted in the sense that they only consider blinded data or do not provide any flexibility to adapt the trial based on unblinded data except in relation to a go/no-go decision.

A further potential for adapting the design occurs when certain aspects of a trial are changed based on external data. For example, it may be that the trial was designed based on only rudimentary knowledge of the variance of the primary endpoint, and additional information from external sources regarding the variance may become available as the trial is ongoing. If the information is that the variance used in the sample size calculation is too small, then the trial is underpowered and a revised sample size calculation can be undertaken based on this new information for the variance and the sample size adjusted upwards. This does not compromise the validity of the study provided the blind is completely maintained. From a regulatory point of view, it is always better to have such considerations pre-planned. Hopefully, we would know at the design stage that new information on the variance would become available during the conduct of the trial, and this reconsideration of sample size based on this could then be pre-planned. Unfortunately, if this is not the case, then there is always the suspicion from regulators that the sample size is being reconsidered as a consequence of some unblinding, and it is often difficult to dispel those concerns completely.

16.1.3 Flexible adaptations

We will call the adaptations that build in additional amounts of flexibility as *flexible adaptations*, and these will be the main focus of our considerations in this chapter. There are many different types of adaptation that are possible, but for our purposes in this book, we will focus primarily on two settings that are the most common.

Firstly, we will consider the reassessment of sample size at an interim time point based on unblinded data where we actually compare the treatments, calculate a p-value at the interim point and resize the trial based on that interim result.

Secondly, there is the seamless phase II/III trial where we start by considering several dose levels and placebo in the dose-finding phase II part and where the plan is to take a reduced number of dose levels (often one) through to the phase III part. At the end of the study, all of the data from the phase II part and from the phase III part is used in the evaluation of statistical significance as a basis for a confirmatory claim.

16.2 Minimising bias

16.2.1 Control of type I error

As we have discussed at various points in this book, it is a requirement in general in a clinical trial to control the potential for the type I error at 0.05. It will be better in this chapter to consider one-sided tests in which we would control at a type I error rate for a one-sided comparison of 0.025. The rules are unchanged when we look at non-inferiority studies (Section 12.4) where again the type I error, falsely concluding non-inferiority when in truth the new treatment is inferior, is controlled at 0.025. The requirement to control the type I error for an adaptive design is one essential element that underpins the validity of the adaptation.

CHMP (2007): 'Reflection Paper on Methodological Issues in Confirmatory Clinical Trials Planned with an Adaptive Design'

'A minimal prerequisite for statistical methods to be accepted in the regulatory setting is the control of the pre-specified type I error ...'.

Consider a simple example. Suppose in a blood pressure lowering placebo-controlled trial we are looking to detect a difference of 4 mmHg in the mean change from baseline between the two groups. Assuming a standard deviation of 8 mmHg, a sample size of 86 per group will give 90 per cent power to detect such a change. In the planned interim analysis, after 43 patients per group have provided data on the primary endpoint, a change of only 3 mmHg is observed. Is it valid to increase the sample size to 151, which gives a power of 90 per cent to detect a difference of 3 mmHg, continue to the end of the study and then use a conventional analysis and p-value calculation to compare the groups? The short answer is no – it is not. It has been shown (see, e.g. Proschan, Lan and Wittes (2006), Section 11.4) that such a procedure potentially more than doubles the type I error rate – you might say that we are *chasing* a significant result!

There is however a statistical solution to this problem that does preserve the type I error, and this is associated with calculating one-sided p-values (p_1 and p_2, respectively) from the two parts of the trial, before and after the adaptation, and combining them in a particular way. There are several different ways of combining; we will primarily use a method that derives from *Fisher's combination test* (Bauer and Köhne, 1994), and this involves simply multiplying the p-values together. If the product $p_1 \times p_2 \leq 0.0038$, we have statistical significance overall at the one-sided 0.025 level. The result on which this test is based is that, under the null hypothesis either in a superiority trial or in a non-inferiority trial, $-2 ln p_1 p_2$ follows a chi-square distribution on 4 degrees of freedom. An example of this procedure is given in Example 16.1 in the context of a non-inferiority study.

> **Example 16.1** Acute treatment of moderate to severe depression with hypericum extract WS 5570
>
> Szegedi *et al.* (2005) report a randomised double-blind non-inferiority trial of hypericum extract WS 5570 versus paroxetine as the active control treatment. The primary endpoint was the change from baseline in the 17-item Hamilton Depression Scale (17-HAMD). The pre-specified non-inferiority margin was set at 2.5 points on the 17-HAMD for the difference in the means. A total of 100 patients were recruited into a part 1 and the data analysed at that point giving a p-value for non-inferiority of 0.084. As set down earlier in order to achieve statistical significance at the end of the trial using Fisher's combination test, the product of the part 1 and part 2 p-values for non-inferiority, $p_1 p_2$, needed to be ≤0.0038, and for this to be achieved, the requirement was that p_2 should be ≤0.045. A total of 150 patients recruited into stage 2 gave 80 per cent power, assuming a true difference between the treatments of zero points, to demonstrate non-inferiority with this adjusted significance level of 0.045. The data at the end of the study gave statistical significance for non-inferiority with $p_1 p_2 \leq 0.0038$ and a positive confirmatory conclusion that hypericum extract WS 5570 is non-inferior to paroxetine was made.

A second method for combining the p-values from the two parts of the study is best expressed in terms of combining the corresponding z-scores. Recall from Section 3.3.3 that the z-score which is equal to the signal/standard error ratio, leads directly to the p-value. The *inverse normal method* (Lehmacher and Wassmer, 1999) calculates an overall z-score as an *average* of the z-scores (z_1 and z_2, respectively) from each of the two parts as follows:

$$z = \frac{z_1 + z_2}{\sqrt{2}}$$

This combined z-score is then used to obtain the one-sided p-value for the trial as a whole with the conventional cut-off of 0.025 for statistical significance.

It is important to note that these p-value calculations are valid, irrespective of the adaptation made at the interim point. There are however some constraints. In particular, the methods used to obtain the p-values (and z-scores) must be pre-specified.

16.2.2 Estimation

In conjunction with a modification to the usual way that we calculate statistical significance in an adaptive trial, there are also issues with the way we estimate the magnitude of the treatment benefit and confidence intervals for that treatment benefit. It is not correct, for example, just to look at the difference between two mean values for the trial as a whole and calculate a conventional 95 per cent confidence interval for the true difference around this estimated value in a trial that includes a flexible adaptation. If we were to do that, then the estimate would be a biased estimate of the true difference, and the 95 per cent confidence interval would not have its usual 95 per cent coverage interpretation; it would not contain the true difference 95 per cent of the time. Controlling the properties of the estimation procedures, that is bias and correct coverage, is not straightforward. There are procedures available but they are complex. Regulators and the clinical community in general are not simply concerned with statistical significance, but are also very interested in the clinical benefit measured in terms of treatment differences, so that they can appropriately judge the benefit–risk trade-off. This is an issue that requires considerable statistical expertise.

CHMP (2007): 'Reflection Paper on Methodological Issues in Confirmatory Clinical Trials Planned with an Adaptive Design'

'Corresponding methods to estimate the size of the treatment effect and to provide confidence intervals with pre-specified coverage probability are required in addition to the presentation of the P-value'.

16.2.3 Behavioural issues

Controlling the type I error rate and providing correct methods for estimation are of course required in order to produce valid confirmatory conclusions. However, these are not the only aspects of an adaptive design that need to be carefully handled. A further issue that is equally important is the control of the dissemination of information regarding the data at the interim point on which an adaptation has been based and indeed the nature of that adaptation. The CHMP in their guideline talks about the importance of confidentiality of interim results. If the results of the interim analysis are revealed to personnel involved in the studies, to investigators or even to patients, then this could cause bias in various aspects of the study from that point on. Potential sources of bias include recruitment of subtly different types of patients following a positive *trend* at the interim stage, specific changes in the administration of the intervention, endpoint assessment and so on. Of course, these concerns regarding dissemination and operational bias are not just confined to adaptive designs but also more widely to any clinical trial containing an interim unblinded look at the data. Regulators have the opportunity to ask (or to undertake in the case of the FDA) for an analysis of data before and after an interim analysis to check for consistency. Any inconsistencies will seriously undermine their confidence in drawing clear conclusions.

CHMP (2007): 'Reflection Paper on Methodological Issues in Confirmatory Clinical Trials Planned with an Adaptive Design'

'Studies with interim analyses where there are marked differences in estimated treatment effects between different study parts or stages will be difficult to interpret. It may be unclear whether the estimated treatment effects differ just by chance, as a consequence of the intentional or unintentional communication of interim results, or for other reasons. This problem can be even greater if the study design has been changed as a result of an interim analysis'.

FDA (2010): 'Guidance for Industry. Adaptive Design Clinical Trials for Drugs and Biologics'

'Of particular concern are situations in which the estimates of the treatment effect obtained before and after the design modification differ substantially. Inconsistent treatment effect estimates among the stages of the study can make the overall treatment effect estimate difficult to interpret'.

Example 16. 2   The 2NN study

This was an open-label, parallel-group, randomised trial in patients with chronic HIV-1 infection reported by van Leth *et al.* (2004). The primary endpoint was treatment failure, a composite endpoint based on virology, disease progression or therapy change. Initially, patients were randomised equally to one of the following three groups:

1 N_1 – nevirapine (once daily)

2 E – efavirenz

3 N_1 + E – combination of nevirapine (once daily) and efavirenz

Five months into the trial (388 patients randomised), another study showed that the effectiveness of nevirapine was related to the minimum concentration, and so the trial was adapted to include a fourth arm – nevirapine twice daily (N_2). Further, the randomisation ratio was changed so that randomisation to N_1, E, N_1 + E and N_2 was in the ratio 1:2:1:2. The final sample size was 1216, and in the final analysis, data from before and after the adaptation were combined. Is this appropriate and supported by the data? The adaptation was driven by external data although note that the trial was not a blinded trial. In the treatment groups that were used throughout the study, the following failure rates together with 95 per cent confidence intervals were seen (Table 16.1).

The issue here is the lack of homogeneity in the results before and after the change. In particular, there is a 12.2 per cent absolute difference between nevirapine (once daily) and efavirenz before the design change, and there is virtually no difference between these two arms after the change. No explanation of why this had occurred was given in the publication. This lack of consistency would cause regulators major concerns.

Table 16.1 Failure rates in the 2NN study

	Before addition of 4th arm (%)	After addition of 4th arm(%)
N_1	46.6 (37.8, 55.5)	39.3 (29.1, 50.3)
E	34.4 (26.3, 43.2)	39.4 (33.5, 45.5)
N_1 + E	51.6 (42.5, 60.6)	55.4 (44.1, 66.3)

As a final point, it should be noted that statistical methods of themselves cannot correct for this operational bias; if it is present, then its impact is unmeasurable.

FDA (2010): 'Guidance for Industry. Adaptive Design Clinical Trials for Drugs and Biologics'

'Because operational bias is a non-statistical source of bias, statistical methods cannot correct or adjust for this bias'.

16.2.4 Exploratory trials

Our concerns regarding the lack of control of the type I error rate have been expressed in the context of confirmatory studies. From a regulatory perspective, there is less concern in this regard in exploratory studies, for example, in phase II proof-of-concept and dose selection trials. Nonetheless, the potential for inflating the false positive rate is still present in those trials, and care must be taken in relation to internal decision making to avoid drawing conclusions that are overly optimistic.

FDA (2010): 'Guidance for Industry. Adaptive Design Clinical Trials for Drugs and Biologics'

'Care should be taken in their design and interpretation so that the limited amount of data, adaptive design elements, or multiple endpoints of an exploratory study do not give rise to unwarranted certainty that can lead to poor choices in areas such as dose, patient population, study endpoints'.

16.3 Unblinded sample size re-estimation

16.3.1 Product of *p*-values

Re-estimating sample size based on unblinded data at an interim point has already been introduced in Section 16.2.1. In this setting, the trial data from the first part of the trial, observed difference between the treatment groups and possibly the within-group standard deviations, are used in the calculation of the final sample size for the study. This may be done because the observed treatment difference, at the interim point is smaller than that anticipated in the sample size calculation or it may be the initial sample size calculation did not specify a target treatment difference to be detected, or there may be some other reason. In Example 16.1, which was a non-inferiority trial, the sample size of 100 patients was chosen based on a significance level for the test for non-inferiority of 0.20. It was argued that this would support a trend in favour of non-inferiority and continuation of the trial because of promising results. In fact, the *p*-value for non-inferiority was 0.084. This is good news and well below the required significance level. The final sample size was then chosen to give adequate power for statistical significance at the 5 per cent level for Fisher's combination test. We could, as an alternative, have used a different test based on the inverse normal method provided that had been the pre-specified methodology.

16.3.2 Weighting the two parts of the trial

The before and after tests give equal weight to the two parts of the trial; the individual p-values, p_1 and p_2, carry the same weight when multiplied together in Fisher's combination test. Similarly, in the inverse normal method, the separate z-scores from the two parts of the trial are given equal weight in the test. This particular property of the tests for adaptive designs is one of the reasons why some commentators have concerns about the efficiency of such designs. In the usual (non-adaptive design) analysis of data, each patient is given equal weight. For example, if there had been 50 patients randomised to group A before the adaptation and 100 patients randomised to group A after the adaptation, then those 150 patients would, ignoring the adaptation, contribute equally to the calculation of the mean for that group with $\bar{x} = \frac{\Sigma x}{150}$ and contribute equally to the calculation of the p-value for the treatment comparison. In the usual analysis for the adaptive design however, this does not happen, and in this example, the 100 patients in group A recruited after the adaptation would collectively only be given the same weight as the 50 patients recruited before the adaptation. In short, in this example a patient recruited after the adaptation is given only half of the weight of a patient recruited before the adaptation.

This flies in the face of certain fundamental statistical principles for the analysis of data, and although it may seem a particularly technical point, it does have implications for the power of these adaptive designs to detect treatment differences (or to establish non-inferiority if that is the objective). A further issue concerns the estimated treatment benefit and the associated confidence interval. Should we use simply the conventional mean values and the difference between those, or should we incorporate the same weighting that has been used in the p-value calculation? In Section 16.2.2, we argued that the former approach is biased. The FDA is clearly concerned about the potential confusion here when presenting trial results associated with the estimated treatment effect:

FDA (2010): 'Guidance for Industry. Adaptive Design Clinical Trials for Drugs and Biologics'

'Differential weighting, however, can lead to some difficulties in interpreting the final analysis. ... This could lead to an estimate of the treatment effect that is different from the estimate when all patients are given equal weight, with resulting confusion regarding the amount of benefit demonstrated'.

There is a way around the issue of unequal weighting in the calculation of p-values, and the interested reader is referred to the work of Mehta and Pocock (2011). This modified method, in which certain restrictions are applied with regard to the choice of the final sample size, is however not without controversy, as set down in a commentary on that paper by Emerson, Levin and Emerson (2011).

16.3.3 Rationale

Under what circumstances might one be interested and willing to increase the sample size at an interim stage in this way? There are two aspects. Firstly, one could envisage a situation where budget constraints result in conducting a trial with only modest size, perhaps with a level for the power less than ideal for a confirmatory study. Results at an interim look however may be promising enough to support additional investment in the project and an increase in the sample size. Secondly, if indeed the observed treatment difference was lower than anticipated and one were increasing the sample size because of that then it would be necessary to argue that the observed treatment benefit in the trial as a whole was going to be worthwhile from a clinical relevance point of view.

16.4 Seamless phase II/III studies

16.4.1 Standard framework

The standard framework for phase II and phase III is displayed in Figure 16.1. The white space between the two phases provides time for the analysis of data (both efficacy and safety), reflection, planning, discussions with authorities, etc., and decisions regarding how to move forward with phase III are built on those considerations.

In an adaptive framework, this space is lost (Figure 16.2) and algorithms covering all of the possible actions that usually take place at the end of phase II need to be well defined for a seamless transition to work in practice. It is a tall order, and some would say too tall! The challenge is setting down in a structured way the breadth of the possible adaptations: are we looking to reduce the three doses down to two or to just a single dose or is that to be left open, is that decision to be made purely on efficacy grounds perhaps because we have no concerns about safety or is it going to be a combination of efficacy and safety, and is there the potential to modify the inclusion/exclusion criteria to focus on a subgroup where

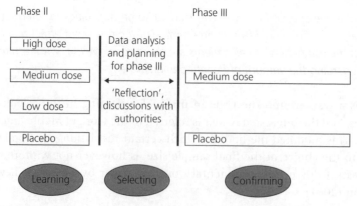

Figure 16.1 Traditional framework for phase II/III

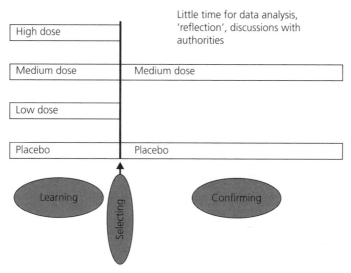

Figure 16.2 Adaptive design for seamless phase II/III

the benefit–risk is optimal or at least to exclude some patients where the benefit–risk balance is unfavourable? Usually, these kinds of considerations are precisely what fill the *'white space'* in the conventional approach.

16.4.2 Aspects of the *p*-value calculation

In the case where we are looking to take forward only one dose into the phase III part of the trial, the *p*-value calculation for the second part is just based on the usual two-group comparison. The *p*-value calculation for the first part however is not straightforward. In Section 16.3.1, where we were considering simply an increase in sample size, this was not an issue; the *p*-value for the first part was again based on the comparison between the two treatments. In our example however, we have three active treatment groups plus placebo. You might think it valid to go back and use the *p*-value that compares the chosen dose with placebo from the first part of the trial, but it is not. This would be 'cherry-picking' from the *p*-values across the three doses versus placebo. Alternatively could this be a *p*-value that is based on the maximum difference between the active groups and placebo (Dunnett's test (Dunnett, 1955)), or should it be a *p*-value for a test that identifies whether there is a trend for improved efficacy as the dose level increases or some other *p*-value? This will have to be pre-specified, but more than that, these alternative *p*-values will mean that the null hypothesis we are testing in part 1, before the adaptation, is different from the null hypothesis that we are testing in part 2, after the adaptation. The combined *p*-value will as a consequence be a *p*-value that relates to two distinct null hypotheses, albeit both associated with the efficacy of the active treatment. An additional possibility that has been discussed in applications is to have the *p*-value in part 1 testing a null hypothesis based on a surrogate endpoint with the *p*-value for part 2 connected to the clinical endpoint. In each of these cases, interpretation of the *p*-value is problematic.

If we take forwards, say, two doses into part 2, then we need to decide also at the interim point how we are going to calculate the p-value(s) (potentially we have two since we are comparing each dose with placebo) for this second part. Several possibilities exist and this compounds the problem of which of these sets of p-values (from part 1 and part 2) we use in the combination.

16.4.3 Logistical challenges
There are a number of logistical challenges that need to be overcome if a seamless trial is to be successful, and these are discussed by Maca *et al.* (2006). Some of these problems are listed below, and the reader should refer to Maca *et al.* who offer ways of dealing with them:

- The endpoint on which decisions relating to the adaptation are to be based needs to be an endpoint that becomes available in a short period of time. Otherwise, the trial will run on in terms of recruitment, and efficacy data in dosage groups that are not taken forwards in part 2 will be wasted.
- Drug supply could be difficult in that the choice regarding the dose for part 2 will need to be made at a particular point in time with supplies then available immediately.
- It is almost inevitable that the sponsor will need to be involved in the decision making at the interim point; it is too difficult to give a watertight algorithm to an IDMC or another body that covers all eventualities. This conflicts with the need to control the dissemination of results.

16.5 Other types of adaptation

16.5.1 Changing the primary endpoint
We have already mentioned in Section 16.4.2 the possibility of using a surrogate endpoint as the basis for the p-value calculation in the first part of the trial and the clinical endpoint in the second part. From a statistical point of view, the issue of changing the primary endpoint at the adaptation is another version of this. The p-value from part 1 of the trial would be based on the predefined primary endpoint, while the p-value for part 2 would be based on the new primary endpoint chosen at the point of the adaptation. A statistical test based on the combination of the p-values from the two separate parts of the trial is still valid in the sense of providing a broad test of treatment effect, but given that the endpoints in the two parts of the trial are different and hence the null hypotheses in the two parts of the trial are different, there is a major problem of interpretation. If we see a statistically significant result, what does this mean in terms of treatment benefit? The CHMP is particularly uncomfortable with this aspect.

CHMP (2007): 'Reflection Paper on Methodological Issues in Confirmatory Clinical Trials Planned with an Adaptive Design'

'The mere rejection of a global hypothesis combining results from different endpoints will not be sufficient as proof of efficacy'.

Just to reiterate, there is one aspect that is a common theme running through the statistical principles that we are following. It may seem acceptable, having chosen a more appropriate primary endpoint in part 2, to go back and calculate a standard *p*-value for this new primary endpoint for the trial as a whole, ignoring the adaptation. What is the problem with doing that? It is all to do with cherry-picking. Presumably, the endpoint that has been chosen to be primary at the adaptation point will have been chosen because it shows promise in part 1 of the trial, maybe the *p*-value associated with it is quite small with a trend towards statistical significance, and there lies the problem. We have introduced bias into the analysis of the trial overall with a part 1 *p*-value that is chosen because it is small.

Other manifestations of this same problem with the primary endpoint include:
- Changing the order in a pre-specified hierarchy of endpoints
- Promoting a secondary endpoint to become primary
- Removing or adding a component to a primary composite endpoint
- Defining a *responder* and using this as the basis for a primary endpoint rather than the pre-specified continuous endpoint

These considerations will also apply to secondary endpoints if these are to be structured, for example, to provide confirmatory conclusions in a hierarchy.

16.5.2 Focusing on a sub-population

Focusing on a sub-population could be a case of adapting inclusion/exclusion criteria in a way that changes the nature of the population being studied or taking the decision at the point of adaptation to restrict further recruitment to a well-defined subgroup. In either case, the two *p*-values, one from part 1 of the trial and one from part 2 of the trial, will relate to different populations, and a test based on a combination of those *p*-values would be difficult to interpret.

16.5.3 Dropping the placebo arm in a non-inferiority trial

We discussed in Section 12.5 and elsewhere in Chapter 12 that including a placebo arm in a non-inferiority study can be of value in terms of providing a basis to evaluate assay sensitivity. Expected differences between each active treatment and placebo may be such that relatively few patients would be needed for those comparisons with more patients needed to establish the non-inferiority of the experimental treatment compared to the active control. In an adaptive design, there would be an opportunity to terminate recruitment to the placebo arm at the interim stage and from that point on recruit only into the two active groups.

In principle, this should not cause problems provided the trial is planned carefully, although there are risks attached. The comparisons of each active arm to placebo would need to be focused on the part 1 data only where those comparisons are based on simultaneous randomisation into the two groups; it would not be correct to use all patients recruited into the active groups for comparison with placebo. The non-inferiority evaluation though would use all data from the active groups from the trial as a whole. The risk here relates to the nature of the patients recruited.

CHMP (2007): 'Reflection Paper on Methodological Issues in Confirmatory Clinical Trials Planned with an Adaptive Design'

'It is well known that clinical trials do not recruit random samples of potential patients. It might be that different types of patients would be recruited into a two-arm trial comparing an experimental treatment with placebo, a three-arm trial including experimental, reference and placebo arms, and a two-arm, non-inferiority, trial comparing the experimental with the reference treatment (e.g. placebo-controlled trials may include a patient population with less severe disease compared to a trial including active treatments only). The treatment effect may then differ to an extent that may make the combination of results from different stages impossible where the placebo arm has been stopped'.

To help prevent such issues from an operational point of view would complicate the running of the trial with concealment of the decision taken at the interim. As the regulators go on to say, a better approach from the outset here could be to run a standard study with an unbalanced randomisation, for example, 2:2:1, with fewer patients randomised to placebo.

16.6 Further regulatory considerations

16.6.1 Impact on power

We have focused primarily on using statistical methods of analysis that control the type I error. Adaptive designs however can also impact the type II error and power in ways that may not be immediately apparent as a consequence of rushing through phase II too quickly without proper consideration of dose level, target population, etc.

FDA (2010): 'Guidance for Industry. Adaptive Design Clinical Trials for Drugs and Biologics'

'Adaptive design methods, however, also have the potential to inflate the Type II error rate for one or more hypotheses. An example of this is a study that begins with multiple doses (or populations or other study features) and that early in the study is adaptively *modified to eliminate all but one or two doses to be continued to the study's end. This study risks failing to demonstrate treatment effects by making erroneous choices based on interim results that are very variable because of the limited amount of early study data. If this risk is not considered by study planners, an apparently efficient adaptive design study can mislead the drug development program and result in program failure, when it might have succeeded had there been better adaptation choices made'.*

In part, this goes to the crux of the problem. There is a tendency to try to move through phase II and into phase III too quickly without due consideration of the best dose, the most appropriate endpoint and the nature of the optimum target population.

16.6.2 Non-standard experimental settings

There are some therapeutic settings where it is acceptable to make a regulatory application based on a single phase III confirmatory study. In this situation, data from a phase II study can often provide some element of independent confirmation of efficacy; having a combined phase II/phase III study would compromise that independence. Regulators recommend that adaptive designs not be considered in such cases.

CHMP (2007): 'Reflection Paper on Methodological Issues in Confirmatory Clinical Trials Planned with an Adaptive Design'

'... a major prerequisite for an application with one pivotal trial in phase III has always been that a sufficient body of evidence from phase II is already available so that phase III can be limited to simply replicating these findings in an independent setting'.

An exception to this however is in the study of orphan diseases where the availability of patients is limited. Logistically in such situations, it may be difficult to run an extensive phase II trial followed by an even more extensive phase III. There is an acceptance of these difficulties by regulators and the use of adaptive designs in these cases.

CHMP (2007): 'Reflection Paper on Methodological Issues in Confirmatory Clinical Trials Planned with an Adaptive Design'

'Investigation of drugs for the treatment of orphan diseases is a difficult task and specific requirements apply. A single phase II/phase III combination trial may be justified if such an approach is more efficient to display the totality of available information that can be derived from a limited number of patients'.

The CHMP makes a more general point somewhat linked to this and other difficult experimental situations where the use of adaptive designs would meet with less regulatory resistance.

CHMP (2007): 'Reflection Paper on Methodological Issues in Confirmatory Clinical Trials Planned with an Adaptive Design'

'Instead, adaptive designs would be best utilized as a tool for planning clinical trials in areas where it is necessary to cope with difficult experimental situations'.

We have covered general aspects of adaptive designs in this chapter. When using such designs, it is important to proceed with caution. An ill-judged adaptive design can actually slow down the development process and lead to increases in costs when the trial fails to provide confirmatory evidence as a consequence of its adaptive structure. Many would argue that standard group sequential designs coupled with tight control of multiplicity, without the accompanying risks of ending up with a trial that does not have a robust interpretation, are the better option.

CHAPTER 17

Observational studies

17.1 Introduction

17.1.1 Non-randomised comparisons

It is widely accepted that the randomised controlled trial has the potential to provide the best evidence for the effectiveness of a new treatment. There can be some special circumstances however where conducting a randomised trial is problematic and where an external control group can be used as a basis to evaluate efficacy and safety. Such non-randomised studies however are susceptible to a range of different biases and in this chapter we will explore the nature of those biases and how to address them from a statistical point of view. It should be pointed out at a very early stage though that if a randomised controlled study is possible, ethically and logistically, then this is the design that should be used. Only if such a design is not possible should the alternative of a non-randomised study be considered.

The focus here is primarily on confirmatory phase III and late phase II studies. In early phase II, it is perfectly possible to run studies without a control group, for example, by simply looking at change from baseline on active treatment only, to give an early impression of the potential for treatment efficacy. The findings coming out of such studies however cannot be confirmatory for efficacy, but may provide information on which considered choices can be made to guide the development programme in relation to endpoints, inclusion criteria and other aspects of trial design.

17.1.2 Study types

In evaluating an experimental intervention in the non-randomised setting, the control group may be chosen either historically, based on a group of subjects who have been treated retrospectively with an alternative intervention, or concurrently where some subjects receive the experimental intervention, while the remaining subjects receive the alternative intervention. An example of a historically controlled study is in the treatment of severe hepatic veno-occlusive disease described by Richardson *et al.* (2012). These authors pointed out that although using historical controls was not ideal, the absence of any other effective

---

Statistical Thinking for Non-Statisticians in Drug Regulation, Second Edition. Richard Kay.
© 2015 John Wiley & Sons, Ltd. Published 2015 by John Wiley & Sons, Ltd.

medication in this life-threatening condition limited the options for a randomised study, and the approach with a historical control group was viewed as the best approach both ethically and practically. A total of 102 patients were assigned to receive the experimental treatment, defibrotide, while a medical review committee was tasked with selecting a control group with baseline characteristics in line with the inclusion/exclusion criteria set down for recruitment into the defibrotide treatment programme. Defibrotide was designated an orphan medicine by the EMA in 2004, and this study was part of the evidence for efficacy and safety submitted to the EMA, who recommended authorisation for defibrotide in 2013.

As an example of a concurrent control group, Bellingan *et al.* (2013) report a phase II study evaluating the efficacy and safety of intravenous interferon-beta-1a in relation to respiratory distress syndrome mortality. The treated group consisted of 37 patients, while the non-randomised concurrent control group contained of 59 patients who entered the study but who did not receive treatment either because of delays in obtaining informed consent or because of recruitment during 14-day safety windows where recruitment was stopped for the group receiving intravenous interferon-beta-1a for ongoing safety evaluation.

Deeks *et al.* (2003) provide a taxonomy of non-randomised studies. Two of these, labelled *concurrent cohort study* and *historical cohort study*, are the two most common non-randomised designs used in the pharmaceutical industry. There are other designs that can also be useful under certain circumstances. A *case–control study*, discussed later in this chapter, can provide information on for example, the safety of a medicine following authorisation. Rosiglitazone was approved in the EU in 2000 and in the USA in 1999 for the treatment of type II diabetes mellitus, but marketing authorisation was withdrawn in the EU in 2010 based on increasing risk of cardiovascular outcomes. The evidence for this increased risk came from a range of observational studies, including several case–control studies.

Another type of non-randomised study is the *cross-sectional study*. In such a study, a large cohort of subjects is identified and subjects are asked, at a specific point in time, to provide information on numerous risk factors and health outcomes. Cross-sectional studies provide a basis for assessing association but cannot provide information on causation. As an example, suppose that data from such a study showed an association between drinking milk and peptic ulcer. Can we conclude that drinking milk causes peptic ulcer? No, we cannot. This association could be the result of other relationships. For example, it could be that peptic ulcer sufferer's drink milk to relieve their symptoms, or it could be that drinking milk is more likely among farm workers who have greater exposure to pesticides and it is the pesticides that cause peptic ulcer. There are a host of possible explanations for this association, and the cross-sectional study cannot distinguish between them. This type of study is less used in the pharmaceutical industry as it cannot provide information on how treatment affects outcome although in principle it can be the basis for generating hypotheses.

The ICH E2E (2005) *Note for Guidance on Planning Pharmacovigilance Activities* lists these three study types, cohort (both retrospective and prospective), case–control and cross-sectional studies, as potential designs for use in pharmacovigilance.

17.1.3 Sources of bias

The major problem with non-randomised, externally controlled trials is bias.

ICH E10 (2001): 'Note for Guidance on Choice of Control Group in Clinical Trials'

'Inability to control bias is the major and well-recognised limitation of externally controlled trials and is sufficient in many cases to make the design unsuitable.... Blinding and randomization are not available to minimize bias when external controls are used'.

The main sources of bias in such studies (Deeks *et al.*, 2003) are as follows:
- Selection bias
- Attrition bias
- Detection bias
- Performance bias

Selection bias is caused by systematic differences in the baseline characteristics of the two groups being compared. In a randomised trial, it is the randomisation itself that takes care of this bias. Any baseline imbalances under those circumstances are simply due to chance, not so in the non-randomised case, where such differences can (and do) frequently undermine the ability of the study to reach a valid conclusion. Note that some authors use the term selection bias to refer to the biased selection of the sample of subjects to be included in the study from the population defined by the inclusion/exclusion criteria. Here, we are using the term only to refer to the biased allocation of subjects to the treatment groups.

Attrition bias occurs as a result of dropout. This type of bias can also occur in randomised trials but is likely to be less of an issue than in a non-randomised study where the follow-up information on subjects in the control group could well be less rigorous than in the experimental treatment, especially when this group is constructed retrospectively.

Detection bias is a consequence of the lack of standardisation in assessing outcomes between the treatment groups. In a blinded randomised trial, outcome assessment is by definition standardised. In an open randomised study, there is however the potential for a greater amount of detection bias, which should be controlled by protocol. In a non-randomised study, such bias is likely to be even greater.

Finally, *performance bias* occurs if there is a lack of consistency in the application and recording of the interventions. In a randomised study, this should not happen under a tight protocol.

In order to have a successful non-randomised comparison, it is essential to address each of these sources of bias and to design the study in such a way that their potential impact is minimised. It is also important, especially with selection bias, to employ statistical methods that additionally help to account for the sources of bias. We will discuss this issue further in Section 17.3.

17.1.4 An empirical investigation

Deeks *et al.* (2003) undertook an interesting exercise to investigate the impact of selection bias in using both concurrent and historical controls. These investigations were based on two large randomised multi-centre trials. The first trial was the International Stroke (IS) trial, which looked at the use of aspirin and heparin in the treatment of ischemic stroke. Patients were randomised into one of four treatment groups: placebo, heparin alone, aspirin alone and finally heparin plus aspirin. The efficacy outcome considered by these authors was dead or dependent at six months, and for the purposes of their investigations, they combined across the heparin groups and compared those patients taking aspirin (with or without heparin), considered as the treated group, with those not taking aspirin (with or without heparin), considered as the control group. The second trial was the European Carotid Surgery (ECS) trial, which evaluated the benefits of carotid endarterectomy in relation to stroke prevention, and the primary outcome for the ECS trial was death or major stroke.

For the IS trial these authors undertook a resampling (simulation) exercise to mimic the conditions that would be present firstly in a concurrent cohort study and secondly in an historical cohort study. In addition, they undertook corresponding resampling exercises to mimic conventional randomised trials. This trial recruited almost 20,000 patients in 467 centres in 36 countries. Fourteen geographical regions were constructed as a basis for the resampling, and the data were also split according to the date of recruitment to give *early recruits* (recruited up to and including 15 January 1995) and *late recruits* (recruited after 15 January 1995).

A concurrent cohort study was then constructed by sampling data from the treated group in one region and comparing with data sampled from the control group in another region (chosen at random). A corresponding randomised controlled trial was constructed for comparison purposes by sampling data from the treated group in one region and comparing with data sampled from the control group in that same region.

Similarly, a historically controlled trial was constructed by comparing data sampled from late recruiters in the treated group in a particular region with data sampled from early recruiters in the control group in the same region. A corresponding randomised controlled trial was constructed for comparison by sampling data from late recruiters in the treated group in one region and comparing with data sampled from late recruiters in the control group in that same region.

For each treatment group, samples of size 100 were used (giving a study sample size of 200), and the sampling for the concurrent control and the corresponding randomised control and for the historical control and the corresponding randomised control settings was repeated 1000 times for each of the 14 regions. In each of the four settings and for each of these 14,000 (=14×1000) studies, the odds ratio (OR) was calculated, aspirin versus no aspirin, and the distributions of these ORs were analysed.

The procedure for the ECS trial was similar, but as this was a smaller trial, only 8 regions were chosen (rather than 14) with group samples of size 40 (rather than 100). For further details of the set up for these and other evaluations, the reader is referred to the paper by Deeks *et al.* (2003). The randomised comparisons in these simulations can be considered to be giving unbiased results, and in what follows, we will compare the results from those comparisons with the results from the comparisons from the concurrently controlled studies and from the historically controlled studies.

For these analyses note that an OR <1 is indicating a benefit for the experimental treatment compared to control, while an OR >1 is indicating a harmful effect. Also note that the results reported by Deeks *et al.* (2003) and repeated here do not relate to the original analyses reported in the publications for these trials. What we are reporting here and what these authors undertook is an empirical investigation of only parts of the data for the sole purpose of investigating bias in non-randomised studies.

17.1.5 Selection bias in concurrently controlled studies: An empirical evaluation

The mean OR for the 14,000 concurrently controlled studies simulated from the IS trial data set was 0.91. The mean OR for the corresponding 14,000 randomised controlled trials was also 0.91, indicating no bias on average. This is what was expected given that, in the concurrently controlled simulation, one of the studies will be comparing treated patients from Region 4 with control patients from Region 11 for example, while another study will be comparing treated patients in Region 11 with control patients in Region 4, and on average, these will give the same *results* as the randomised comparisons that would compare treated patients in Region 4 with control patients in Region 4 and similarly for Region 11. The variation though was much greater for the concurrently controlled studies. The standard deviation for the log of the OR (*ln*OR) was 0.85 across the concurrently controlled studies compared to only 0.34 for the randomised trials, and this has implications for the numbers of spurious results. For the randomised comparisons, 7 per cent gave statistical significance ($p<0.05$) in favour of aspirin, and 2 per cent gave statistical significance in favour of no aspirin, compared to 29 per cent and 21 per cent, respectively, for the concurrently controlled comparisons. If we take the randomised comparisons as being reflective of the true situation in this investigation, then the concurrently controlled comparisons are giving many more significant results than we would expect, in both directions.

The results for the ECS data set however were somewhat different. The mean ORs were again in close agreement, but in this example, the standard deviations were also approximately equal, 0.69 for the concurrently controlled studies and 0.68 for the randomised trials, as were the percentages of studies giving statistically significant results in both directions.

17.1.6 Selection bias in historically controlled studies: An empirical evaluation

For the evaluation of the bias in historically controlled studies, Deeks *et al.* reported a mean OR of 0.88 for the 14,000 simulated historically controlled studies based on the IS trial data compared to a mean of 0.89 for the randomised controlled trials. Again, we see no bias in this particular case. There was however again a difference in the standard deviations (on the *ln*OR scale) with values of 0.44 for the historically controlled studies and 0.35 for the randomised trials. Although this difference was not as marked as that for the concurrently controlled trials, it still resulted in a larger number of significant findings in the historically controlled studies compared to the randomised setting. For the randomised trials, there were 9 per cent statistically significant results in favour of aspirin and 2 per cent in favour of no aspirin compared to 16 per cent and 4 per cent, respectively, for the historical studies. Again, we see more spurious findings for the historically controlled trials.

The results for the ECS trial data again gave a rather different picture. The mean OR for the randomised controlled trials was 1.23, while the mean OR for the historically controlled studies was only 1.06, indicating a strong bias on average. The randomised trials are suggesting an average 23 per cent increase in the odds for death or major stroke with treatment compared to only 6 per cent for the corresponding odds for the historically controlled trials. Again, do note that these findings are not reflective of the true situation with this treatment in this setting; we are simply reporting a simulation exercise to evaluate the properties of historical controls compared to randomised controls. The standard deviations for *ln* OR were similar for the randomised controlled and historically controlled studies, 0.83 and 0.85, respectively, but the difference in the mean OR values resulted in slightly more positive findings for carotid endarterectomy in the historical controlled studies compared to the randomised controlled trials (6 per cent vs. 4 per cent statistically significant results) and fewer negative findings (10 per cent vs. 12 per cent statistically significant results).

17.1.7 Some conclusions

This resampling exercise indicates the unpredictability of results when using both concurrently controlled studies and historically controlled studies compared to the randomised setting.

For the concurrently controlled studies, we saw no bias on average and this was a consequence of the way in which the resampling was undertaken, but the increased variability associated with the OR in the case of the IS data and the corresponding increase in the number of statistically significant results indicate that at the study level we would tend to produce many more statistically significant findings than we would were we to conduct a randomised study in the same setting. This is one manifestation of selection bias. The comparability of the patients in the two treatment groups in a concurrently controlled study is not guaranteed, and it is these differences in comparability that are causing increases in the numbers of statistically significant findings. The authors did not see this bias in the ECS study probably because the patients recruited across regions were more comparable.

For the historically controlled studies, again, there was no bias on average and only a small increase in the variability for the OR in the case of the IS data, but this increase did result in more statistically significant findings compared to the randomised trials. There was however bias on average for the ECS data set with a reduced OR across the historically controlled studies. Selection bias in historically controlled studies is a consequence of underlying time trends in the characteristics and behaviour of patients in the trial and in the changing trial conditions and so on and in the case of the ECS data these trends worked against treatment differences.

These findings have clear implications for the way in which non-randomised studies of this kind are conducted. It is essential that the subjects assigned to treatment and control groups are comparable and are treated within a common environment as much as possible. This is more likely to achieve in a concurrently controlled study compared to a historically controlled study.

17.2 Guidance on design, conduct and analysis

17.2.1 Regulatory guidance

When should non-randomised comparative studies be considered? There appear to be several situations:

- When the scientific and clinical community strongly believes that the test therapy is superior to all other available therapies. Under these circumstances, it would be extremely difficult to conduct a randomised study that would attract sufficient investigators who would be willing to recruit patients into the study.
- When the course of disease is highly predictable based on clinical evidence.

ICH E10 (2001): 'Note for Guidance on Choice of Control Group in Clinical Trials'

'An externally controlled trial should generally be considered only when prior belief in the superiority of the test therapy to all available alternatives is so strong that alternative designs appear unacceptable and the disease or condition to be treated has a well-documented, highly predictable course'.

- In orphan indications where the population size is limited and using for example, a historical control group may be the only way to gain enough statistical power to demonstrate a treatment difference.

CHMP (2006): 'Guideline on Clinical Trials in Small Populations'

'Although internal controls are the preferred option for comparative trials, under exceptional circumstances external controls may be acceptable. Historical controls (using patients treated with "current" therapies, or not treated at all) might, in some circumstances (even if not routinely), be acceptable to demonstrate efficacy, safety, ease of administration and so on, of a new treatment'.

The ICH E10 guideline includes comments on the control of bias and associated requirements for successful non-randomised studies:

- The study endpoint or endpoints should be objective.
- The persuasiveness of findings from non-randomised studies is greater when there is a high degree of statistical significance and much larger estimated differences than we would normally expect from a randomised trial.
- Covariates influencing outcome should be well characterised. We will talk in Section 17.3 about adjusting for baseline covariates to help account for selection bias, and having well-established predictors of outcome is necessary for this to be helpful.
- The control group and the experimental treatment group should be highly comparable in terms of all relevant baseline factors and concomitant treatments received.
- When no clear control group is available, it is of value to study a range of possibilities and to show superiority of the experimental treatment to the most favourable control group.
- It can be useful to involve an independent set of reviewers to reassess endpoints in a blinded way. It can also be useful to involve an independent committee in selecting the control group, again working in a blinded way, but this time blind to outcome. The defibrotide example discussed in Section 17.1.2 had such a group.

17.2.2 Strengthening the Reporting of Observational Studies in Epidemiology

The Strengthening the Reporting of Observational Studies in Epidemiology (STROBE) initiative began in 2004 and was reported in 2007 (von Elm *et al.*, 2007). This initiative developed recommendations for the accurate and complete reporting of observational studies covering the three main study designs, cohort, case–control and cross-sectional designs. These recommendations are provided in terms of a 22-item checklist, some of which are general, while others are specific to the type of design. The authors are clear to point out that STROBE does not provide guidance on design and conduct. Nonetheless, following the checklist for reporting the design, conduct and results of a study will help researchers to think through some important aspects of those aspects. The authors also point out that STROBE is not a tool for assessing the quality of observational studies. Tools for assessing quality are available and the reader is referred to Deeks *et al.* (2003) and Viswanathan *et al.* (2013) for more details.

17.3 Evaluating and adjusting for selection bias

17.3.1 Baseline balance

Selection bias will result in imbalances in known and unknown baseline factors. In a randomised trial, the randomisation itself protects against imbalance, at least in large studies. Methods as discussed in Chapters 5 and 6, in particular ANCOVA, can be used to adjust for any imbalances that do occur in relation to known and measured baseline factors. In a non-randomised study, there will be greater baseline imbalances, and one key aspect of assessing the validity of such a study is an evaluation of the balance of baseline factors across the experimental and control groups. It is only of course possible to undertake this evaluation for known factors that have been measured in patients in both treatment groups. This is one of the drawbacks of a non-randomised study compared to a randomised study. In a randomised study, there is a guarantee that factors that have not been measured will on average be balanced across the groups. In non-randomised studies, we can only assess balance for those factors that have been measured.

How should we best do this? It is tempting to use *p*-values at baseline to identify factors that are statistically significantly different between the treatment groups and maybe then adjust for those. We have already indicated that this is of no value in randomised studies, 5 per cent of such tests will be significant purely by chance. See Section 6.8 for further discussion on this point. Such significance testing is also of little help in non-randomised studies. There may be important factors, unbalanced at baseline, that are highly predictive of outcome but yet give non-significant *p*-values. This could be because the imbalance is only modest yet very important clinically, while the sample size is not large enough to give sufficient power to detect statistical significance. Conversely, we could see statistically significant differences for a factor that has no impact on patient outcome, in which case the imbalances are irrelevant and will not influence our ability to obtain a valid treatment comparison. As discussed in Section 9.2, *p*-values tell us nothing about magnitude, and it is the magnitude of the difference, and whether this is for a factor that predicts outcome, that determines if that difference is relevant.

The best way to evaluate baseline imbalances is to consider these from a clinical perspective. The focus should be on those factors that are likely to influence outcome, and clinical judgment is then required to assess whether any observed imbalances could potentially undermine the validity of the treatment comparisons.

17.3.2 Adjusting for imbalances using stratification and analysis of covariance

In Chapter 5, we presented a detailed development of methods for adjusting or stratifying the analysis to account for baseline imbalances in randomised trials. These same techniques can also be used in non-randomised studies. The limitation of these methods, in that only a small number of baseline factors can be included, was raised in Section 6.1. In non-randomised studies, it is very likely that we are dealing with imbalances that not only are more severe but are also affecting several important predictors of outcome. The ANCOVA methods detailed in Chapter 6 are better equipped to deal with many baseline factors, and it is these methods that potentially have greater value in non-randomised comparisons. Section 6.5 dealt with continuous (and score) endpoints and this is where the ANCOVA technique was introduced. In Section 6.6, we covered non-continuous endpoint types, in particular logistic regression, which is a methodology that enables corrections to be made for baseline imbalances when the endpoint is binary. Finally, in Section 13.5, we presented methods for adjustment when the endpoint is time to event. The proportional hazards model enabled us to adjust for multiple factors for endpoints of this kind. So to recap, in any non-randomised study, we will usually be looking to adjust for a range of baseline factors, and it is ANCOVA (continuous, score endpoints), logistic regression (binary and ordinal endpoints) and the proportional hazards model (time-to-event endpoints) that provide the most useful approaches.

17.3.3 Propensity scores

Propensity score methods were first introduced by Rosenbaum and Rubin (1983) and provide an alternative way to adjust for baseline factors, especially where these are large in number. D'Agostino (1998) presents an extensive discussion of the technique when used for comparing a treated group to a non-randomised control group. The methodology is best presented through an example.

Austin and Mamdani (2006) undertook a comparison of different propensity score methods in a study evaluating the use of statins in reducing all-cause mortality in patients discharged from hospital who had been admitted previously with a diagnosis of acute myocardial infarction (MI). The cohort of patients consisted initially of 11,524 individuals admitted to hospitals in Ontario, Canada, with a diagnosis of acute MI between 1 April 1999 and 31 March 2001. Of these, 1137 died during hospitalisation and 1283 were excluded from further consideration due to incomplete data on baseline factors collected during hospitalisation. A total of 9104 were therefore included in the analysis. Of these, 3049 (33.5 per cent) were prescribed statins on discharge, while 6055 were not. The objective of the analysis was to evaluate the effectiveness of statins to reduce three-year mortality. This was not a randomised study, and it may well be that the statins were prescribed only for certain kinds of patients as decided by the physician treating the patient at the time of discharge. Without considering any kind of adjustment for baseline imbalances, the three-year mortality among patients receiving statins was 14.2 per cent compared to 25.3 per cent for those patients who did not receive statins with an OR of 0.49 and $p<0.0001$. This result is highly statistically significant with almost a 50 per cent reduction in the odds of dying within three years. However, there is selection bias potentially influencing this result caused by differences in known (and unknown) factors measured at baseline. Data was available on 24 baseline factors including age, gender, presenting characteristics (shock, acute chronic heart failure/pulmonary oedema), acute MI risk factors (family history, diabetes, etc.), co-morbidities (angina, cancer, etc.), vital signs on admission (diastolic and systolic blood pressure, heart rate, respiratory rate) and finally laboratory parameters (white blood count, haemoglobin, etc.).

The basic idea behind the propensity score is to estimate the probability that a patient would receive a statin (as opposed to not receiving a statin) based on these baseline factors. We will denote this quantity by

$$\text{Prob}\left(\text{patient with baseline characteristics } x_1, x_2, \ldots, x_{24} \text{ receives a statin}\right)$$

Here x_1 denotes age, x_2 denotes whether the patient is male or female and so on through all the 24 baseline factors. To give a flavour of how this is done, let's suppose we were adjusting for just two factors, gender and whether or not a patient was diabetic, and consider the (artificial) data set down in Table 17.1.

In this hypothetical example, overall, 1190 patients received statins and 2500 did not. We have split the data down according to the two baseline factors: gender and diabetic/non-diabetic. Of the 590 male diabetics, only 210 received a statin that is 36 per cent, so the probability that a male diabetic receives a statin is 0.36. Similarly, the probabilities associated with the other factor combinations are given in the final column. This probability is what we term the *propensity score* – it is the probability of receiving the intervention. So across the whole dataset, each patient has a propensity score that differs from patient to patient depending on their baseline characteristics. With lots more baseline factors to account for, it is not possible to divide the data up according to all combinations of baseline factors and do what we did in Table 17.1, but the principle is the same. With lots of baseline factors, we do this by building a logistic regression model for

Table 17.1 Constructing propensity scores based on two characteristics (hypothetical)

	Statin	Non-statin	Total	Probability (patient receives statin)
Male, diabetic	210	380	590	210/590 = 0.36
Male, non-diabetic	660	1200	1860	660/1860 = 0.35
Female, diabetic	90	300	390	90/390 = 0.23
Female, non-diabetic	230	620	850	230/850 = 0.27
	1190	2500		

the probability of receiving the intervention. See Section 6.4 for a little more discussion on logistic regression. In this logistic model, the **outcome** variable is the binary variable that takes the value 1 if the patient receives the statin and 0 if the patient does not receive the statin. Fitting this model then gives a propensity score for each and every patient in the sample as the probability that that particular patient, with baseline factors $x_1, x_2, ..., x_{24}$, would have received a statin. This probability assignment has been based on which patients are more or less likely to receive a statin according to the patterns in the data. In a randomised study, each of these probabilities is equal to 0.50 as a result of the randomisation; every patient has a 50/50 chance of receiving the experimental treatment! In a non-randomised study however, investigator or patient preferences or both will take these probabilities away from 0.50.

So, how do we now use these propensity scores? Well, there are several possibilities. Firstly, we could compare the statin and non-statin patients in terms of their three-year mortality rates by stratifying by the propensity score. So, for example, we divide all of the patients according to their values of the propensity score, <0.20, ≥0.20 but <0.40, ≥0.40 but <0.60, ≥0.60 but <0.80 and ≥0.80, to create a structure as in Table 17.2. The n's in the table refer to the numbers of patients within each category.

Stratifying by the propensity score produces subsets of statin and non-statin patients with similar propensity scores, and what a stratified analysis does is to calculate a treatment difference for each of these subsets. So in our hypothetical example, there would be five such treatment differences and the stratified analysis then averages these (as in Section 5.2). The basic idea is that patients with the same (or similar) propensity score have the same (or similar) probability to receive a statin, and whether or not they do is simply *chance*. What we have effectively done is to mimic a randomised setting where each patient within each of these 5 strata has a similar probability to get the experimental treatment. It is fairly standard practice to use five groupings. These groupings can be based on a fixed split of the propensity score as in Table 17.2 or chosen according to the quintiles across both groups combined. So the first subset includes those patients

Table 17.2 Stratified analysis by propensity score (hypothetical)

Propensity score	Statin	Non-statin
<0.20	$n=30$	$n=180$
≥0.20 but <0.40	$n=38$	$n=150$
≥0.40 but <0.60	$n=62$	$n=121$
≥0.60 but <0.80	$n=144$	$n=63$
≥0.80	$n=205$	$n=26$
Total	479	540

Table 17.3 Analysis of the statin observational study by propensity score and other methods

	OR	p-value
Unadjusted	0.49	<0.0001
Model-based adjustment using 24 factors	0.75	<0.0001
Stratified by quintiles of the propensity score	0.77	0.0003
Model-based adjustment using the propensity score	0.84	0.0033
Matching on propensity score	0.85	0.037

who have the lowest 20 per cent of propensity scores, the second subset includes the next 20 per cent of patients according to their propensity scores, and so on with the fifth subset containing the 20 per cent with the highest scores.

This stratified analysis has adjusted for propensity score, but this is not the only way to adjust. A second approach uses the propensity score as a covariate in its own right in an adjusted (model-based) analysis, and finally, a third approach takes each patient in the statin group and matches to a patient in the control group with a propensity score that is the closest. The two resulting groups (by definition of the same size) are then compared using a simple two-group test (such as the chi-square test). Table 17.3 shows the ORs from each of these three methods for the statin example together with the OR from the simple comparison without adjustment, and also an analysis that uses all 24 of the baseline factors in an adjusted (model-based) analysis (Austin and Mamdani, 2006).

It is noticeable that all of the adjusted analyses give ORs that are closer to 1 compared to the unadjusted analysis. This indicates that the unadjusted analysis is overestimating the benefit of statins in reducing the three-year mortality. Each of the adjusted analyses is giving an OR between 0.75 and 0.85, indicating between a 15 per cent and 25 per cent reduction in the odds for death within three years. All of the results are statistically significant at the 5 per cent level, but the matching method has a much less significant p-value. This is as a result of using a reduced sample size. The matching method, matched on a 1 to 1 basis, so that the number of patients used in that analysis was simply double the sample size in the statin group. This gave an overall sample size that was only around 67 per cent of the sample size used for the other adjustment methods resulting in a loss of power.

17.3.4 Different methods for adjustment: An empirical evaluation

Deeks *et al.* (2003) undertook an empirical investigation of the ability of these methods to adjust in both the concurrently controlled studies and the historically controlled studies to bring the results back in line with the results of the randomised studies. They used those studies that were sampled previously in their evaluation of selection bias and described in Section 17.1. As these authors point out, these methods of baseline adjustment are looking to achieve, through analysis, what could not be achieved by design.

A total of 10 relevant baseline factors, in terms of factors that were viewed as potentially predicting outcome, were considered for the IS trial, while 7 factors were considered for the ECS trial. For the IS trial, these included sex, age, atrial fibrillation (yes/no), infarct visible on CT scan, etc., while for the ESCT trial, factors included sex, age, previous MI, degree of stenosis, etc. For our purposes, we will consider the unadjusted analysis and then only a subset of the adjustment methods considered by Deeks *et al.* (2003), namely:

- Logistic regression adjusting for all baseline factors
- Propensity score adjustment based on 5 strata
- Propensity score adjustment based on using the score as a covariate
- Propensity score adjustment-based matching

The results of these investigations into methods of adjustment are contained for the concurrently controlled studies in Table 17.4 for the IS study and Table 17.5 for the ECS study. Similar tables for the historically controlled studies are Table 17.6 for the IS data and Table 17.7 for the ECS data. Note that in each case the results for the randomised control and for the unadjusted analysis have already been discussed in Sections 17.1.5 and 17.1.6. The main issues centre around whether the methods of adjustment have improved on the unadjusted methods in terms of bringing the results in line with the unbiased results from the randomised studies. In each evaluation, it is the number of significant findings that tell us how much more likely we are to be deceived compared to the *true* situation as reflected by the randomised study results.

Table 17.4 Comparison of methods of adjustment for baseline imbalance: Concurrently controlled studies resampled from the IS trial

Method	% of studies with $p < 0.05$	
	Benefit	Harm
Randomised control	7	2
Unadjusted	29	21
Logistic regression	23	18
Propensity score; stratified	19	15
Propensity score; logistic regression	19	15
Propensity score; matched	15	12

Source: Deeks *et al.*, 2003. Reproduced with permission from National Institute for Health Research.

Table 17.5 Comparison of methods of adjustment for baseline imbalance: Concurrently controlled studies resampled from the ECS trial

Method	% of studies with $p < 0.05$	
	Benefit	Harm
Randomised control	3	5
Unadjusted	3	6
Logistic regression	4	6
Propensity score; stratified	5	3
Propensity score; logistic regression	5	3
Propensity score; matched	2	6

Source: Deeks et al., 2003. Reproduced with permission from National Institute for Health Research.

Table 17.6 Comparison of methods of adjustment for baseline imbalance: Historically controlled studies resampled from the IS trial

Method	% of studies with $p < 0.05$	
	Benefit	Harm
Randomised control	9	2
Unadjusted	16	4
Logistic regression	13	3
Propensity score; stratified	9	2
Propensity score; logistic regression	9	2
Propensity score; matched	7	2

Source: Deeks et al., 2003. Reproduced with permission from National Institute for Health Research.

In Table 17.4 for the IS data, we see that there are statistically significant findings in 9 per cent of the randomised studies, 7 per cent in favour of aspirin (benefit) and 2 per cent against (harm), while the unadjusted analysis for the concurrently controlled studies gave a total of 50 per cent, 29 per cent in favour of aspirin and 21 per cent against. All of the adjustment methods improve on the unadjusted analyses. The biggest improvement comes from the propensity score adjustment-based matching, which gives a total of 27 per cent statistically significant studies, split 15 per cent in favour of aspirin and 12 per cent against.

Table 17.7 Comparison of methods of adjustment for baseline imbalance: Historically controlled studies resampled from the ECS trial

Method	% of studies with $p < 0.05$	
	Benefit	Harm
Randomised control	4	12
Unadjusted	6	10
Logistic regression	12	14
Propensity score; stratified	12	10
Propensity score; logistic regression	12	10
Propensity score; matched	5	10

Source: Deeks et al., 2003. Reproduced with permission from National Institute for Health Research.

Table 17.5 presents results for the concurrently controlled studies based on the ECS trial data. A total of 8 per cent of the randomised studies gave statistically significant results, 3 per cent showing a benefit for carotid surgery and 5 per cent showing harm. In this case, as was seen in Section 17.1.5, the unadjusted analyses actually performed in a similar way, showing little bias in this case. Here, all of the adjusted methods seem to leave things pretty much unchanged although it is the propensity score-matched analyses that are closest to the randomised analyses (and the unadjusted analyses).

Table 17.6 presents the results for the adjusted analyses for the historically controlled studies for the IS data. The unadjusted analyses gave 20 per cent statistically significant studies, 16 per cent in favour of aspirin and 4 per cent against. This compared to only 11 per cent for the randomised studies, 9 per cent in favour and 2 per cent against. The propensity score adjustment methods worked well here in terms of correcting the results of the analyses to be in line with the randomised studies with little to choose between them.

Table 17.7 presents the analyses for the ECS trial data. Here, there were 16 per cent of studies giving statistically significant results for the unadjusted analyses, 6 per cent in favour of carotid surgery and 10 per cent against. This contrasted slightly with the randomised studies where 4 per cent showed a benefit and 12 per cent showed harm. Each of the adjustment methods made things worse compared to the unadjusted analyses with the exception of the propensity score adjustment-based matching method where the results were closest to those for the randomised studies.

17.3.5 Some conclusions

This empirical investigation has given somewhat mixed results firstly in terms of the value of adjustment in correcting for selection bias and secondly, of the adjustment methods considered, which one gives the best results. For the IS trial, all the methods of adjustment considered improved on the unadjusted analyses, but it was the propensity score method that used matching that made the biggest improvement and indeed for the historically controlled studies brought the results back in line with those from the randomised studies.

For the ECS trial, the results for the unadjusted analyses were already similar to those for the randomised studies and little was gained through adjustment. In some cases, in particular for the historically controlled studies, some adjustment methods made things worse although again the propensity score method based on matching appeared to be that approach that gave results most similar to the unadjusted analyses and hence closest to the results from the randomised studies. It was argued earlier that it was the homogeneity in patient characteristics and probably the standardisation of the environment in which patients were treated across the regions in the ECS trial that resulted in the unadjusted analyses being close to the randomised analyses for the concurrently controlled studies.

It is difficult based on these specific empirical investigations to make general recommendations, but two points are worth making:

- When comparability between the two groups is achieved, adjustment does not appear to be useful. As mentioned earlier in this section, comparability is likely easier to achieve with a concurrent control group rather than with a historical control group,
- When comparability between the groups cannot or has not been achieved, then adjustment using propensity scores based on matching seems to be the preferred approach,

17.4 Case–control studies

17.4.1 Background

The purpose of this section is to comment on some statistical aspects associated with case–control studies. Case–control studies have a long history, and such a study (Doll and Bradford-Hill, 1950) was the basis for establishing the causal effects of smoking on lung cancer. In this example, the cases were subjects with the disease that is being investigated, lung cancer, while controls were those subjects without the disease.

In general, each case is matched to one or more controls on the basis of sex, age and possibly geographical location (e.g. each case may be matched to a control from the same GP practice). Controls can be thought of as subjects who do not have the disease under study, but had they had the disease, then they would have been included as cases. The disease under study is considered in this case as the *outcome*. We now ascertain for each case and each control whether or not they have the *attribute* (smoking in the earlier example) that we are

Table 17.8 Case–control study investigating smoking and lung cancer (hypothetical data). One control to each case

	Lung cancer	No lung cancer	Total
Smoker	170	50	220
Non-smoker	30	150	180
Total	200	200	400

investigating. Research suggests that between one and four controls per case can be used depending on practicality. More controls will to a certain extent increase the power, but this should not be at the expense of choosing controls who are not good matches as that will have the opposite effect and weaken the size of the effect we are trying to establish. Table 17.8 provides some hypothetical data for the smoking example for illustrative purposes.

In this example, 200 cases were chosen and there was a 1 to 1 matching to give 200 controls. Of the 200 cases, 170 were smokers, while 30 were non-smokers. For the 200 controls, 50 were smokers, while 150 were non-smokers. The OR for lung cancer is calculated as

$$OR = \frac{170/50}{30/150} = 17$$

Note that odds for the smokers, the attribute we are investigating, go as the numerator, while the odds for the non-smokers provide the denominator. This is a large OR and would give a highly statistically significant result. In the original investigation (Doll and Bradford-Hill, 1950) for the males, there were 649 cases (lung cancer) and 649 controls (no lung cancer). Among the cases, 647 were smokers and 2 were non-smokers, and among the controls, 622 were smokers, while 27 were non-smokers. The OR was 14.04 with $p = 0.00000064$! For the females (60 cases and 60 controls), the OR was less dramatic (OR = 2.47) but nonetheless statistically significant, $0.01 < p < 0.02$. These authors clearly established through this case–control study that there was a causal effect of smoking on lung cancer. The Doll and Bradford-Hill study was conducted at 20 London hospitals, and these hospitals were asked to include all cases of lung cancer. Each case was matched with a control patient with a disease other than cancer who was of the same sex, closely comparable in terms of age (within a five-year age band) and from the same hospital or, if this was not possible, from a neighbouring hospital. This study remains the classic example of a well-designed and well-conducted case–control study.

One critical aspect of a case–control study is the population from which the controls are taken. There has been considerable discussion over many years about the risk of soft tissue sarcoma following exposure to phenoxy herbicides and chlorophenols, and a number of case–control studies have been conducted.

See Smith and Christophers (1992) for a general discussion. In some studies, controls have been taken from the general population, while in others, the controls have been patients with other cancers. It may be that those studies with controls from the general population overestimate the risk because of poor recall regarding exposure, while studies using controls with other cancers underestimate the risk if phenoxy herbicides and chlorophenols are linked to other cancers. The true risk may be somewhere between the two.

Nowadays, within the pharmaceutical industry, case–control studies are used primarily within the context of safety evaluation and pharmacovigilance. In these settings, the serious side effect of interest is the outcome, while the drug being evaluated is the attribute. As mentioned earlier, a series of such studies were conducted to investigate the risk of cardiovascular adverse effects associated with rosiglitazone in patients with type II diabetes.

17.4.2 Odds ratio and relative risk

In Section 4.5, we discussed both odds ratios and relative risks and drew the distinction between the two. We also discussed the difficulties in interpreting odds ratios as opposed to relative risks. In this section, we will explore this distinction again in the context of a case–control study. Looking at the data in Table 17.8, we can at least in theory think in terms of calculating a relative risk, that is, the risk of lung cancer among smokers divided by the risk of lung cancer among non-smokers. This relative risk is $RR = \dfrac{170/220}{30/180} = 4.64$. Suppose however that we have decided to have, for example, two rather than one matching controls for each case. The data would then be as in Table 17.9.

In this case, the relative risk is $RR = \dfrac{170/270}{30/330} = 6.93$. The relative risk has changed merely as a result of choosing a different design, two controls to each case as opposed to one control per case. This is clearly unsatisfactory and is indeed why relative risks should not be used in case–control studies. We must remember that this is not a randomised comparison with subjects randomised to be smokers or non-smokers and we do not have control over the

Table 17.9 Case–control study investigating smoking and lung cancer (hypothetical data). Two controls to each case

	Lung cancer	No lung cancer	Total
Smoker	170	100	270
Non-smoker	30	300	330
Total	200	400	600

proportions of these types of subjects in the study. The odds ratio for Table 17.9 however is $OR = \dfrac{170/100}{30/300} = 17$, unchanged from the odds ratio from Table 17.8. The odds ratio is unaffected by changing the ratio of controls to cases. This is one of the main reasons behind the importance and usefulness of the odds ratio as a suitable statistic for the evaluation of binary data in that in some settings it is not possible to calculate a relative risk. A further point to make is that with large sample sizes and rare events, the relative risk and the odds ratio take similar numerical values (see Section 4.5.6), and in many case–control studies, we are in this situation. It is then often possible to calculate the odds ratio, but then for ease of interpretation, talk in terms of relative risk and risk reduction/increase.

CHAPTER 18

Meta-analysis

18.1 Definition

Meta-analysis is a formal way of bringing together the results from separate studies to provide an overview regarding a particular treatment or intervention. More generally, the phrases statistical or systematic review/overview are sometimes used to describe an analysis of this kind. Meta-analysis, however, should not be confused with pooling. *Pooling* is a related procedure that simply puts all the data together and treats the data as if they came from a single study. Meta-analysis does not do this; it recognises study-to-study variation and indeed looks to see if the data from the different studies are giving a consistent answer. Meta-analysis is to be preferred to pooling as Example 18.1 illustrates.

Example 18.1 Success rates in removing kidney stones

This non-randomised investigation (Julious and Mullee, 1994) compared open surgery with percutaneous nephrolithotomy in removing kidney stones. Table 18.1 presents the data separately for patients presenting with small stones (<2 cm diameter) and for patients with larger stones (≥2 cm in diameter).

Table 18.1 Contingency tables for kidney stones

Stone diameter <2 cm	Success	Failure	Total
Open surgery	81 (93%)	6	87
Percutaneous nephrolithotomy	234 (87%)	36	270

Stone diameter ≥2 cm	Success	Failure	Total
Open surgery	192 (73%)	71	263
Percutaneous nephrolithotomy	55 (69%)	25	80

Statistical Thinking for Non-Statisticians in Drug Regulation, Second Edition. Richard Kay.
© 2015 John Wiley & Sons, Ltd. Published 2015 by John Wiley & Sons, Ltd.

It is clear from each of these tables that open surgery is more successful than percutaneous nephrolithotomy (success rates are 93 per cent vs. 87 per cent for small stones and 73 per cent vs. 69 per cent for large stones), irrespective of the size of the kidney stone.

Now however consider pooling the data (Table 18.2).

Table 18.2 Combined data

Diameter <2 cm and ≥2 cm combined	Success	Failure	Total
Open surgery	273 (78%)	77	350
Percutaneous nephrolithotomy	289 (83%)	61	350

This table suggests that percutaneous nephrolithotomy has a higher success rate (83 per cent vs. 78 per cent) than open surgery, but we are being fooled; it is the reverse that is true. The pooled table is misleading and it is the separate tables that are the basis of a correct interpretation. We are being misled because of two things: firstly, patients with small stones do better than patients with larger stones, and secondly, patients with small stones tend to receive percutaneous nephrolithotomy. The overall high success rate on percutaneous nephrolithotomy is primarily due to the fact that in the main the patients who received percutaneous nephrolithotomy were those presented with small kidney stones.

This phenomenon, known as *Simpson's paradox*, illustrates the dangers of simple pooling. A meta-analysis approach for these data would retain the separate tables and compute a treatment difference for the patients with small stones and a treatment difference for patients with larger stones. These two differences would then be *averaged* to give a valid overall treatment difference.

Example 18.2 Adverse event rates (hypothetical)

In two randomised trials, each with 300 patients, comparing two active treatments in terms of the incidence of a particular adverse event, the data were as follows (Table 18.3):

Table 18.3 Adverse event rates in two trials

Treatment A	Treatment B	Difference
10.0% ($n=100$)	8.0% ($n=200$)	2.0%
3.5% ($n=200$)	2.0% ($n=100$)	1.5%

Pooling the data gives an overall adverse event rate on treatment A of 5.7 per cent, compared to 6.0 per cent on treatment, a pooled difference (A – B) of –0.3 per cent with a higher rate on treatment B. This is clearly misleading since in each trial there is a higher adverse event rate on treatment A, and a more appropriate measure of the treatment difference is given by the average absolute difference of 1.75 per cent.

Example 18.2 (hypothetical data) illustrates how these problems with pooling could occur with data on adverse events within the context of randomised comparisons.

It is recognised that the studies usually being combined in a meta-analysis will not all be identical and will not all have the same protocol. The dosages may be different, the precise definition of the endpoints may be different, treatment duration may differ, the nature of both the treatment and the comparator may be different and so on. Clearly, the more specific the research question being addressed by the meta-analysis, the more closely the studies must match, but the breadth of the studies that are combined will depend on the breadth of the question being asked.

18.2 Objectives

Meta-analysis is used in numerous different ways and both within and outside of the regulatory setting.

The technique can provide a quantification of the current state of knowledge regarding a particular treatment both in terms of safety and efficacy. The *Cochrane Collaboration* uses the methodology extensively to provide systematic overviews of treatments in particular therapeutic areas and to answer general health questions.

In a similar way, meta-analysis can be a useful way to combine the totality of data from studies in relation to a particular treatment, perhaps as the basis for a marketing campaign.

Combining studies can also very effectively increase power for primary or secondary efficacy endpoints or for particular subgroups. Individual studies are unlikely to be powered for secondary endpoints and subgroups, and meta-analysis can be a way of increasing power in relation to these. For primary endpoints, increasing the power in this way will improve precision (reduce the standard error) and give narrower confidence intervals enabling clinical benefit to be more clearly understood. In evaluating safety issues, it may well be that there is simply not enough information in any single trial and a meta-analysis is better able to make comparative inferences and identify safety problems. This is a useful approach within an integrated safety evaluation at the regulatory submission stage but also useful retrospectively when safety concerns arise.

A more recent area of application for meta-analysis is in the choice of the non-inferiority margin, Δ. As mentioned in Section 12.7, Δ is often chosen as some proportion of the established treatment effect (over placebo), and meta-analysis can be used to obtain an estimate of that treatment effect and an associated confidence interval.

Combining studies can be useful in resolving apparently conflicting results. For example, Mulrow (1994) reported a meta-analysis of trials of intravenous streptokinase for treatment in acute myocardial infarction. The complete analysis involved a total of 33 trials reported between 1959 and 1988, and Mulrow presented a *cumulative meta-analysis* that combined the trials chronologically over time. Of the eight trials reported between 1959 and the end of 1973, five gave odds ratios that favoured intravenous streptokinase (two were statistically significant), while three trials gave odds ratios favouring control (none were statistically significant). In one sense, there was a confusing picture emerging with six negative/inconclusive trials out of the first eight conducted. The meta-analysis combination at that point in time, however, gave a clear result, with an odds ratio around 0.75 in favour of streptokinase and a highly significant *p*-value of 0.0071.

The technique can also address whether or not the studies provide a consistent result, and exploring heterogeneity is a key element of any meta-analysis.

In the applications that follow, we will focus on the combination of clinical trials although the methodology can also apply more widely in an epidemiological setting.

18.3 Statistical methodology

18.3.1 Methods for combination

Each trial that is to be included in the meta-analysis will provide a measure of treatment effect (difference). For continuous data, this could be the mean response on the active treatment minus the mean response in the placebo arm. Alternatively, for binary data, the treatment effect could be captured by the difference in the cure rates, for example, or by the odds ratio. For survival data, the hazard ratio would usually be the measure of treatment difference.

Assume that we have decided on the best measure for the treatment effect. If this is expressed as a difference, for example, in the means, then there will be an associated standard error measuring the precision of that difference. If the treatment effect is captured by a ratio, for example, an odds ratio or a hazard ratio, then there will be an associated standard error on the log scale, the standard error of the log odds ratio or the standard error of the log hazard ratio.

Again, whichever measure of treatment effect is chosen, the meta-analysis combination proceeds in a standard way. We average the treatment effect over the m studies being combined. This is not the straight average, but a weighted average, weighted according to the precision of each individual study, and this precision is captured by the standard error. This is very similar to what we did in Section 5.2 when we adjusted the analysis for comparing treatments for baseline factors. In our development here, stratum is replaced by study. For study i, let d_i

be the treatment effect with associated standard error se_i. The overall estimate of the treatment effect is then

$$d = (w_1 d_1 + w_2 d_2 + \cdots + w_m d_m) / (w_1 + w_2 + \cdots + w_m)$$

where $w_i = 1/se_i^2$. Essentially weighting by the inverse of the standard error in this way is weighting primarily by the sample size so that the larger, more precise studies are given more weight.

If the treatment effect in each of the individual trials is the difference in the mean responses, then d represents the overall adjusted mean difference. If the treatment effect in the individual trials is the log odds ratio, then d is the overall adjusted log odds ratio and so on. In the case of overall estimates on the log scale, we generally antilog this final result to give us a measure back on the original scale, for example, on the odds ratio scale. This is similar to the approach we saw in Section 4.5.5 when we looked at calculating a confidence interval for an odds ratio. Again note that for ratios we work on the log scale because that is the scale on which we have a formula for the standard error.

18.3.2 Confidence intervals

The methods of the previous subsection give us a combined estimate, d, for the treatment effect. We now need to construct a confidence interval around this estimate. This initially involves obtaining a standard error for d, which is given by

$$se = \frac{1}{\sqrt{w_1 + w_2 + \cdots + w_m}}$$

From this, it is easy to obtain a 95 per cent confidence interval for the overall treatment effect as $(d - 1.96se,\ d + 1.96se)$.

If this confidence interval is on the log scale, for example, with the odds ratio and the hazard ratio, then both the lower and upper confidence limits should be converted by using the antilog to give a confidence interval on the original odds ratio or hazard ratio scale.

18.3.3 Fixed and random effects

The *fixed effects model* considers the studies that have been combined as the totality of all the studies conducted. An alternative approach considers the collection of studies included in the meta-analysis as a random selection of the studies that have been conducted or a random selection of those that could have been conducted. This results in a slightly changed methodology, termed the *random effects model*. The random effects model allows the true treatment effect to be different for the different trials. For example let θ_1 be the true difference in the cure rates in trial 1, θ_2 be the true difference in trial 2 and so on to trial m with a true difference in the means of θ_m. The model then assumes that the *m* different values

θ_1, θ_2, etc. are drawn from a normal distribution with mean θ and variance τ^2. The random effects model implicitly allows for study-to-study variation, and the resulting analysis provides estimates of the overall mean θ and the variance τ^2. The mathematics for fixed and random effects models is a little different, and the reader is referred to Fleiss (1993), for example, for further details. The net effect of using a random effects model is to produce a different estimate for the overall treatment effect and a slightly more conservative analysis with wider confidence intervals. Both approaches are valid and useful.

18.3.4 Graphical methods

An extremely useful addition to the formal method for combining the studies is to represent the data from the individual studies, together with the combination, in a *forest plot*. Example 18.3 displays this kind of plot. Note that the confidence intervals in Figure 18.1 are not symmetric around the estimated hazard ratio. This is because confidence intervals for hazard ratios and odds ratio and indeed ratios in general are symmetric only on the log scale and once the endpoints of the interval are transformed back onto the ratio scale, symmetry is lost. Sometimes, we see plots where the *x*-axis is on the log scale, although the scale will be calibrated in terms of the ratio itself, and in this case, the confidence intervals will appear symmetric.

The studies with the highest precision are those with the narrowest confidence intervals, and usually, these aspects of the different trials are emphasised by plotting squares at the estimated values whose size is related to the precision within that trial. Each square has area proportional to the weight, w_i, given to study i in the meta-analysis. Recall that this is closely related to the sample size of the study. This helps visually to identify those studies that are providing the most precise information; these are the ones with the most prominent squares. The diamond provides the overall combined result.

18.3.5 Detecting heterogeneity

A key element of any meta-analysis is to look for heterogeneity across the studies. This is akin to looking for treatment-by-factor interactions in an adjusted analysis. Here, we are looking for treatment-by-study interactions. This can be done by calculating Cochran's Q statistic (Cochran, 1954):

$$Q = w_1(d_1 - d)^2 + w_2(d_2 - d)^2 + \cdots + w_m(d_m - d)^2$$

and comparing the resulting value with the χ^2_{m-1} distribution to obtain a *p*-value. If the individual studies are giving very different results so that the d_i values are not comparable, then, on average, the differences $d_i - d$ will be large and Q will be statistically significant on the χ^2_{m-1} scale. A significant *p*-value, and again we would usually use 0.10 as the indicator for statistical significance for interactions, tells us that there is trial-to-trial heterogeneity. Unfortunately, this test lacks power, and even a large amount of heterogeneity, especially if there are

Example 18.3 Meta-analysis of adjuvant chemotherapy for resected colon cancer in elderly patients

Sargent *et al.* (2001) undertook a fixed effects meta-analysis of seven phase III randomised trials, involving a total of 3351 patients, that compares the effects of fluorouracil plus leu-covorin (five trials) or fluorouracil plus levamisole (two trials) with surgery alone in patients with stage II or stage III colon cancer.

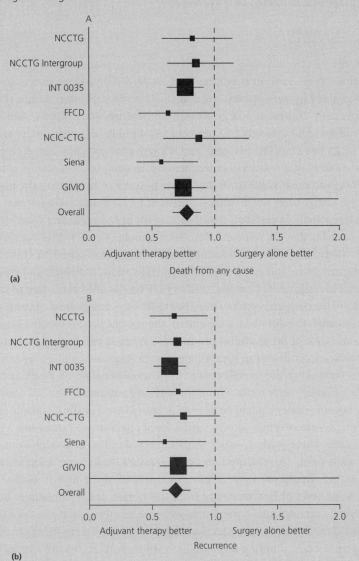

(a)

(b)

Figure 18.1 Hazard ratios and 95 per cent confidence intervals for (a) death from any cause and (b) recurrence, by treatment group. Source: Sargent DJ, Goldberg RM, Jacobson SD, MacDonald JS, *et al.* (2001). A pooled analysis of adjuvant chemotherapy for resected colon cancer in elderly patients. *NEJM*, **345**, 1091–1097. Reproduced by permission of Massachusetts Medical Society.

only a small number of studies, can easily go undetected with this test. Higgins *et al.* (2003) have developed a related statistic, or index, ℓ^2 that takes values between 0 per cent and 100 per cent with 0 per cent denoting no heterogeneity and increasing values indicating increasing heterogeneity. If there is no heterogeneity, then it can be shown that on average the Q statistic will be $m-1$ (recall that m is the number of studies being combined). The ℓ^2 statistic is expressed as a percentage and is related to Q as follows:

$$\ell^2 = 100 \times \frac{Q - (m-1)}{Q}$$

If Q is close to $m-1$, then ℓ^2 will be close to zero. The convention is to replace negative values by zero so that the statistic is always positive and in the range 0–100 per cent. If there is a large amount of heterogeneity, then Q will be large and ℓ^2 will increase towards 100 per cent. As a guide, Higgins *et al.* suggest that values of 25 per cent, 50 per cent and 75 per cent indicate, respectively, low, moderate and high amounts of heterogeneity. In analyses, it is common to quote ℓ^2 together with the p-value from the Q statistic but to rely more on the numerical value of ℓ^2 rather than the p-value in terms of picking up heterogeneity.

If heterogeneity is detected, it will be important to investigate what is causing this. It may be that in some studies, for example, those recruiting only older patients, there is a different treatment effect when compared to those studies recruiting across the full age range. Such considerations may already be built into the overall investigation. Typically, studies may be classified according to the characteristics of the patients recruited into the studies, the dosage level of the treatment being evaluated, the duration of treatment, the specific drug if the meta-analysis is looking at a class of drugs and so on. In these cases, it will be necessary to divide up the studies according to an appropriate classification and conduct separate meta-analyses, comparing the overall results from these separate analyses and indeed evaluating homogeneity again within the separate analyses.

One possible strategy might be to use Cochran's Q-test or the ℓ^2 statistic (or both) in order to decide whether to stay with a fixed effects model or to use a random effects model where study-to-study variation is built into the model. Some practitioners in relation to retrospective meta-analyses addressing specific safety or health settings would use random effects models all of the time in order to allow at least some level of heterogeneity from the outset. It is still possible however, even within a random effects meta-analysis, to see heterogeneity but at a different level. Recall that in a random effects model there is an underlying true treatment effect in each study, differing from study to study, with an overall average of θ. It could be that there is an additional level of heterogeneity with the studies recruiting only older patients having a different θ from those recruiting across the age range. In such cases, even with random effects modelling, it will be important to separate out these two groups of studies to further investigate heterogeneity.

18.3.6 Robustness

Within any meta-analysis, some trials will be larger than others, and because of the way the trials are combined, the larger trials, that is, those that have higher precision, will tend to dominate. It is helpful therefore to assess the robustness of the overall conclusion by omitting maybe the largest study (or studies) to see if the result remains qualitatively the same. If it does, then the result is robust. If it does not, then the robustness of the result is drawn into question as it is being driven by the largest trial (or trials).

18.3.7 Rare events

In meta-analyses dealing with safety issues, for example, based on the occurrence of a specific serious adverse event, it is often the case that the number of events in the individual trials being combined is low. At the extreme, it may be that there are no events in one or both groups in a particular trial. If the number of events in the control group is zero in a trial, then the relative risk and the odds ratio are not defined. If the number of events in the control group is not zero while the number of events in the experimental group is greater than zero, then the relative risk and the odds ratio are both zero. In either case, it is not possible to include these studies routinely in the analysis when using the relative risk and odds ratios as summary measures. Using the risk difference is a little better provided that both groups do not have zero counts. Omitting studies with zero counts causes bias. A large study where the event counts are zero in both groups is conveying the information that the experimental treatment in that trial is not increasing the incidence of the event and to exclude that study from the meta-analysis is potentially leading to an overestimation of the extent of the safety problem.

A simplistic way to account for these zero values is to include a continuity correction to the data in that study. This typically involves adding 0.5 to each of the four counts (group 1, patients with the SAE, patients without the SAE; group 2, patients with the SAE, patients without the SAE) in the 2×2 contingency table for that trial. This is effectively adding a patient into each treatment group and splitting them 50:50 across the two outcome categories, event/no event. This is a common, albeit ad hoc, *fudge factor* that enables the maximum amount of information to be included in the final meta-analysis. There are alternative ways of dealing with this problem, but these are beyond the scope of this discussion. The interested reader is referred to Bradburn *et al.* (2007).

18.3.8 Individual patient data

When conducting a retrospective meta-analysis, it may be that trials are combined on the basis of summary statistics from publications and summary trial reports without access to the underlying individual patient data. Within a regulatory submission of course this is not an issue but outside of that it often is. Access to the patient-level data is much better for two main reasons. Firstly, it can help to achieve consistency for the analysis as a whole in terms of defining the primary endpoint in a precise way, constructing analysis sets in a consistent way, using methods for dealing with missing data that are the same for every trial, having a common approach to defining and excluding protocol violators from the analysis and so on. Secondly, it enables more sophisticated methods of analysis using regression models that enable a wider range of approaches to be considered for the analysis. Having access to individual patient data is always better; there are no exceptions to this rule.

18.4 Case study

It will be useful to review the methods that have been described already in this section through a case study. This case study will also be of value in cementing some of the ideas that are to follow. Tang *et al.* (2007) report a meta-analysis looking at the use of calcium or calcium plus vitamin D supplementation in preventing fractures and bone loss in people over 50 years of age. The 16 randomised controlled trials that were eventually included in the meta-analysis for the binary endpoint of fracture (yes/no) are displayed in Figure 18.2 and combined in terms of the relative risk for fractures. Note that one trial, the RECORD study, is included twice. There were four treatment groups in this study including calcium alone, calcium plus vitamin D and placebo, and the two relative risks that were included in the analysis were for the calcium versus placebo comparison and for the calcium plus vitamin D versus placebo comparison. In fact, including the placebo group twice is incorrect. The relative risks being combined are not independent since the placebo group appears in both, and this violates one of the assumptions on which the methods for combination are based. Simply combining the two active groups giving a single calcium or calcium plus vitamin D group and calculating a single relative risk would have been a better approach. Despite this shortcoming, we will use this example to highlight some of the methodological points already made. It is worth noting that the authors were able to obtain individual patient data and did not have to rely on summary statistics from the trials on which to base their meta-analysis.

The *x*-axis is on the log scale, and consequently, the confidence intervals displayed are symmetric around the observed relative risk. The overall relative risk is 0.88 with 95 per cent confidence interval 0.83 to 0.95 and a highly statistically significant *p*-value of 0.0004. There is strong evidence for this analysis that calcium and calcium in combination with vitamin D prevent fractures in this over 50s population. Heterogeneity was assessed using Cochran's Q statistic that gave a non-significant *p*-value of 0.20, and the value of ℓ^2 was 20 per cent, suggesting a low level of heterogeneity. Despite this, the authors choose to use a random effects model for the meta-analysis, and it is the results of this model that are set down in Figure 18.2 for the combination. These authors also defined a set of 12 variables for subgroup analyses and divided the data up according to,

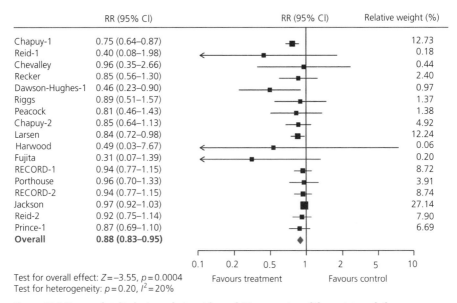

	RR (95% CI)		RR (95% CI)	Relative weight (%)
Chapuy-1	0.75 (0.64–0.87)			12.73
Reid-1	0.40 (0.08–1.98)			0.18
Chevalley	0.96 (0.35–2.66)			0.44
Recker	0.85 (0.56–1.30)			2.40
Dawson-Hughes-1	0.46 (0.23–0.90)			0.97
Riggs	0.89 (0.51–1.57)			1.37
Peacock	0.81 (0.46–1.43)			1.38
Chapuy-2	0.85 (0.64–1.13)			4.92
Larsen	0.84 (0.72–0.98)			12.24
Harwood	0.49 (0.03–7.67)			0.06
Fujita	0.31 (0.07–1.39)			0.20
RECORD-1	0.94 (0.77–1.15)			8.72
Porthouse	0.96 (0.70–1.33)			3.91
RECORD-2	0.94 (0.77–1.15)			8.74
Jackson	0.97 (0.92–1.03)			27.14
Reid-2	0.92 (0.75–1.14)			7.90
Prince-1	0.87 (0.69–1.10)			6.69
Overall	**0.88 (0.83–0.95)**			

Test for overall effect: $Z = -3.55$, $p = 0.0004$ Favours treatment   Favours control
Test for heterogeneity: $p = 0.20$, $I^2 = 20\%$

Figure 18.2 Forest plot displaying relative risks and 95 per cent confidence intervals for occurrence of fractures in studies contained in the meta-analysis. Source: Tang BMP, Eslick GD, Nowson C, *et al.* (2007). Use of calcium or calcium in combination with vitamin D supplementation to prevent fractures and bone loss in people aged 50 years and older: a meta-analysis. *The Lancet*, **370**, 657–666. Reproduced with permission from Elsevier.

for example, sex, previous fractures (yes/no), clinical setting (community/institutionalised), age (50–69, 70–79, ≥80) and so on. They then undertook separate meta-analyses within each subgroup producing separate relative risks together with a *p*-value for study-by-factor interactions based on comparing those relative risks. Several of these were statistically significant. For example, the relative risks for the three age groups were 0.97 (50–69 age group), 0.89 (70–79 age group) and 0.76 (≥80 age group) with a *p*-value for interaction of 0.003. This is a quantitative interaction (see Section 5.4.2), and in each of the age categories, calcium/calcium plus vitamin D is having a beneficial effect according to the relative risks although the effect seems to be greater for the older patients. There were several other statistically significant interactions, but all were quantitative in nature and calcium and calcium in combination with vitamin D were seen to have a beneficial effect across the population as a whole.

18.5 Ensuring scientific validity

18.5.1 Planning

In order to ensure that a meta-analysis is scientifically valid, it is necessary to plan and conduct the analysis in an appropriate and rigorous way. It is not sufficient to retrospectively go to a bunch of studies that you like the look of and stick them together!

Ideally, the meta-analysis within a regulatory submission should be pre-planned as part of the development plan, and the rules regarding which trials are to be combined and in what way set down in advance of running the trials.

The CPMP (2001) *Points to Consider on Application with 1. Meta-Analysis; 2. One Pivotal Study* indicates that it is good practice to write a protocol for the meta-analysis:

'When a meta-analysis is included in an application it should be performed in accordance with a protocol ...'.

This document then goes on to list the issues that should be covered by that protocol:

- Objective of the meta-analysis
- Criteria for inclusion/exclusion of studies
- Hypotheses and endpoints
- Statistical methods
- Approaches to ensure consistent quality of the studies and how to handle poor quality studies
- Evaluating homogeneity and robustness

Writing a protocol in this way is important for a meta-analysis that is pre-specified within a development plan, but, in order to ensure its integrity, it is maybe even more critical when an analysis is performed retrospectively within a regulatory submission.

A meta-analysis to address an emerging safety issue or to address a general therapeutic issue also requires very careful planning. The first step in any such analysis is to clearly define the research question. For the case study outlined in Section 18.4, the research question was to assess *'the effect of calcium, or calcium in combination with vitamin D supplementation, on osteoporotic fractures and bone-mineral density, in adults aged 50 years and older'*. Having set down a clear research question, the second step is to specify search criteria to find the trials that are potentially relevant to that question and to define study eligibility criteria, methods of data extraction and finally the methods for statistical analysis.

The search criteria will involve searching electronic databases such as Medline, Embase and the Cochrane Database of Systematic Reviews while also looking for unpublished and ongoing trials. The study eligibility criteria will often restrict trials to be included to those with a control group, those giving treatment at a certain target dose over an appropriate period of time as well as those specifying in a precise way the patient population being studied. Data extraction is often undertaken by at least two individuals independently with disagreements resolved through discussion.

The research question itself will usually have set down what the endpoints of interest are, at least in an approximate way. Specifying the statistical methods will involve defining those endpoints in a clear way and also the summary measures that are to be used for measures of treatment effect. Further points that need consideration include whether the analysis will use fixed effects or random effects (or both), how to assess heterogeneity and robustness, the extent of the subgroup analyses and finally how to deal with any specific problems such as rare events.

18.5.2 Assessing the risk of bias

Many publications based on meta-analysis talk in terms of the methodological quality of the trials that are to be included in the analysis possibly excluding those that fail to meet certain quality standards. In the past, it has been common to use checklists for the assessment of quality. More recently, the emphasis has been on assessing the risk of bias. A new tool for assessing the risk of bias has been developed by the Cochrane Collaboration (Higgins *et al.*, 2011) and is summarised in Table 18.4.

Various forms of bias are listed in this table with a description of the source of that bias. In assessing the potential for bias, each of these items is assessed as being low risk, high risk or risk unclear. Trials that have a high risk of various biases may well be excluded from the meta-analysis. Further, and as part of the evaluation of robustness, it might also be appropriate to also exclude some trials on the basis of a potential for bias from some sensitivity-type analyses.

18.5.3 Publication bias and funnel plots

One particular issue concerns meta-analyses based upon data obtained through a literature search. It is certainly true that a study that has given a statistically significant result is more likely to be reported and accepted for publication; so if we only focused on published studies, then we would get a biased view of the totality of the available studies. Eggar and Smith (1998) discuss various aspects

Table 18.4 Cochrane Collaboration's tool for assessing risk of bias

Bias domain	Source of bias	Assess as low, unclear or high risk of bias
Selection bias	Random sequence generation	Inadequate generation of a randomised sequence
Selection bias	Allocation concealment	Inadequate concealment of allocations before assignment
Performance bias	Blinding of participants and personnel	Knowledge of allocated interventions by participants and personnel during study
Detection bias	Blinding of outcome assessment	Knowledge of the allocated interventions by personnel assessing outcome
Attrition bias	Incomplete outcome data	Amount, nature or handling of incomplete outcome data
Reporting bias	Selective reporting	Selective outcome reporting
Other bias	Anything else	Bias due to problems not covered elsewhere

Source: Adapted from Higgins JPT, Altman DG, Gotzsche PC, *et al.* (2011). The Cochrane Collaboration's tool for assessing risk of bias in randomised trials. *BMJ*, **343**, d5928. Reproduced with permission from BMJ Publishing Ltd.

of this *publication bias* and its causes. There have been many calls over the years for registries of studies to be set up, and in early 2005, the European Federation of Pharmaceutical Industries and Associations (EFPIA), the International Federation of Pharmaceutical Manufacturers & Associations (IFPMA), the Japan Pharmaceutical Manufacturers Association (JPMA) and the Pharmaceutical Research and Manufacturers of America (PhRMA) issued a joint statement committing to increasing the transparency of research by setting up a Clinical Trial Registry. Although this is a voluntary initiative, most companies are following this guidance and registering their clinical trials. The registry is maintained by the National Library of Medicine in the USA and can be found at www.clinicaltrials. gov. In theory, this makes it possible to identify all studies sponsored by the industry and potentially avoid any publication bias.

There is a graphical technique available, introduced by Eggar *et al.* (1997), called a *funnel plot*, which helps to detect the presence of publication bias by plotting the treatment effect (e.g. the difference in the means or the odds ratio) in each study on the *x*-axis against the sample size on the *y*-axis. Smaller studies will tend to give more variable results in terms of the observed treatment difference, while the larger studies should give more consistent results. The resultant plot with all studies included should then appear like a funnel with the wide part of the funnel at the bottom and the narrow part of the funnel at the top of the plot. If, however, there is publication bias, then the non-significant studies, very often those with smaller sample sizes, will be under-represented, and either the lower left-hand part of the plot or the lower right-hand part of the plot, depending on how the active compared to placebo difference is measured, will be missing. Once this has been detected, then it can be compensated for in the statistical analysis. Visually inspecting the funnel plot in this way is somewhat informal, although the technique can provide some reassurance regarding the absence of publication bias. However, it is not a substitute for relentlessly tracking down all of the studies and all of the data.

Figure 18.3 is a funnel plot for the case study described in Section 18.4 (Tang *et al.*, 2007). Note that the funnel is sketched on for guidance; this is not the result of some curve-fitting exercise. Inspection of the plot suggests that there is an absence of small studies with log risk ratio above zero. These would be studies where the risk ratio is greater than 1, studies in which calcium and calcium plus vitamin D supplementation is increasing the fracture risk. The key issue now is, does it make a difference, in the sense that were such studies, presumably conducted but not published, included, would that negate the overall meta-analysis result? One way to address this point is to calculate the *fail-safe number* (Rosenthal, 1979), that is, the number of studies out there with a risk ratio of 1 or with a risk ratio giving a statistically significant result against calcium and calcium plus vitamin D, that would be needed to negate the statistically significant result in favour of calcium and calcium plus vitamin D in the meta-analysis. In the case study, approximately 100 studies with a risk ratio of 1 or 22 studies with a statistically significant

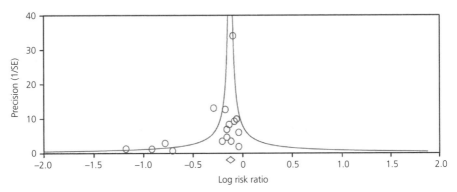

Figure 18.3 Funnel plot for meta-analysis of trials. Source: Tang BMP, Eslick GD, Nowson C, *et al.* (2007). Use of calcium or calcium in combination with vitamin D supplementation to prevent fractures and bone loss in people aged 50 years and older: a meta-analysis. *The Lancet*, **370**, 657–666. Reproduced with permission from Elsevier.

but negative result for calcium and calcium plus vitamin D would be needed to negate the overall effect. Tang *et al.* (2007) conclude that it is very unlikely that such unpublished studies exist and therefore that their results were not materially affected by publication bias.

18.5.4 Preferred Reporting Items for Systematic Reviews and Meta-Analyses

The Preferred Reporting Items for Systematic Reviews and Meta-Analyses (PRISMA) statement (Liberati *et al.*, 2009) provides recommendations for the reporting of a meta-analysis in the form of a checklist. Although this statement does not directly talk about the planning and conduct of a meta-analysis, it does in fact say a lot about these issues. For example, the statement talks in detail about searches, providing a clear rationale for conducting the meta-analysis including specifying the research question, describing the study selection or eligibility criteria, data extraction and assessing the risk of bias. Anyone planning to conduct a meta-analysis should read this statement in detail.

18.6 Further regulatory aspects

In a regulatory setting, a pre-planned meta-analysis is always going to be more convincing. Often however, a meta-analysis will only be envisaged either part way through a development plan or at the end of the trial activity once the submission is being put together. It is interesting to note that within the regulatory context, meta-analysis has frequently caused problems for regulators:

> *'Meta-analysis has long been a source of regulatory discomfort, mostly because of the poor quality of some meta-analyses submitted in applications for licences'* (Lewis, 2002).

The regulators do however, recognise that pre-planning is not always possible.

CPMP (2001): 'Points to Consider on Application with 1. Meta-Analysis; 2. One Pivotal Study'

'A retrospective specification when the results from all or some of the studies are known should be avoided ... There are, however situations where the need for a meta-analysis becomes apparent after the results from some or sometimes all studies are known. This is the case when there is a need to put seemingly conflicting results into perspective, or in the exceptional situation where a meta-analysis seems to be the only way to provide reliable proof of efficacy'.

It is still important even in this retrospective setting to write a protocol so that the meta-analysis can be performed as objectively as possible. The CPMP Points to Consider paper lists the prerequisites that are needed for such a retrospective analysis.

CPMP (2001): 'Points to Consider on Application with 1. Meta-Analysis; 2. One Pivotal Study'

'Prerequisites for a retrospective meta-analysis to provide sufficient evidence for a claim include:
- Some studies clearly positive
- Inconclusive studies showing positive trends in the primary variable
- No statistically significant heterogeneity
- Pooled 95 per cent confidence interval well away from zero (or unity for odds ratios, or the pre-defined margin for non-inferiority trials)
- A justification that a biased selection of studies and/or endpoints is unlikely
- A sensitivity analysis demonstrating robustness of the findings

For meta-analyses where these requirements are not fulfilled it will prove difficult to get a regulatory acceptance'.

CHAPTER 19

Methods for the safety analysis and safety monitoring

19.1 Introduction

19.1.1 Methods for safety data

The majority of the statistical methods we have developed and presented in this book have been focused on the evaluation of efficacy data. In this chapter, we will consider methods that relate to the analysis of safety and tolerability data. We will start by looking at the routine analysis and presentation of safety data within a single clinical trial and more broadly within the regulatory package as a whole. We will then go to discuss methods for safety monitoring and pharmacovigilance post-approval.

In some circumstances, there may be specific safety and tolerability parameters that within the confirmatory structure of the trial. For example, in an oncology study, we may be interested in assessing the potential for a drug to reduce the rate of Common Terminology Criteria (CTC) Cancer Therapy Evaluation Program (2006) grade 3/4 neutropenia associated with a standard chemotherapeutic regimen. This may well be the main focus of the trial or at least an important secondary consideration. In this case, there is a specific hypothesis to test, and this binary endpoint would be something that is incorporated into the confirmatory testing strategy and would be treated in exactly the same as would an efficacy endpoint. But this is not what we are discussing primarily in this chapter. Here, our attention will be on gaining an overview of the totality of the safety information in order to identify specific safety signals and concerns to allow evaluation of the benefit–risk ratio both at time of approval and beyond. *P*-values in this setting convey little information and indeed can be misleading and as such are not recommended. Non-significant *p*-values may simply be because the event rate overall for a particular adverse event (AE) is low and hence the power to detect differences is small. But even a rare very serious AE can have major implications if it occurs more frequently in the experimental group. Statistically significant *p*-values on the other hand may be a consequence of multiplicity. We could well be looking at several thousand distinct AEs together with other safety parameters, and significant *p*-values will inevitably occur purely by chance. We do however sometimes calculate 95 per cent confidence intervals, but these are

Statistical Thinking for Non-Statisticians in Drug Regulation, Second Edition. Richard Kay.
© 2015 John Wiley & Sons, Ltd. Published 2015 by John Wiley & Sons, Ltd.

not to be used to make formal inferences in the statistical significance sense. These intervals are there to provide information on the potential magnitude of effect that is supported by the data.

ICH E9 (1998): 'Note for Guidance on Statistical Principles for Clinical Trials'

'In most trials the safety and tolerability implications are best addressed by applying descriptive statistical methods to the data, supplemented by calculation of confidence intervals wherever this aids interpretation. It is also valuable to make use of graphical presentations in which patterns of adverse events are displayed both within treatment groups and within subjects'.

Note the final point here on the use of graphical presentations and this will be a particular focus in this chapter.

We will use the following terms in our discussions:
- *Safety* – the medical risk of the product (drug, device, treatment) to the subject
- *Tolerability* – the degree to which the subject can tolerate the adverse effects of a product (drug, device, treatment)
- *Benefit* – the established therapeutic efficacy of a product (drug, device, treatment)
- *Risk* – the probability of being harmed by the product (drug, device, treatment)
- *Harm* – the extent of damage caused by the product (drug, device, treatment)

19.1.2 The rule of three

ICH E1 makes several statements about what would normally be expected in terms of characterising AEs within the clinical trial programme through to phase III.

ICH E1 (1995): 'Population Exposure: The Extent of Population Exposure to Assess Clinical Safety'

'It is expected that short-term event rates (cumulative 3-month incidence of about 1%) will be well characterized. ... The safety evaluation during clinical drug development is not expected to characterize rare adverse events, for example, those occurring in less than 1 in 1000 patients'.

Suppose that the incidence of a particular AE occurring with a certain drug is 1 per cent. If we were to study $n=300$ patients receiving that drug, then the probability that we would see no events is $0.99^{300}=0.049$. It follows that the probability that we would see at least one patient suffering the event is $1-0.049=0.951$, around 95 per cent in percentage terms. This type of calculation leads to the probabilities in Table 19.1.

Table 19.1 Number of patients needed according to incidence rate

Probability	Incidence				
	1%	0.5%	0.1%	0.05%	0.01%
95%	300	600	2,995	5,990	29,956
80%	161	313	1,608	3,128	16,094

The probabilities in this table give measures of our ability to detect an AE according to its incidence. So, for example, if we are dealing with a rare AE with an incidence of only 0.1 per cent (1 in 1000), then we would need a trial (or trials) recruiting 2995, almost 3000, patients in order to have a 95 per cent probability of detecting its presence. Turning this around, it follows that if in a trial of 3000 patients we did not see a certain AE, then we can be 95 per cent confident that its incidence is less than 1 in 1000. This leads to the *rule of 3* (Jovanovic and Levy, 1997); if you fail to see a particular AE in a trial with n patients, then we can be 95 per cent confident that the incidence of that AE is less than $3/n$.

The recommendations coming out of the ICH E1 guidance for the size of the safety database are as follows:

- It is usually sufficient to have safety data on 300 to 600 patients treated for 6 months. Should be adequate to characterise patterns of AEs over time,
- To gauge longer-term AEs, safety data are needed on 100 patients for 12 months. Note that according the rule of 3, if a particular AE is not seen, then we have reasonable assurance (95 per cent) that the incidence is less than 3/100 (3%).

Further details on these and other recommendations are contained in that guidance.

19.2 Routine evaluation in clinical studies

Within the context of a single clinical trial, the analyses of safety and tolerability will usually be based on the safety set. In Section 7.2, we defined the full analysis set and the per-protocol set, and these were the analysis sets on which analyses of efficacy were undertaken. The *safety set* is defined as the set of subjects who have received at least one dose of the study medication.

ICH E9 (1998): 'Note for Guidance on Statistical Principles for Clinical Trials'

'For the overall safety and tolerability assessment, the set of subjects to be summarized is usually defined as those subjects who received at least one dose of the investigational drug'.

This analysis set will on many occasions coincide with the FAS, but not always. In addition, the make-up of the treatment groups in the FAS may differ from the make-up in the safety set. For example, a subject who is randomised to receive treatment A but receives treatment B by mistake could well be included in group A for the analysis of efficacy in order to comply with the randomisation but would be included in group B for the analysis of safety and tolerability.

19.2.1 Types of data

The kinds of data that we collect in order to evaluate the safety and tolerability of a product include AEs and serious adverse events (SAEs), data on laboratory parameters, ECGs and vital signs.

AEs and SAEs will be classified based on the Medical Dictionary for Regulatory Activities (MedDRA). This dictionary is organised by System Organ Class (SOC) and then divided into High-Level Group Terms, High-Level Terms, Preferred Terms (PTs) and finally Lower-Level Terms. Data presentations in tabular form usually only use the SOC and the PT as a basis for classification. In some cases, there may be *AEs of special interest* that have been identified as being potentially associated with the drug/disease under study, possibly because of early phase data for the drug or simply because of experience of drugs within that same class. These need to receive special attention, and this is possibly one area where formal inference associated with a pre-specified hypothesis and the calculation of a *p*-value is justified. There is a substantial clinical overlap across individual PTs in the MedDRA system, and some grouping of the terms may be needed to get a full picture of a particular area of concern. We will not however address this grouping issue further in our discussions.

In all clinical trials and development plans, there will be the routine collection of a range of laboratory parameters, both clinical chemistry and haematology in serum, with associated normal ranges with possibly some parameters obtained via a urinalysis. Normal ranges can be age and gender specific and can also differ according to the laboratory performing the testing. The list of parameters measured will depend on the disease setting. A specific issue of concern with all drugs is the potential for liver damage as indicated by values for the liver transaminases, alanine transaminase (ALT) and aspartate transaminase (AST). Raised levels of these parameters can be a precursor of acute liver damage and failure. *Hy's law* is now widely used to signify altered liver function with the potential to cause a fatal drug-induced liver injury (DILI) and is defined in the FDA guideline (FDA, 2007) on Drug-Induced Liver Injury as cases where there is:

- A 3-fold or greater elevation above the upper limit of the normal range (ULN) for ALT or AST.
- Elevation of the serum total bilirubin of 2-fold or greater than the ULN without any findings of cholestasis (serum alkaline phosphatase $>2 \times$ ULN).
- No other reason for these increases such as the presence of hepatitis or pre-existing liver disease can be found.

Electrocardiography (ECG or EKG) provides information on the electrical activity of the heart, and the QT interval when prolonged is associated with increased risk of ventricular arrhythmia and potentially sudden death. The QT interval is usually corrected for heart rate and denoted QT_C. There are more sophisticated methods of correction, namely, Bazett's formula (QT_B) and Fridericia's formula (QT_F). The QT interval, corrected for heart rate, has separate normal ranges for males and females, but in data analysis, it is the change from baseline that is generally the focus. Increases of 30 ms and 60 ms are considered as levels for concern.

Finally, vital signs include body temperature, heart rate, systolic and diastolic blood pressure (sBP and dBP) and possibly respiratory rate. Acceptable ranges for each of these parameters are available and vary with age, although these ranges tend not to be used formally in analysis in the same way for example, that normal ranges for laboratory parameters are.

19.2.2 Adverse events

AEs and SAEs are usually summarised by SOC and PT in tables reporting incidence (both absolute and percentage). Incidence is expressed as the number of subjects suffering the event divided by the number of subjects in that treatment group. Note that incidence is not usually expressed in terms of the number of events divided by the number of subjects; if a subject suffers two headaches during the course of the trial, then this subject will only count once in the calculation of incidence. These incidences are calculated for the individual PTs but are also totalled for each SOC. At that level though, there is the potential for some double counting. For example, the SOC gastrointestinal disorders contain the events nausea and vomiting as separate PTs. If a patient suffers three bouts of nausea and vomiting on two occasions, then they would be counted once for the PT nausea, once for the PT vomiting and once for the SOC gastrointestinal disorders.

It is also not uncommon to produce similar tables for *AEs related to study medication* according to the information on relationship to treatment provided by the investigator and for *severe AEs* according to predefined levels of severity.

If the duration of treatment differs between the treatment groups, then simple calculation of incidence may not be a sound basis on which to compare treatments in relation to AEs. Duration may differ by design for example, where one treatment is given for a fixed period of time, while the other treatment can continue through to the end of the study. This differential exposure can happen in oncology trials where the standard chemotherapeutic regimen is given say, for six 3-week cycles, while in the experimental arm the add-on treatment continues until disease progression. Duration may also differ at the subject level where subjects withdraw from treatment for safety reasons. In both of these

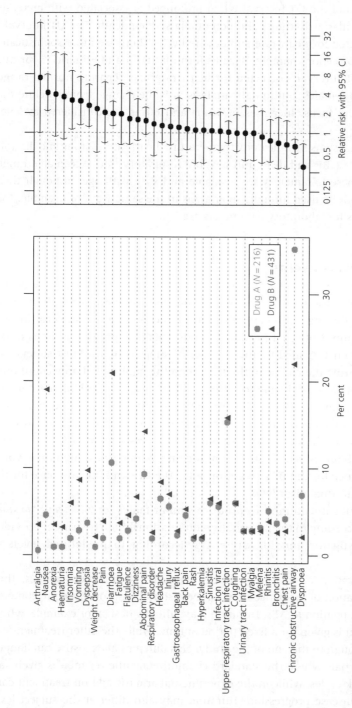

Figure 19.1 Most frequent on-therapy events ordered by relative risk. Source: Amit O, Heidberger RM and Lane PW (2008) 'Graphical Approaches to the Analysis of Safety Data from Clinical Trials' *Pharmaceutical Statistics*, **7**, 20–35. Reproduced with permission from John Wiley & Sons.

cases, it can be of value to calculate incidence rates in addition to the incidence itself. This would be defined as follows:

$$\text{Incidence rate} = \frac{\text{number of subjects suffering the event}}{\text{total exposure}}$$

Total exposure expressed in years, would be calculated by summing up the exposures for all subjects in that treatment group. It may also be of value when dealing with rare events to multiply this rate by 1000 to express it as the rate per 1000 subject-years. It is possible when considering rates in this way to replace the *number of subjects suffering the event* in the numerator above by the *number of events suffered over all subjects*. This would account for multiple occurrences of an event. Whether this is appropriate or not depends on the context.

While tables are extremely important and useful, it can be of value to provide some graphical presentation of the differences in incidence rates for the commonly occurring events. Figure 19.1 is an example of such a display and is taken from Amit *et al.* (2008). The events listed down the left-hand side are those occurring most frequently in the experimental group. The circles and triangles on the left-hand side of the display are the incidences by treatment group. The right-hand side of the display shows the relative risks with 95 per cent confidence intervals. The events are ordered according to the value of the relative risk. AEs for which there is an increased risk are immediately apparent. In some cases, for example, when there are zero events of a particular type in the control group, it may be preferable to plot the risk difference rather than the relative risk; with a zero observed risk in the control group, the relative risk is not defined. Ordering according to relative risk or risk difference is the natural ordering in these cases, but ordering by absolute risk in the experimental arm or absolute risk in both arms combined might also be appropriate.

We mentioned earlier that there may be events of special interest, and in addition to presenting possibly separate tables that provide information for only these events, it can be useful to look at the time to an event (or the onset of an event) of special interest. This will give information not only on the frequency of these events in the treatment groups but also on whether the event occurs earlier in one of those groups. Figure 19.2 is taken from Solomon *et al.* (2005) who report on a retrospective evaluation of an increased cardiovascular risk associated with celecoxib for the prevention of colorectal adenomas. Patients were randomised to two doses of celecoxib (200 mg or 400 mg twice daily) or placebo, and the endpoint evaluated was a composite of death from cardiovascular causes, myocardial infarction, stroke or heart failure. This investigation was evaluating a particular hypothesis as a consequence of there being heightened awareness of the possibility that COX-2 inhibitors could be associated with increased cardiovascular risk, and for this reason, a formal *p*-value comparison was undertaken to test this hypothesis. The Kaplan–Meier plots of time to the composite event and the statistically significant *p*-value of 0.01 comparing the

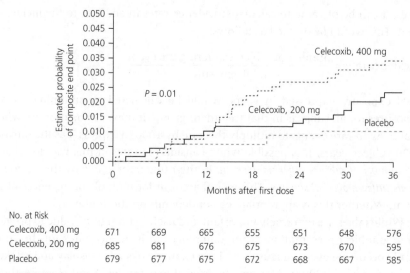

No. at Risk

Celecoxib, 400 mg	671	669	665	655	651	648	576
Celecoxib, 200 mg	685	681	676	675	673	670	595
Placebo	679	677	675	672	668	667	585

Figure 19.2 Kaplan–Meier plots for time to composite safety endpoint. Source: Solomon S, McMurray JJV, Pfeffer MA, *et al.* (2005). Cardiovascular Risk Associated with Celecoxib in a Clinical Trial for Colorectal Adenoma Prevention. *NEJM* **352**, 1071–1080. Reproduced by permission of Massachusetts Medical Society.

three groups collectively clearly show that there is an increased risk associated with celecoxib and that this is dose related.

19.2.3 Laboratory data

The most useful tabular presentations for laboratory data are shift tables. These tables display numbers of subjects in the treatment groups separately who move from having values within/outside the normal range at baseline to having values outside/within the normal range at each visit. A graphical version of this table would be a series of scatter plots, one for each visit, with the baseline value on the *x*-axis and the corresponding value at the visit on the *y*-axis with vertical and horizontal lines drawn at the upper and lower limits of the normal range as shown in schematic form in Figure 19.3.

   Points within the box formed by those horizontal and vertical lines (Region A) would correspond to patients with values that start within the normal range and remain within the normal range at the visit. Values in Region B correspond to patients whose values start within the normal range but then go above the upper limit if normal at the visit. Patients in Region C also had a value within the normal range at baseline, but their value at the visit fell below the lower limit of normal. The graphical version however could only work in a straight-forward way if the normal range was the same for the study as a whole. If there were separate normal ranges for males and females, then the graphs would need to be produced by sex. If there were different normal ranges for different centres in the study, then these graphs would need to be modified by standardising the measurements across centres (and for males and females if

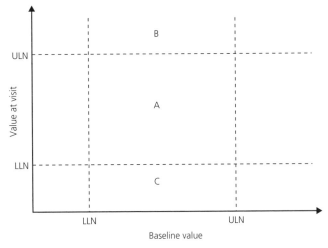

Figure 19.3 Schematic for baseline and visit values in a shift plot for a typical laboratory parameter. Note: LLN, lower limit of normal; ULN, upper limit of normal

required). If LLN and ULN represent the lower and upper levels of the normal range, the standardised measurement, y, is then

$$y = \frac{x - \text{LLN}}{\text{ULN} - \text{LLN}}$$

where x is the observed laboratory value. This gives a transformed laboratory value that will be between 0 and 1 when the actual laboratory value is within the normal range, will be greater than 1 when the untransformed value is above the ULN and will be less than 0 when the untransformed value is below the LLN. The horizontal and vertical lines in Figure 19.3 would then be drawn at 0 and 1.

It is often the outliers that are of interest in relation to laboratory data and graphical displays can highlight these. Figure 19.4 taken from Amit *et al.* (2008) displays data on AST (labelled ASAT in the graph) using box plots (Section 2.2.5) at baseline and by on-treatment visit. The especially large values are easily seen at each visit in this plot. In the right-hand panel, there is also a plot of the maximum on-treatment value. Horizontal lines have been drawn as reference lines at $2 \times \text{ULN}$. In plots for other laboratory parameters, it may be more appropriate to draw lines at LLN and ULN. Note that the units on the y-axis are in terms of proportions of the upper limit of normal. This is in effect using y in the earlier formula with LLN = 0. Figure 19.4 also contains the numbers of subjects at each visit and the numbers of subjects in each group with values above twice the upper limit of normal. Restricting these plots to the subgroups of subjects with values within the normal range at baseline can be useful in highlighting interesting trends. Certain laboratory parameters display highly skewed distributions, and it can sometimes be difficult to plot values on a linear scale while maintaining separation of the individual points at the lower numerical

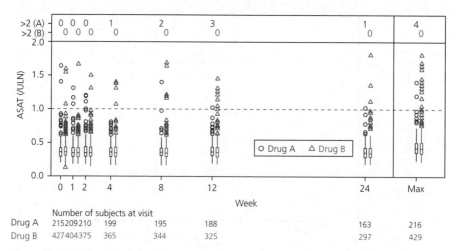

Figure 19.4 Distribution of AST by time and treatment. Source: Amit O, Heidberger RM and Lane PW (2008). Reproduced with permission from John Wiley & Sons.

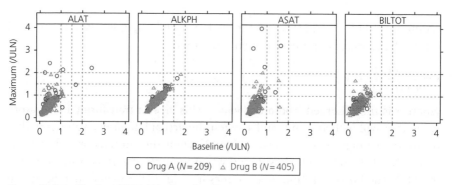

Figure 19.5 Trellis plot of LFT shifts from baseline to maximum by time. Note: ALAT, ALKPH and ASAT, the clinical concern level is 2 ULN; BILTOT, the CCL is 1.5 ULN; where ULN is the upper level of normal range. Source: Amit O, Heidberger RM and Lane PW (2008). Reproduced with permission from John Wiley & Sons.

end of the scale. In these circumstances, it can be advantageous to plot parameter values on the log scale. Judgement is needed to decide when to do this.

As we have mentioned the liver transaminase parameters invariably get special attention, and it is the maximum values through the study period that are of particular concern. We have already seen in Figure 19.4 a representation of one of these parameters. It is useful also to look at these parameters as a group. Figure 19.5 taken from Amit *et al.* (2008) shows alkaline phosphatase (ALKPH) and total bilirubin (BILTOT) in addition to AST and ALT (labelled ASAT and ALAT, respectively, in this figure) again using values for these parameters expressed as proportions of the upper limit of normal. All data are presented in these plots and not just those for subjects with normal values at baseline, and the figure presents bivariate plots of maximum value versus baseline value with lines on the plots at ULN,

1.5 × ULN and 2 × ULN. Each of these component plots is similar to Figure 19.3 but now focusing on the maximum value post-baseline. The concerning data points are those that lie in the upper left-hand quadrants corresponding to subjects whose values at baseline are within the normal range but whose values post-baseline go above ULN, 1.5 × ULN and 2 × ULN.

19.2.4 ECG data

The analysis of the QTc interval will usually focus on two aspects:
- Overall increase in the average value through the study
- Exceeding thresholds that are of particular concern

Tables showing median values through time, numbers of subjects exceeding the threshold values of 450 ms, 480 ms and 500 ms, and numbers of subjects with change from baseline >30 ms and >60 ms, which are the concerning values as set down in the CHMP guidance (CHMP, 2005), give the information that is of interest. Box plots as shown in Figure 19.6, also taken from Amit *et al.* (2008), can address both aspects visually: trends over time and numbers exceeding threshold values. This plot is looking at change from baseline but a similar plot could be produced for the absolute values. The horizontal line within each box is the median value, and this is provided for each treatment group and for each visit. These values can additionally be joined across time within each group to help pick up trends. Note that trends are much easier to identify in a plot than in a table especially when a comparison between treatment groups is needed. It is important that evaluation of such trends is based on such a comparison as regression towards the mean can give a false impression for any one group in isolation. Regression towards the mean in this context would occur if only subjects with normal (low)

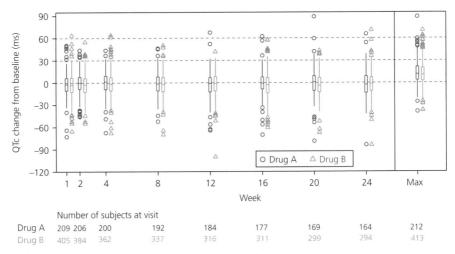

Figure 19.6 Box plot of change from baseline in QTc by time and treatment.
Note: Increase <30 ms 'Normal', 30–60 ms 'Concern', >60 ms 'High'. Source: Amit O, Heidberger RM and Lane PW (2008). Reproduced with permission from John Wiley & Sons.

values for the QTc interval were recruited into the study as there would be a tendency for these to increase over time as a result of random fluctuations.

Looking at absolute values rather than change from baseline in the plots would enable numbers above absolute thresholds to be seen. To avoid having to produce too many plots, it would also be possible to augment the change from baseline plots with numbers exceeding those absolute thresholds at each visit.

19.2.5 Vital signs

Tables and plots for vital signs would be similar to those for the QTc interval. Both change from baseline and absolute values would be of interest, and we would focus on average trends compared between treatment groups, and in addition, the numbers of subjects with values outside of what could be considered *normal*. For body temperature, anything above 38.5 °C would indicate fever. For blood pressure, the norms are 80 mmHg for dBP and 120 mmHg for sBP. Heart rate is very much age dependent and even within age brackets can vary enormously from subject to subject so that looking at extremes in terms of change from baseline may be of greater value. Similar comments apply for respiratory rate.

19.2.6 Safety summary across trials

The methods for presenting AE and SAE data covered earlier in this section in relation to single clinical trials can also be used across a collection of trials within the context of a regulatory package by simply totalling over the trials. Some considerations will need to be given however to dose level and duration of treatment with tables separated accordingly. Note that with dose level this would also apply to a single trial. Data for the collection of trials within the package will be more extensive, and this will also allow individual data tabulations and plots within subgroups of patients, for example, males/females, <65/≥65 years and so on. We discussed in Section 18.1 the dangers of simply pooling data over separate studies and that doing so can be misleading under some circumstances. The same applies here and we need to be cautious especially if we have unbalanced randomisation in some studies, very different populations being studied in different trials and with varying rates of AEs between those trials. As discussed in that earlier section, the preferred approach to pooling would be a meta-analysis. We also discussed in Section 18.3.7 the problem of rare events, and in many analyses of SAEs, both prospective and retrospective, this problem can arise. We will discuss a specific example of the meta-analysis-type approach in Section 19.5.1 where we look at methods for safety monitoring post-approval.

Given that the trials within the package are likely to differ somewhat in their design, it would not usually be useful to provide tables and graphs that look at individual visits in relation to laboratory parameters, ECGs and vital signs. Here, it will be better to focus on maximum changes from baseline in each of the studies and collectively summarise those across all trials or across groups of trials that had similar design.

There will also be focus, in the summary of safety, on specific issues that arise during the course of the programme. For example, if liver toxicity has been an issue, then in addition to the tables and graphs for the liver transaminases, there would be a presentation of the numbers of Hy's law cases possibly looking also at time to occurrence in Kaplan–Meier curves.

19.2.7 Specific safety studies

At the approval stage and as a condition for approval, the sponsor may be requested to conduct a safety study in order to better characterise the incidence rates for specific AEs. This could be a randomised study but more likely would be an open-label single group study potentially involving an external control group. We have discussed observational studies in Chapter 17, but for the moment, let's consider what statistical arguments might be brought to bear in order to choose an appropriate sample size. As an example, suppose that the incidence rate for a particular event in the target population is generally around 2 per cent and there is concern that this rate may increase to an unacceptably high level, say, 10 per cent on the new experimental treatment. If the safety study was to be in a single group receiving the experimental treatment, then we would need to calculate the sample size needed to rule out an incidence rate on the experimental treatment of 10 per cent with, for example, 90 per cent power. Assuming a true rate on the experimental treatment of 4 per cent, a sample size of 200 will satisfy these conditions with a 2.5 per cent type I error. The analysis approach here is based around non-inferiority where the margin is set at 10 per cent, and we are looking to show that the incidence rate on the experimental treatment is below that level. With the data in hand, we would calculate a one-sided 97.5 per cent confidence interval for the rate, θ. If the upper endpoint is below 10 per cent, then we have ruled out an increase to that level.

19.3 Data monitoring committees

Data Monitoring Committees (DMCs) (DSMCs, DSMBs) are tasked with reviewing accumulating safety data in order to protect the safety of the subjects in the study. We have already spoken about the responsibilities of such committees in Section 14.4 and also the things they might look at from a safety point of view in Section 14.3. Here, we will further consider the kinds of safety data that they should be looking at and the form in which those data should be presented.

The tables and graphs that are reviewed by DMCs will be in line with those already discussed earlier in this chapter. In fact, it is often the case that the sponsor will provide the table templates that are the basis for the safety tables for the final clinical study report (CSR) to the independent statistician who will produce those same tables for the DMC in an ongoing way. Graphs are especially useful and enable the committee to gain an overview of evolving trends and safety concerns quickly.

It has to be accepted that although some data cleaning will have occurred, this will only be cursory and the tables and graphs will not be 100 per cent clean. Committee members should not be too alarmed at seeing discrepancies across the tables and graphs, although if these were to be substantial, they might want to ask questions about the cleaning process. There is always a conflict between wanting data that is timely and wanting data that is clean; the adage 'do you want it now or do you want it clean' applies! The data supplied to the DMC will come from the clinical database, which will be based on data collected on the case report forms (CRFs). There will be a delay in getting the data from the CRFs to the clinical database (although with electronic data capture the time for this should be short), cleaning the data in the database, sending those data through to the independent statistician and finally producing the tables and graphs and delivering these to the DMC members. These then need to be reviewed by the committee who then meets to discuss their content and issues arising. All of this takes time and it may well be that the data are several months out of date by time the committee comes to review them. In light of this, it is of value to at least have the SAE data more current. These data will come from the safety database and will be supplied by the sponsors Drug Safety Group and should be completely up to date. There may be some analysis in terms of summaries and descriptive statistics to be undertaken by the independent statistician, but essentially these data will be available to the DMC in real time. It could also be the case that the members of the committee have been receiving individual SAE reports in an ongoing way.

The DMC will usually only be reviewing tables and graphs that contain descriptive statistics. If however there are events of special interest, then some more formal analysis may be required. P-values can be produced periodically and form part of the evaluation of those events at the meetings of the DMC. Multiplicity is an issue if these p-values are calculated repeatedly, and this must be borne in mind when interpreting them, although the main concern with safety is not so much the false positive (falsely concluding that there is a signal); it is more the false negative (missing a signal) that we are worried about. It is possible to set up more formal stopping rules that protect the type I error at some pre-specified value, but in my experience these are rarely used.

19.4 Assessing benefit–risk

19.4.1 Current approaches

Balancing benefits and risks is a key element of the regulatory evaluation of all new products, and both the EMA and FDA use structured approaches for that evaluation. The EMA structure has been set down in the CHMP Day 80 Assessment Report template under a series of headings:

- Benefits
- Beneficial effects
- Uncertainty in the knowledge about the beneficial effects
- Risks
- Unfavourable effects
- Uncertainty in the knowledge about the unfavourable effects
- Balance (*between beneficial effects and unfavourable effects*)
- Importance of favourable and unfavourable effects
- Benefit–risk balance
- Discussion on the benefit–risk assessment

The FDA recognised the shortcomings of benefit–risk evaluation and set up a review with an associated implementation plan (FDA, 2013), which will be reported in 2017. Their initial review has led to the adoption of a benefit–risk framework with structure as set down in Table 19.2.

Neither of these frameworks uses any formal way of numerically combining the evidence for therapeutic benefit with the evidence for risk or harm. Each of those aspects is kept separated and their balance assessed intuitively through extensive discussion and consideration.

The CHMP in 2008 adopted a Reflection Paper on benefit–risk assessment methods (CHMP, 2008) and set up a Benefit–Risk Methodology Project to review the existing approach with a view to developing new methodologies. In a series of Work Packages (EMA, 2010, 2011a, 2011b, 2012), they evaluated a number of those methodologies, and this led to the adoption of multi-criteria decision analysis (MCDA) as the quantitative model for the assessment of benefit–risk. This methodology, which includes specific numerical ways of combining the evidence for benefit and risk in a formal way, will be described in the next section.

19.4.2 Multi-criteria decision analysis

Work Package 4 of the EMA Benefit–Risk Methodology Project sets down the MCDA methodology from the point of view of the regulatory assessment team. There are four steps and these are displayed in Figure 19.7.

Table 19.2 FDA benefit–risk framework

Decision factor	Evidence and uncertainties	Conclusion and reasons
Analysis of condition		
Current treatment options		
Benefit		
Risk		
Risk management		
Benefit–risk summary assessment		

Note: The first two factors are therapeutic area specific, while the final three factors relate to the drug.

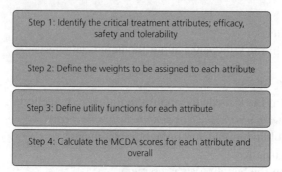

Step 1: Identify the critical treatment attributes; efficacy, safety and tolerability

Step 2: Define the weights to be assigned to each attribute

Step 3: Define utility functions for each attribute

Step 4: Calculate the MCDA scores for each attribute and overall

Figure 19.7 Steps in the calculation of MCDA scores

Step 1 of this approach sets down the efficacy benefits, termed favourable effects, and risks and harms, termed unfavourable effects, as a list of attributes with associated estimated effects. The example that follows is based on Caprelsa (300 mg) in the treatment of inoperable thyroid cancer and is adapted from Work Package 4, which used this as one of a series of hypothetical examples. The attributes and estimated effects below were taken from a single phase III placebo-controlled trial but more generally would be based on the totality of confirmatory evidence from the regulatory package as a whole:

- Favourable effects
  - Primary endpoint, progression-free survival (PFS): median = 30.5 months versus 19.3 months on placebo
  - Secondary endpoint, objective response rate (ORR): proportion of complete or partial responders = 45 per cent versus 13 per cent on placebo
- Unfavourable effects
  - Diarrhoea CTC grades 3–4: 10.8 per cent versus 2.0 per cent on placebo
  - QTc-related CTC grades 3–4: 13.4 per cent versus 1.0 per cent on placebo
  - Infection CTC grades 3–4: 49.8 per cent versus 36.4 per cent on placebo

The recommendation is to choose at most around 8 to 10 attributes, and these should encompass the key efficacy endpoints and those unfavourable effects that are relevant to the benefit–risk balance.

Step 2 involves giving weightings to the various attributes in stages that reflect their importance to the benefit–risk balance. These weights are subjective and will be chosen based on discussions within the assessment team. Sensitivity analyses to be discussed later will look at how the final benefit–risk balance is affected by changing these weights. Given the regulatory emphasis on safety, weights of 40 per cent and 60 per cent were assumed for efficacy and safety, respectively. Within the efficacy attributes, weights of 75 per cent for PFS and 25 per cent for ORR were assigned to reflect their relative importance, and within safety, the assigned weights were 20 per cent for diarrhoea, 40 per cent for QTc and 40 per cent for infections. Combining these weights gives relative importance weights as follows:

- PFS: $40\% \times 75\% = 30\%$
- ORR: $40\% \times 25\% = 10\%$

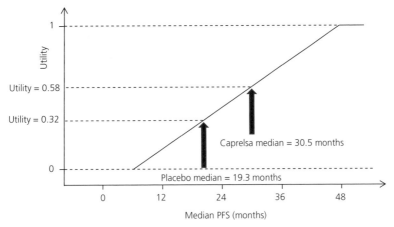

Figure 19.8 Utility values for PFS

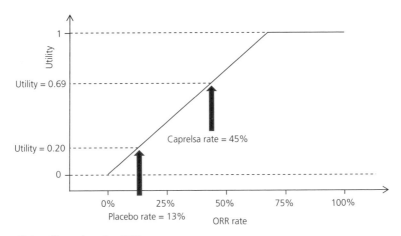

Figure 19.9 Utility values for ORR

- Diarrhoea: $60\% \times 20\% = 12\%$
- QTc: $60\% \times 40\% = 24\%$
- Infections: $60\% \times 40\% = 24\%$

Note that these weights add up to 100 per cent.

Step 3 requires the assignment of *utility* values to each of the attributes. These reflect the value to be placed on treatment differences of various orders of magnitude. For PFS, a median of below 6 months is viewed as being of little clinical value, and a median greater than 48 months is considered theoretically very unlikely. Figure 19.8 is a reflection of possible utility values. Again, this element of the model is subjective and would be formulated through a discussion with clinical experts in the field. The observed median PFS on Caprelsa is 30.5 months, giving a utility of 0.58, and the median PFS on placebo is 19.3 months, giving a utility of 0.32. Note that the higher the utility, the better.

Figure 19.9 provides a corresponding utility function for ORR. The assumption here is that an ORR of up to 0.65 is theoretically possible and the utility is a

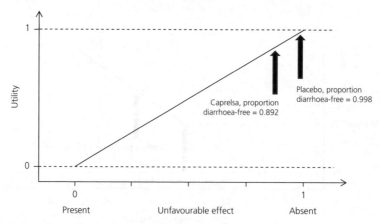

Figure 19.10 Utility values for unfavourable effects – diarrhoea

linear function of the ORR up to that value. According to the utility function, Caprelsa has a utility value of 0.69 and placebo a utility value of 0.20.

In step 4, we calculate the MCDA utility scores. The overall MCDA score, $SFE_{Caprelsa}$, for the favourable effects of Caprelsa is then

$$SFE_{Caprelsa} = 30\% \times 0.58 + 10\% \times 0.69 = 24.3$$

For placebo, the MCDA score is

$$SFE_{Placebo} = 30\% \times 0.32 + 10\% \times 0.20 = 11.6$$

The utility function for each of the unfavourable effects will be assumed to be linear taking the value 1 if the effect is absent and 0 if the effect is present (Figure 19.10). Again, higher values are better. We then use the incidence rates to calculate the utility values.

In order for larger values to correspond to desirable effects as for PFS and ORR, we will actually calculate 1 minus the incidence rate, which is the incidence rate for absence of the effect, so for each of the effects of interest, the utility values are:
- Caprelsa
  - Diarrhoea $= 1 - 0.108 = 0.892$
  - QTc $= 1 - 0.134 = 0.866$
  - Infections $= 1 - 0.498 = 0.502$
- Placebo
  - Diarrhoea $= 1 - 0.002 = 0.998$
  - QTc $= 1 - 0.001 = 0.999$
  - Infections $= 1 - 0.364 = 0.636$

The MCDA scores for the unfavourable effects are then

$$SUFE_{Caprelsa} = 12\% \times 0.892 + 24\% \times 0.866 + 24\% \times 0.502 = 43.5$$

$$SUFE_{Placebo} = 12\% \times 0.998 + 24\% \times 0.999 + 24\% \times 0.636 = 51.2$$

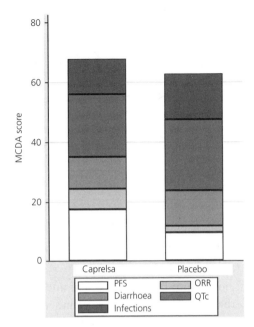

Figure 19.11 Stacked bar graph for MCDA scores

The total MCDA scores are then the sums corresponding to the favourable and unfavourable effects giving final scores of 24.3+43.5=67.8 for Caprelsa and 11.6+51.2=62.8 for placebo. The fact that the Caprelsa score is higher than the placebo score indicates a positive benefit–risk balance for Caprelsa. These scores are usually placed into a stacked bar graph as in Figure 19.11 to allow comparisons of the overall scores but also how the individual components make up those scores.

Clearly, there are several components of the MCDA model that have an element of subjectivity. In particular, the differential weights attached to the favourable and unfavourable effects, 40 per cent and 60 per cent, respectively in the example, may differ between regulators and payers on the one hand and physicians and patients on the other. Physicians and patients are possibly going to give more weight to the favourable effects arguing that the unfavourable effects can be managed. Changing these weights will change the MCDA scores. Greater weight given to the favourable effects, and corresponding less to the unfavourable effects, will usually favour the experimental treatment if it is efficacious. In the earlier example, assigning 50 per cent to both favourable and unfavourable effects gives an MCDA score of 66.7 to Caprelsa and 57.2 to placebo, an even greater benefit–risk balance. Figure 19.12 displays the sensitivity of the results to the chosen weights.

The positive benefit–risk balance is only lost if one is prepared to give a weight of 28.7 per cent or less to the favourable effects. The sensitivity of the overall scoring to the weights assigned to the separate attributes within the favourable and unfavourable effects can be explored in a similar way by changing those weights. There are commercial software packages available that apply this methodology. The EMA in their example uses Hiview Version 3 (available at www.catalze.co.uk).

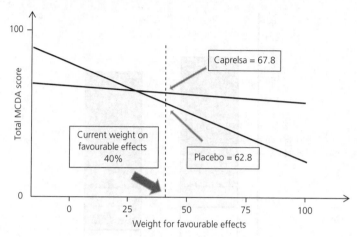

Figure 19.12 Sensitivity analyses for favourable–unfavourable weightings

For the moment, no account has been taken of uncertainly in the estimated treatment benefits, that is, the median PFS values and the ORRs, and the observed frequencies of undesirable effects, that is, the frequencies of CTC grade 3–4 diarrhoea, QTc prolongation and infections. A full sensitivity analysis will involve changing the estimated treatment differences and seeing what impact that has on the benefit–risk balance. It is straightforward to show that the difference in the MCDA scores (Caprelsa – placebo) is given by

$$\text{MCDA}_{\text{Caprelsa}} - \text{MCDA}_{\text{Placebo}} = 40\% \left\{ 75\% \times \left(\frac{m_C - m_{Pl}}{42} \right) + 25\% \times \left(\frac{\text{ORR}_C - \text{ORR}_{Pl}}{0.65} \right) \right\}$$
$$+ 60\% \left\{ 20\% \times \left(D_{Pl} - D_C \right) + 40\% \times \left(\text{QTc}_{Pl} - \text{QTc}_C \right) + 40\% \left(\inf_{Pl} - \inf_C \right) \right\}$$

where m_C and m_{Pl} are the median PFS values for Caprelsa and placebo, ORR denotes the objective response rates and D, QTc and inf are the incidence rates of CTC grade 3–4 diarrhoea, QTc prolongation and infections, respectively. Note that it is 1 minus the rates for the unfavourable effects that is used in the MCDA score calculation, and this is why the differences between those incidence rates in this equation are calculated by taking the Caprelsa incidence rate away from the placebo incidence rate, whereas for the favourable effects differences are taken by subtracting the placebo value away from the Caprelsa value. It might then be of interest, for example, to see what the impact would be if the actual difference in the PFS medians had been smaller than the observed 11.2 months. Undoubtedly, taking the difference in the medians much lower would remove the positive benefit–risk balance, but these aspects need to be explored in light of the sampling variation around the observed difference.

As mentioned the MCDA methodology contains certain subjective elements; the choice of which favourable and unfavourable effects to focus on, the weights assigned to those effects and finally the utility functions. We can of course evaluate the robustness of the conclusions by varying each of these aspects, but nonetheless, these elements of subjectivity have resulted in criticism of the technique. It is also the case that regulators, payers, clinicians and patients may all have quite difference views on which favourable and unfavourable effects are important, what weights should be placed on these and the utility functions to be assigned. In a sense, this criticism is understandable but in my view a little misplaced. The evaluation of the benefit–risk balance is subjective anyhow, and again, different people view this balance differently. At least with the MCDA method the various subjective elements are out in the open and can form a sound basis for discussion.

The MCDA methodology has been discussed earlier from the point of view of assessing benefit–risk (favourable–unfavourable effects) within a regulatory submission. This same technique can also be used for internal decision making within a company, perhaps for deciding which dose to take forwards from phase II to phase III where a corresponding trade-off between benefits and undesirable effects is needed. It can also be used to compare a product with a competitor product to allow better positioning in the marketplace.

19.4.3 Quality-Adjusted Time without Symptoms or Toxicity

Another method, *quality-adjusted time without symptoms or toxicity (Q-TWiST)*, is used in oncology and balances benefits in terms of overall survival (OS) against the toxic effects of treatment and disease progression. The method was introduced by Glasziou, Simes and Gelber (1990) and is now used widely in oncology settings as a combined efficacy/ quality of life measure of benefit. The method gives positive weight to increasing survival time that is free from both the toxic effects of treatment and progression.

The basic idea is to consider the time from randomisation in a clinical trial as consisting of three components labelled TOX, TWiST and REL. TOX measures the duration of toxicity as the time that the patient is suffering CTC grade 3 or 4 events, TWiST is the duration of survival that is free of toxicity and is prior to disease progression, and REL is the duration of time following progression or relapse. The mean values of each of these quantities are calculated from the patient data in each group. The mean value for TOX is the duration of toxicity up to progression or death for each patient. This duration may be zero if the patient does not suffer any CTC grade 3 or 4 events or may consist of two (or more) distinct periods if the patient suffers an event (or several events) over separate periods of time.

The mean values for PFS and OS are calculated from the Kaplan–Meier curves and represent restricted means over the complete follow-up period. There is a mathematical result that states that the mean survival time, for example, is equal to the area under the Kaplan–Meier curve for OS. This is only strictly true if that Kaplan–Meier curve comes down to meet the x-axis at zero. If it does not, then the area is not defined since the Kaplan–Meier curve for later time points simply stays flat and above zero. So in practice, what we do is to artificially bring the curve vertically down to zero at the maximum follow-up time. In a 48-week study for example, this would then happen at week 48. The mean that comes out of this calculation is a *restricted mean*, the mean value where the maximum value for each patient is set equal to 48 weeks in this example. This is fine in practice and allows us to compare treatments over the 48-week period. The mean for PFS is calculated from the Kaplan–Meier curve for that endpoint in the same way. There are three mean values for each treatment group, mean time with toxicity, mean PFS and mean OS, and based on these, we can calculate the duration of TWiST and the duration of REL as follows:

Duration of TWiST = mean PFS – mean time with toxicity

Duration of REL = mean OS – mean PFS

We then attach a utility to each of these states, u_{TOX}, u_{TWiST} and u_{REL}. Generally, we put $u_{TWiST} = 1$ as that is the best state (time without symptoms and toxicity) and give u_{TOX} and u_{REL} values below 1 1. The so-called *base case* often puts $u_{TOX} = u_{REL} = 0.5$; this says that one day in TWiST has the same value as two days in either the TOX or REL states. Sensitivity, or *threshold*, analyses will vary the values of these utilities to evaluate the robustness of the conclusions.

A Q-TWiST analysis will calculate the value of Q-TWiST for each of the treatment groups and look at the difference where

Q-TWiST = u_{TOX} × duration TOX + duration TWiST + u_{REL} × duration REL

A positive difference for an experimental treatment indicates a positive quality-adjusted survival for that treatment. The bootstrap method (Section 3.2.4) can be used to obtain confidence intervals for this difference and also give a *p*-value based on the ratio of the Q-TWiST difference divided by the bootstrap standard error. Example 19.1 provides an application of this methodology.

Example 19.1 Panitumumab plus best supportive care versus best supportive care in patients with wild-type KRAS metastatic colorectal cancer

Wang *et al.* (2011) report a Q-TWiST analysis in a comparison of panitumumab plus best supportive care (BSC) versus BSC in patients with wild-type KRAS metastatic colorectal cancer (mCRC). The mean durations (in weeks) in the various health states were 3.47, 13.26 and 9.35 for TOX, TWiST and REL in the panitumumab group and correspondingly 1.09, 8.01 and 16.15 in the BSC alone group. Note that the mean time with toxicity was greater in the experimental arm as might be expected. The mean time in the preferred state without symptoms or toxicity (TWiST) was however also greater for the experimental treatment, while the mean time in the relapse state was less. In the base case, the balance was such that there was a Q-TWiST advantage of 3.03 weeks with a 95 per cent bootstrap confidence interval of (0.86, 5.20). This difference was statistically significant; note that the confidence interval excludes 0. These authors also collected data on a quality of life scale (EQ-5D) and used that to derive utility weights of 0.60, 0.77 and 0.63 for the TOX, TWiST and REL states in the experimental arm and corresponding weights equal to 0.44, 0.66 and 0.64 in the BSC only arm. Note here that the utility weights were allowed to differ across treatment groups. Using these weights, the advantage of panitumumab+BSC over BSC alone in terms of Q-TWiST was 6.5 weeks (12.3 weeks vs. 5.8 weeks). A threshold analysis showed a numerical advantage for panitumumab except for some cases where the REL state was given a utility weight of 1. A utility weight of 1 for the REL state, as well as for the TWiST state, is not distinguishing the REL state in terms of quality of life from the TWiST state and this to a certain extent could be viewed as being unrealistic.

The Q-TWiST approach gives a broad-based measure for the balance between a specific favourable effect, prolonging life, and the unfavourable effects of toxicity and relapse. Clinicians find that this measure has intuitive appeal in that it down weights days living with toxicity and relapse.

19.5 Pharmacovigilance

19.5.1 Post-approval safety monitoring

Following regulatory approval for a drug, adverse drug reactions (ADRs) will be reported in a variety of different ways to the regulatory authorities. In Europe, the EMA for example, has set up the EudraVigilance Data Analysis System that stores data generated through spontaneous case safety reports of individual ADRs and enables stakeholders to analyse those data using various statistical techniques. We are looking here for *signals*, that is, early hints at *unintended drug effects*. In this section, we will be focusing on one particular approach to signal detection, the *proportional reporting ratio (PRR)*. This is the most frequently used measure and is the recommended approach in the EudraVigilance Expert Working Group guidance on the use of statistical signal detection methods within their system (EMA, 2008). Before going on to discuss the PRR, it is worth mentioning one or two other statistical techniques that can be of value in post-approval safety monitoring.

It may be that information comes to light which generates a hypothesis about safety concerns for a particular drug. In these settings, it can be of value to conduct a systematic review and meta-analysis to test out this hypothesis. Prochaska and Hilton (2012), for example, report on an evaluation of the risk of cardiovascular SAEs associated with varenicline use for tobacco cessation. Concern had been expressed for some time regarding this issue and one other systematic review had hinted at the potential for a problem. Prochaska and Hilton included a meta-analysis of 22 double-blind, placebo-controlled trials and reported a trend for increased risk in those subjects taking varenicline, although this increase was not statistically significant ($p=0.11$). The event of interest in this analysis was rare, and across all trials involving a total of over 9000 subjects, there were only 52 subjects with cardiovascular SAEs. A total of 8 of the trials reported no cardiovascular SAEs across both groups, while a further 8 trials reported no events in one or other treatment group. The low event rates make the statistical analysis more challenging. See Section 18.3.7 for discussion on this issue. The 8 trials with zero events were excluded from the meta-analysis. For the 8 trials that had zero counts in one of the treatment groups, a continuity correction was applied and 0.5 was added to each of the 4 counts in the 2×2 contingency table for that trial; so in a hypothetical example where there are 85 patients per group and the four contingency table entries are 0 and 85 in group 1 and 2 and 83 in group 2, 0 becomes 0.5, 2 becomes 2.5, 85 becomes 85.5, and 83 becomes 83.5.

Table 19.3 Contingency table for calculating a PRR

	Event (E)	All other events	Total
Drug (D)	a	b	a+b
All other drugs	c	d	c+d
Total	a+c	b+d	N=a+b+c+d

The MCDA methodology was presented in Section 19.4.2 in the context of balancing benefit and risk at the time of regulatory submission. As more data become available on both efficacy and safety post-approval, it is possible and useful to revisit such an analysis to judge whether the benefit–risk ratio has changed sufficiently to be concerning.

19.5.2 Proportional reporting ratios

The PRR has become a standard metric for the evaluation of safety signals. It is calculated for a drug–event pair and uses ideas associated with the disproportionality of reporting. The basic argument is that if a particular event (E) is indeed more prevalent with a particular drug (D), then that event should be reported more frequently with drug D than with other drugs. Table 19.3 is a 2×2 contingency table based on the number of events E associated with the drug of interest and all other drugs in a pharmacovigilance database. In this table:

- a is the number of subjects taking drug D who suffer the adverse event E.
- b is the number of subjects taking drug D who suffer other adverse events (not E).
- c is the number of subjects taking others drugs (not D) who suffer adverse event E.
- d is the number of subjects not taking drug D who suffer other adverse events (not E).

The PRR is defined as follows:

$$PRR = \frac{a/(a+b)}{c/(c+d)}$$

If event E is more prevalent in patients taking drug D compared to other drugs. then $a/(a+b)$ will be larger than $c/(c+d)$ and the PRR will be much bigger than 1. This is the idea behind the PRR with values above 1 signifying an association between the drug and the event. The formula for the standard error associated with the PRR is expressed on the log scale and is:

$$se\,(ln\text{PRR}) = \sqrt{1/a + 1/c - 1/(a+b) - 1/(c+d)}$$

A 95 per cent confidence interval on the log scale is then

$$\left(ln\text{PRR} - 1.96 \times se, ln\text{PRR} + 1.96 \times se\right)$$

Once this is calculated. the reverse transformation (antilog) can be applied to the ends of the interval to give a 95 per cent confidence interval back on the PRR scale.

The examples contained in Example 19.2 are taken from EMA (2008).

Example 19.2 Calculating PRR

Here. we are looking for an association between a drug D and the event nausea.

Case 1
Suppose that there are 100 reports of patients with AEs for drug D and of these 5 are of nausea. Then

$a = 5, \; b = 95$ and $a + b = 100$

Suppose there are 100,000 reports of patients with AEs for all other drugs in the database (not including drug D) and of these 5,000 are of nausea. Then

$c = 5,000, \; d = 95,000$ and $c + d = 100,000$

In this case, $\dfrac{a}{a+b} = \dfrac{c}{c+d} = 0.05$ and PRR $= 1$ and we do not have a signal that links this drug with nausea. The 95 per cent confidence interval for the PRR in this case is (0.43, 2.35).

Case 2
Suppose that there are 100 reports of patients with AEs for drug D and of these 15 are of nausea. Then

$a = 15, \; b = 85$ and $a + b = 100$

Suppose there are 100,000 reports of patients with AEs for all other drugs in the database (not including drug D) and of these 5,000 are of nausea. Then

$c = 5,000, \; d = 95,000$ and $c + d = 100,000$

In this case, $\dfrac{a}{a+b} = \dfrac{15}{100}, \dfrac{c}{c+d} = \dfrac{5000}{100000}$ and PRR $= \dfrac{0.15}{0.05} = 3$ and we do have a signal that links this drug with nausea. The 95 per cent confidence interval for the PRR in this case is (1.88, 4.79).

The ideas behind the PRR were developed by Evans, Waller and Davis (2001) who suggested that a PRR greater than 2 indicates a drug–event combination that is worthy of further investigation. In addition to the PRR, they suggest two other criteria that should be applied as a guide to the existence of a signal, namely, that there should be at least 3 or more cases of the event E associated with drug D and also that the chi-square (test) statistic in the 2×2 table (Table 19.3) should be at least 4. The chi-square statistic in that table is given by

$$\frac{N \times (a \times d - b \times c)^2}{(a+b)(a+c)(c+d)(b+d)}$$

Note that this statistic was expressed differently $\left(\text{as} \; \sum \dfrac{O - E^2}{E} \right)$ in Section 4.4.1 when we developed the chi-square test based on observed and expected frequencies, but these two quantities are numerically equal. There is a slight variant on this three-item detection system. If the 95 per cent confidence interval is calculated for the PRR, then rather than simply taking the value 2 as the threshold for a signal, we look at the lower end of that confidence interval and an alternative threshold is based on that value being above 1.

Using this method based on these three criteria (with the condition that the PRR be >2, rather than the lower confidence limit above 1), Evans *et al.* examined retrospectively 15 newly marketed drugs in the UK Yellow Card database, which had the highest levels of ADR reporting at that time. The method identified 481 signals. Further evaluation showed that 339 (70 per cent) were known adverse reactions, 62 (13 per cent) were signals that were linked to the underlying disease and 80 (17 per cent) were signals requiring further investigation. Of the 80 new signals identified, many went on to receive a detailed review. Of the 80 signals, 11 signals were in fact for dexfenfluramine that was withdrawn from the market during the period covered by the study.

It is accepted that there are a number of potential biases associated with these methods. The spontaneous reporting system on which the validity of the methodology depends has clear limitations in terms of collecting complete information in an unbiased way.

EMA (2008): 'Guideline on the Use of Statistical Signal Detection Methods in the EudraVigilance Data Analysis System'

'The results of quantitative methods should be interpreted with caution and bearing in mind the limitations of the spontaneous reporting system databases. ... Consequently there is a scientific consensus that SDRs (Signals of disproportionate reporting) identified with quantitative methods should always be medically assessed'.

Also, there will inevitably be over-reporting, in part because of multiplicity, although methods that take account of that are available and these will be briefly discussed in the next section. Despite this and given the development of methods that account for some, but not all of the problems, the PRR methodology has been widely adopted and over the years has proved to be a reliable way to detect safety signals in pharmacovigilance.

19.5.3 Bayesian shrinkage

Some signals detected using PRRs will simply be caused by random fluctuations. Also, there are issues associated with multiplicity when looking at a number of drugs and SAEs in a routine way. To account for these, methods are available (see, e.g., DuMouchel, 1999) that down weight or *shrink* the PRR values. Many methods are available but one common approach is based on an empirical Bayesian method (see Section 15.5). Suppose that there are n drugs and m events reported in the database and an associated $n \times m$ PRR values. The *empirical*

Bayes geometric mean (EBGM) uses the distribution of the observed PRRs as the prior distribution in a Bayesian analysis. This prior, apart from a few extremes, represents random fluctuation (and this represents our *a priori* sceptical view on the distribution of these ratios) and when combined with the PRR for the drug×event of interest (the data in the Bayesian analysis) produces a posterior distribution. The EBGM value is then the geometric mean of this posterior distribution, and this is the adjusted PRR. This will be adjusted (or shrunk) downwards towards 1 as a consequence of the sceptical prior distribution. The posterior distribution is positively skewed, which is why the method is based on geometric means (which behave rather like medians) rather than arithmetic means. It is these adjusted values that we tend to work with for decision making. It is straightforward to calculate a 95 per cent credible interval with a lower limit denoted by EB05 and an upper limit by EB95. Various rules can be applied with regard to what constitutes a signal. For example if EB05 is greater than 1 there is a 95 per cent probability that an increase in the risk of suffering that event with that drug.

CHAPTER 20
Diagnosis

20.1 Introduction

Evaluating diagnostic tests requires measuring performance we will initially review relevant statistical methods. As a start point, we will assume that we have a definitive diagnosis through some gold standard (*standard of truth*) or something very close to that; regulators talk in terms of a *surrogate standard of truth*.

CHMP (2009): 'Guideline on Clinical Evaluation of Diagnostic Agents'

'Surrogate standard of truth: a diagnostic test or a combination of tests or follow-up which has been shown to provide a very good approximation to the true disease state or value of measurement'.

We will then discuss aspects of the design of trials that are looking to develop new diagnostic tests. Throughout the development, we will use a specific example as a case study. De la Taille *et al.* (2011) evaluated the clinical utility of the PCA3 (prostate cancer gene, PROGENSA®) assay in supporting biopsy decisions in prostate cancer. Higher values of the PCA3 score are indicative of the presence of cancer. The study recruited 516 men who recorded serum total prostate-specific antigen (tPSA) between 2.5 ng/ml and 10 ng/ml and were therefore scheduled for initial biopsy.

There are also many situations where a standard of truth or a surrogate standard of truth do not exist, and methods then focus on assessing the agreement between different diagnostic tests. In the final sections, we will look at methods based on the kappa statistic, which can measure the extent of the agreement.

20.2 Measures of diagnostic performance

20.2.1 Sensitivity and specificity

Sensitivity and specificity are the measures that we primarily use in judging the performance of a diagnostic test. Table 20.1 is based on the de la Taille *et al.* data. Initially, these authors used 50 as the cut-off score on the PCA3 scale potentially indicating the presence of cancer.

Statistical Thinking for Non-Statisticians in Drug Regulation, Second Edition. Richard Kay.
© 2015 John Wiley & Sons, Ltd. Published 2015 by John Wiley & Sons, Ltd.

Table 20.1 PCA3 and biopsy results

	Biopsy negative	Biopsy positive	Total
PCA3 < 50	TN = 256	FN = 103	TN + FN = 359
PCA3 ≥ 50	FP = 53	TP = 104	FP + TP = 157
Total	TN + FP = 309	FN + TP = 207	n = 516

TN, true negative; FN, false negative; FP, false positive; TP, true positive; n = total sample size.

Source: Data from de la Taille *et al.* (2001).

The rows relate to the result of the PCA3 assay, while the columns denote the result of the biopsy that definitively tells us about the presence (biopsy positive) or absence (biopsy negative) of prostate cancer. The symbols in the table denote the following:

- TN = true negative. Patients who had PCA3 < 50 and a negative biopsy
- FN = false negative. Patients who had PCA3 < 50 and a positive biopsy
- FP = false positive. Patients who had PCA3 ≥ 50 and a negative biopsy
- TP = true positive. Patients who had PCA3 ≥ 50 and a positive biopsy

Sensitivity is defined as the proportion of (true) positives (those that have cancer) that are correctly diagnosed using the diagnostic test, that is,

$$\text{Sensitivity} = \frac{TP}{FN + TP} = \frac{104}{207} = 0.50 \text{ or } 50\%$$

Of the patients who have cancer, 50 per cent are correctly diagnosed using the diagnostic test.

Specificity is defined as the proportion of (true) negatives (those that do not have cancer) that are correctly diagnosed using the diagnostic test, that is,

$$\text{Specificity} = \frac{TN}{TN + FP} = \frac{256}{309} = 0.83 \text{ or } 83\%$$

Of the patients who do not have cancer, 83 per cent are correctly diagnosed using the diagnostic test.

For a diagnostic test to be effective, both of these measures need to be high. Sensitivity is about the ability of the test to detect the true cases of cancer (true positive rate); we do not want to be missing real cases. Specificity is all about correctly eliminating those patients who do not have cancer (true negative rate).

20.2.2 Positive and negative predictive value

The *positive predictive value* (PPV) is the proportion of true positives among those patients testing positive:

$$PPV = \frac{TP}{FP + TP} = \frac{104}{157} = 0.66 \text{ or } 66\%$$

The *negative predictive value* (NPV) is the proportion of true negatives among those patients testing negative:

$$NPV = \frac{TN}{FN + TN} = \frac{256}{359} = 0.71 \text{ or } 71\%$$

PPV estimates the probability that a patient has the disease given that they have tested positive, while NPV estimates the probability that the patient does not have the disease given that they have tested negative.

20.2.3 False positive and false negative rates

The *false positive rate* (FPR) is the proportion testing positive among those patients who do not have the disease:

$$FPR = \frac{FP}{TN + FP} = \frac{53}{309} = 0.17 \text{ or } 17\%$$

The *false negative rate* (FNR) is the proportion testing negative among the those patients who do have the disease:

$$FNR = \frac{FN}{FN + TP} = \frac{103}{207} = 0.50 \text{ or } 50\%$$

The FPR records the number of false alarms, while the FNR records the number of missed cases. Note that these two quantities are directly related to specificity and sensitivity with FPR = 1 − (specificity) and FNR = 1 − (sensitivity).

20.2.4 Prevalence

In the example taken from de la Taille *et al.*, the proportion of patients with prostate cancer (*prevalence*) is 207/516 = 0.40 or 40 per cent. Suppose we had been assessing the performance of the PCA3 assay (with a cut-off at 50) in a slightly different population, one where the prevalence had been for example 60 per cent. Table 20.2 provides data for this setting. Note that these data are artificial and they have been generated simply by changing the prevalence from 40 per cent to 60 per cent.

Table 20.2 PCA3 and biopsy results, prevalence = 60 per cent

	Biopsy negative	Biopsy positive	Total
PCA3 < 50	TN = 171	FN = 154	TN + FN = 325
PCA3 ≥ 50	FP = 35	TP = 156	FP + TP = 191
Total	TN + FP = 206	FN + TP = 310	n = 516

TN, true negative; FN, false negative; FP, false positive; TP, true positive; n = total sample size.

The values for sensitivity and specificity for the diagnostic test remain unchanged at 50 per cent and 83 per cent, respectively, as do the FPR and FNR. The values for PPV and NPV however change and , with a prevalence of 60 per cent, PPV = 156/191 = 0.82 or 82 per cent and NPV = 171/325 = 0.53 or 53 per cent. These changes reflect the fact that when prevalence increases, we are much more likely to say that the disease is present *a priori* than we are to say that the disease is absent, so the PPV goes up, while the NPV goes down. Sensitivity and specificity are quantities that objectively measure how good the test is. Altman and Bland (1994) discuss the connections between PPV, NPV, sensitivity, specificity and prevalence further.

20.2.5 Likelihood ratio

The so-called *likelihood ratio* (LR) in connection with diagnostic tests is defined as

$$LR = \frac{\text{sensitivity}}{1 - \text{specificity}}$$

This is the ratio of the estimated probability of having a positive diagnostic test result among patients with the disease compared to the estimated probability of also having a positive diagnostic test result among patients who do not have the disease. We want this ratio to be large for a good diagnostic test, and for our case study with a cut-point of 50, the likelihood ratio is equal to 2.9.

20.2.6 Predictive accuracy

If we were simply to look at the *predictive accuracy* (PA) overall, then this would be $PA = \dfrac{TP + TN}{n} = \dfrac{256 + 104}{516} = 0.70$ or 70 per cent. Note that this quantity also depends on prevalence. For the artificial data in Table 20.2 where the prevalence is increased from 40 per cent to 60 per cent, the PA is now only 63 per cent. The reason for this is that this particular PCA3-based test is better at identifying the true negatives than it is at identifying the true positives, and as the prevalence of disease increases, the diagnostic test performs less well overall.

Most of the measures defined in this section are based on proportions, and it is straightforward to obtain standard errors and hence confidence intervals for those proportions as in Section 2.5.2.

20.2.7 Choosing the correct cut-point

The performance of the diagnostic test relies on the cut-off that has been chosen on the underlying continuous scale in order to classify an observed value on that scale as either positive or negative. In the case study, a score of 50 on the PCA3 scale was the chosen cut-point. One issue then is, is this the best cut-point? If we were to change the cut-point how would the performance of the test change? Table 20.3 contains values for sensitivity and specificity using several different cut-points.

Table 20.3 Sensitivity and specificity of the PCA3 assay

Cut-point	Sensitivity (%) (95% CI)	Specificity (%) (95% CI)
20	84 (78, 88)	55 (50, 61)
35	64 (57, 71)	76 (71, 81)
50	50 (43, 57)	83 (79, 87)

Source: Data from de la Taille *et al.* (2011).

The best cut-point will be chosen in order to balance the trade-off between sensitivity and specificity. Are we more concerned about the true positive rate (identifying true cases) with the emphasis on sensitivity or the true negative rate (eliminating negative cases) with the emphasis on specificity?

CHMP (2009): 'Guideline on Clinical Evaluation of Diagnostic Agents'

'In case the test decision is based on a cut-off value the trade-off between sensitivity and specificity requires careful analysis with respect to intended applications of an experimental test and their implications on patient care'.

A cut-point of 35 gives sensitivity of 64 per cent and specificity of 76 per cent, and de la Taille *et al.* argue that this provides the optimal balance between these two measures based on clinical considerations.

20.3 Receiver operating characteristic curves

20.3.1 Receiver operating characteristic

Receiver operating characteristic (ROC) curves plot sensitivity on the *y*-axis against 1– (specificity) on the *x*-axis, as the cut-point (threshold for defining a positive result) is varied. These curves overall provide a summary of the potential for the underlying measure (PCA3 in our example) to form the basis for a good diagnostic test. Figure 20.1, taken from de la Taille *et al.* (2011), shows four ROC curves together with an ROC curve at a line of 45°, which will serve as a reference curve. The PCA3 measure is the basis of one of those curves.

The ROC curve that is the 45° line depicts a diagnostic test that has no discriminating ability. Such a measure, whatever the cut-point chosen, gives a test with 50 per cent sensitivity and 50 per cent specificity; in other words, the test provides a diagnosis based on the toss of a coin. Diagnostic tests that have value will have associated ROC curves that are to the left of the 45° line, and the more to the left, the better.

A numerical measure of the potential of the diagnostic test is given by the *area under the curve* (AUC). For the test to be useful, the AUC will need to be

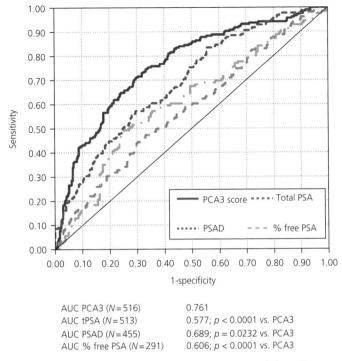

AUC PCA3 (*N* = 516)   0.761
AUC tPSA (*N* = 513)   0.577; *p* < 0.0001 vs. PCA3
AUC PSAD (*N* = 455)   0.689; *p* = 0.0232 vs. PCA3
AUC % free PSA (*N* = 291)   0.606; *p* < 0.0001 vs. PCA3

Figure 20.1 ROC curves for PCA3 and other diagnostic tests. Source: de la Taille A, Irani J, Graefen M, *et al.* (2011) Clinical Evaluation of the PCA3 Assay in Guiding Initial Biopsy Decisions. *Journal of Urology*, **185**, 2119–2125. Reproduced with permission from American Urological Association Education and Research, Inc.

above 0.5, given that a test that assigns based on chance alone achieves that. In theory, it is possible to see the AUC below 0.5; this is a test that systematically provides a wrong diagnosis. In practice, we rarely come across this. The AUC for the PCA3 ROC curve in the case study is 0.761 (de la Taille *et al.*, 2011). It is possible to construct a test of the hypothesis (one sided) that the diagnostic test has AUC at least 0.5 ($H_0 : AUC \leq 0.5$ vs. $H_1 : AUC > 0.5$). Further details of this test are provided in Zhou, Obuchowski and McClish (2002, Chapter 4).

20.3.2 Comparing ROC curves

It is of interest to compare ROC curves based on distinct diagnostic procedures. In addition to the PCA3 assay, de la Taille *et al.* (2011) investigate three other methods, namely, total prostate specific antigen (tPSA), per cent free total specific antigen (%free PSA) and prostate-specific antigen density (PSAD). The AUCs for these alternative measures were 0.577 (tPSA), 0.606 (%free PSA) and 0.689 (PSAD), indicating poorer performance compared to PCA3, and the ROC curves are shown in Figure 20.1.

DeLong, DeLong and Clarke-Pearson (1988) have constructed a non-parametric statistical test that formally compares the different measures through their AUC values. For the data of the case studies, the p-values comparing PCA3 with each of the three other methodologies were <0.001 when comparing with tPSA ($n=513$) and with%free PSA ($n=291$) and 0.023 when comparing with PSAD ($n=455$). These p-values are statistically significant, indicating a significantly improved performance from the PCA3 assay. Note that the n's in brackets here tell us the numbers of patients who gave observations on the particular measure under consideration.

20.4 Diagnostic performance using regression models

It may well be the case that there are variables, such as age, prostate volume, etc., that provide additional information (additional to PCA3) on which to base a diagnosis. Regression modelling allows us to take these additional factors into account and to assess to what extent they improve the performance of the diagnostic test. Conversely, these variables of themselves may provide the basis for a diagnosis. The key question then might be, does PCA3 provide any additional discriminating ability? The variables considered may also include the results of other diagnostic tests, and we are looking to see if the new test provides any additional diagnostic discrimination.

The four variables considered in the modelling exercise for the case study were:

x_1 Age (in years)

x_2 Digital rectal examination (DRE), classified as suspicious or unsuspicious

x_3 PSA

x_4 Prostate volume

A logistic model (Section 6.4) was fitted to the data by de la Taille *et al*. This model used the true outcome prostate cancer/no prostate cancer as the binary outcome with each of these variables plus PCA3 considered as potential x-variables in a model for the odds in favour of having prostate cancer as follows:

$$ln(\text{odds}) = a + b_1 x_1 + b_2 x_2 + \cdots$$

The model is initially fitted to the observed data to obtain estimated values of the coefficients a, b_1, b_2 and so on. Using this fitted model, it is then possible to predict the odds in favour of having prostate cancer based solely on the x-variable values for each and every patient. If these odds are >1, then the model is predicting that the patient has prostate cancer. If the odds are <1, then the opposite prediction – that they do not have prostate cancer – is being made for that patient. This then produces a series of individual patient predictions, and based on these, it is possible to form a 2×2 table as we have seen in Tables 20.1 and 20.2 and to calculate various summary statistics to measure the performance of the model in predicting the outcome. In the discussion here, we will focus on predictive accuracy as a measure of performance although equally one could look at sensitivity and specificity or any other suitable measure. One thing to note is that the prevalence here affects

Table 20.4 Logistic regression analysis of potential diagnostic variables

	Base model		Base model plus PCA3		Base model plus PCA3 (cut-point 35)	
	Coefficient	p-value	Coefficient	p-value	Coefficient	p-value
Age	1.07	<0.001	1.05	0.001	1.04	0.01
DRE	2.30	0.001	2.24	0.003	2.16	0.006
PSA	1.15	0.006	1.15	0.013	1.13	0.013
Prostate volume	0.96	<0.001	0.96	<0.001	0.97	<0.001
PCA3			1.01	<0.001	4.38	<0.001
Predictive accuracy	0.737		0.780		0.792	

Source: Data from de la Taille *et al.* (2011).
DRE, digital rectal examination, classified as suspicious or unsuspicious; PCA3, prostate cancer antigen 3;
PSA, prostate-specific antigen.

only the value of a in the model and not the values of b_1, b_2, etc. and therefore the contribution of each of the variables being considered.

Table 20.4 provides the coefficients of the x-variables together with p-values assessing the statistical significance of each variable in the model. Note again that the coefficients (b_1, b_2, etc.) and the associated p-values are unaffected by the underlying prevalence in the population under study. The *base model* is the model containing the four potential predictors listed earlier in this section. As can be seen, each of those variable coefficients is statistically significantly different from 0, indicating that each variable is providing information as to whether or not a patient has prostate cancer. The overall predictive accuracy of the model for the data of the case study is 73.7 per cent. PCA3, measured on a continuous scale, is then introduced into the model. The coefficient of PCA3 is significantly different from 0 suggesting that this variable is having a significant impact on predicting the outcome in addition to the other variables. The statistical significance of all the other variables in the model is also maintained, and the predictive accuracy with PCA3 in the model increases to 78.0 per cent. Finally, a model is fitted with PCA3 included as a binary variable using 35 as the cut-point. The coding of this variable is 0 if PCA3 < 35 and 1 if PCA3 ≥ 35. Again, all variables in this model are statistically significant, but more importantly, the PA is increased to 79.2 per cent using this model.

The predictive accuracy using PCA3 with 35 as the cut-point without using the logistic modelling and additional variables, calculated as in Table 20.1, was 71.1 per cent. The modelling, where additional information has been included based on the four key variables, age, DRE, PSA and prostate volume, has increased this to 79.2 per cent. It is not uncommon to see increases resulting from a modelling exercise that includes key additional variables and associated diagnostic information. Modelling of this kind can lead to the construction or a *diagnostic index*, which in this case would be the right-hand side of the fitted logistic model earlier. If for a particular patient the value of this index is positive, then this would lead to an odds for prostate cancer >1, while a negative value for the index would lead to an odds for prostate cancer <1.

20.5 Aspects of trial design for diagnostic agents

Trials evaluating new diagnostic tests will usually be within-patient designs with each patient receiving the investigational agent, a comparator agent and a definitive diagnosis that establishes the standard of truth. Inclusion of the comparator agent allows assessment of superiority to that agent or possibly non-inferiority if the investigational agent offers some advantages such as cost, convenience or safety. Usually, it will not be appropriate however to have a full crossover-type design especially if the standard of truth involves some form of invasive procedure such as surgery. The preferred design would be a 2×2 design randomising to either investigational agent followed by comparator agent or comparator agent followed by investigational agent with the definitive diagnosis following on from that. Within the 2×2 portion of the study, it would be important to avoid *information carry-over* so that the second test is evaluated without knowledge of the results of the first test. See Section 1.7 for a discussion on carry-over effects in crossover trials.

Superiority of the investigational agent over the comparator can be established using the logistic regression techniques detailed in the previous section. Here, PCA3 played the role of the investigational agent, while PSA played the role of the comparator agent. Including PSA in the model assessing the additional impact of PCA3 is considering the investigational agent as add-on to an existing diagnostic work-up. If we were looking to replace an existing diagnostic agent by the new agent, perhaps because of cost or safety reasons, then we would be comparing two models, one including PSA (but not PCA3) with one including PCA3 (but not PSA). This latter scenario could also be evaluated by comparing AUCs under the ROC curves using the DeLong *et al.* (1988) method detailed in Section 20.3.2 although this would not be in the presence of the additional 3 variables; age, DRE and prostrate volume.

The methodology using logistic modelling does not directly evaluate sensitivity and specificity, and it may be appropriate to work more closely with these quantities. Indeed, the regulatory guidelines suggest that these measures be considered as co-primary endpoints. Methods that use these measures directly are available but beyond the scope of this book, and the reader is referred to Chen, Hsueh and Liu (2003) for further details. The methods of that paper are primarily focused on demonstrating the non-inferiority of the investigational agent versus the comparator agent, but these methods are easily adapted to deal with superiority by considering the non-inferiority margin to be zero.

When no standard of truth is available, developing new diagnostic agents is more challenging, and it may be necessary to conduct trials that focus on clinical outcomes; does the investigational agent lead to better clinical outcomes when evaluated against the comparator agent?

CHMP (2009): 'Guideline on Clinical Evaluation of Diagnostic Agents'

'Studies assessing patient outcomes may be required if there is no standard of truth to compare to'.

In these circumstances, an evaluation of the agreement between the investigational and comparator agents may be of value. This is the topic of the next section.

20.6 Assessing agreement

20.6.1 The kappa statistic

The kappa statistic developed by Cohen (1960) is a measure of agreement between two diagnostic tests. The tests, for example, may be a radiologist's analysis of an X-ray and a computer analysis of the same X-ray. Neither test is perfect in the sense that neither gives a definitive answer in terms of the tumour being malignant or benign and neither can therefore be considered the standard of truth. There is inevitably going to be some level of agreement purely by chance and the kappa statistic takes account of this chance element in the calculation. Table 20.5 presents some hypothetical data on 94 X-rays with classification in terms of benign/malignant being made by both the radiologist and the computer. There is quite a lot of agreement between the radiologist and the computer. For a total of 61 X-rays, both methods result in a diagnosis of benign, while for 25 X-rays, both give a diagnosis of malignant. There are also some disagreements; 8 in total.

Some of the agreements will occur purely by chance even if both the radiologist and computer are simply guessing at what the diagnosis is. Overall, the radiologist declares benign in 63 out of 94 X-rays (67.0 per cent), while the computer declares benign in 67 out of 94 X-rays (71.3 per cent); there is a slight tendency

Table 20.5 Classification by radiologist/computer in relation to benign/malignant disease

		Computer		Total
		Benign	Malignant	
Radiologist	Benign	61	2	63
	Malignant	6	25	31
	Total	67	27	$n = 94$

n, total sample size.

for the computer to be more likely to result in a diagnosis of benign. If both were diagnosing based on chance, then the proportion of cases that would result in a diagnosis of benign would be $0.670 \times 0.713 = 0.478$. So for 47.8 per cent of the X-rays, there would be an agreed diagnosis of benign by chance. The radiologist declares malignant in 31 out of the 94 X-rays (33.0 per cent), while the computer declares malignant in 27 out of the 94 X-rays (28.7 per cent). By chance, we would then expect them to agree with a diagnosis of malignant on $0.330 \times 0.287 = 0.095$, that is, 9.5 per cent of occasions. Overall agreement will therefore happen purely by chance on $0.478 + 0.095 = 0.572$, that is, 57.2 per cent of occasions. The observed level of agreement is $(61 + 25)/94 = 0.915$, and the *kappa statistic* then measures how much better we are compared to chance alone:

$$\kappa = \frac{0.915 - 0.572}{1 - 0.572} = 0.801$$

Higher values for κ signify better agreement. Landis and Koch (1977) set down various thresholds for an interpretation of the magnitude of this statistic: $\leq 0.20 =$ slight agreement, > 0.20 but $\leq 0.40 =$ fair agreement, > 0.40 but $\leq 0.60 =$ moderate agreement, > 0.60 but $\leq 0.80 =$ substantial agreement and $> 0.80 =$ excellent agreement.

It is possible in theory to get a value for κ that is below zero; this will happen if the level of agreement is worse than chance. Fortunately, this is rarely seen in practice.

It is also possible to obtain a confidence interval for κ in the usual way based on assuming large sample normality for the distribution of the statistic. The standard error formula is

$$se(\kappa) = \sqrt{\frac{p\,(1-p)}{n\,(1-p_e)^2}}$$

where p is the observed proportion of agreements and p_e is the expected proportion of agreements that would be obtained by chance. Note that using this notation the kappa statistic is defined as $\kappa = (p - p_e)/(1 - p_e)$. In the example earlier, $p = 0.915$ and $p_e = 0.572$, giving a standard error of 0.067 and a 95 per cent confidence interval of

$$0.801 \pm (1.96 \times 0.067) = (0.67, 0.93)$$

In practice, if the calculated upper limit of this confidence interval is above 1, it is replaced by 1 in the reported confidence interval.

20.6.2 Other applications for kappa

The kappa statistic is used outside of diagnosis to measure inter-rater and intra-rater agreement. *Inter-rater agreement* is the agreement between two independent raters or observers. *Intra-rater agreement* concerns agreement between separate assessments by the same observer.

In this context, it is not uncommon for an observer to provide an outcome rating on an ordinal rather than a binary scale. For example, two observers may be rating the general health of an individual as poor, fair, good and excellent based on some general guidelines, and as an evaluation of the performance of the guideline and the training given to the observers, it may be necessary to ascertain the level of agreement between the two observers. Not all disagreements however are alike. If one observer records a poor rating for an individual, while the other observer rates that same individual as excellent, then we have major disagreement. Had the second observer given a rating of fair, then maybe that would be not quite so bad. *Weighted kappa* takes account of the level of disagreement by assigning weights to the various disagreement possibilities. One simple way of doing this might be to give a weight of 1 to disagreements that are one category apart, a weight of 2 to disagreements that are two categories apart and a weight of 3 to the most major disagreements, those that are three categories apart. Alternatively, we may view the most major disagreements as very problematic and assign a weight of 4 (or even 5) rather than 3 for that. The interested reader is referred to Altman (1991, Sections 14.3) for further details and formulas for the calculation of weighted kappa.

CHAPTER 21

The role of statistics and statisticians

21.1 The importance of statistical thinking at the design stage

A clinical trial is an experiment, and not only do we have to ensure that the clinical elements fit with the objectives of the trial, but we also have to design the trial in a tight scientific way to make sure that it is capable of providing valid answers to the key questions in an unbiased, precise and structured way. This is where the statistics comes in, and statistical thinking is a vital element of the design for every clinical trial.

The following list of areas where statistical thinking is required is not exhaustive, but is meant to give a flavour of the sorts of things that need to be considered:

- What are the key prognostic factors, and how, if at all, should these be used to stratify the randomisation?
- Should the randomisation be stratified by centre or by some higher-level factor, for example, region or country?
- What are the implications for block size in terms of ensuring balance and to prevent inadvertent unblinding?
- How should we choose primary and secondary endpoints in line with the clinical objectives for the trial?
- What methods can be used to control variability in order to increase precision?
- Which objectives form part of the confirmatory strategy for the trial, and which elements are purely exploratory?
- What statistical testing strategy will provide valid answers to the range of questions being asked, particularly in terms of controlling multiplicity in the confirmatory setting?
- For each of the comparisons being considered, is the focus superiority, equivalence or non-inferiority, and in the latter two cases, how should we choose the non-inferiority margin?
- How will the homogeneity of treatment effect be assessed, and in particular, what subgroups will be evaluated in this regard?

Statistical Thinking for Non-Statisticians in Drug Regulation, Second Edition. Richard Kay.
© 2015 John Wiley & Sons, Ltd. Published 2015 by John Wiley & Sons, Ltd.

- Is it appropriate to build in an interim analysis given the nature of the trial; is this practical, and if so, how should the interim analysis be structured?
- How many patients are needed to provide answers to the questions being asked, and what are the assumptions upon which this calculation is based?
- Do we need to revisit the sample size calculation at some interim stage in the trial?
- What are the implications of the trial procedures on the potential dropout rate and the extent of missing data?
- What impact are the dropouts and missing data likely to have on the definition of analysis sets and in particular our ability to align with the principle of intention-to-treat?
- Overall, will the trial provide an unbiased and precise estimate of the true treatment effect?

These particular points relate to each individual trial, but equally, there will be similar considerations needed at the level of the development plan. In order for the overall, ordered programme of clinical trials to be scientifically sound, there needs to be a substantial amount of commonality across the trials in terms of endpoints, definitions of analysis sets, recording of covariates and so on. This will facilitate the use of integrated summaries and meta-analysis for the evaluation and presentation of the complete programme or distinct parts of that programme and, outside of that, will allow a consistency of approach to the evaluation of the different trials.

At both the trial level and the development plan level, statisticians should take time to review the case report forms (CRFs) to make sure, in particular, that the data being collected will be appropriate for the precise, unambiguous and unbiased measurement of primary and secondary endpoints. Other aspects of the data being collected should also be reviewed in light of the way they will be used in the analysis. For example, baseline data will provide information with regard to covariates to be used in any adjusted analyses, and intermediate visit data may be needed for the use of certain imputations, for example, LOCF, and data recorded for the determination of protocol violations will be used to define the per-protocol set.

21.2 Regulatory guidelines

Statistical thinking and practice are very much determined by the regulatory guidelines that are in place. Primarily it is ICH E9 *Statistical Principles for Clinical Trials*, published in 1998, that sets down the broad framework within which we operate. In 2001, we saw the publication of ICH E10 *Choice of Control Group*, which contains advice on the appropriate choice of concurrent control group and in particular introduces the concept of assay sensitivity (see Section 12.5) in active control, non-inferiority trials.

Since that time, we have seen numerous additional guidelines on specific statistical issues, for example, the European (CPMP/CHMP) *Points to Consider* papers. Both the FDA and the EMA have also issued guidance on various issues. Here are some of the landmarks.

CPMP (2000) Points to Consider on Switching between Superiority and Non-Inferiority

This guideline spelt out the circumstances where it is possible to change the objective of a trial from non-inferiority to superiority if the evidence is sufficiently strong but clearly stated that switching in the opposite direction would generally not be possible (see Section 12.10).

CPMP (2001) Points to Consider on Applications with 1. Meta-Analysis; 2. One Pivotal Study

This guideline defined the role of meta-analysis within a regulatory submission (see Section 18.5.1) and indicated the circumstances where a single pivotal trial might be acceptable as the basis for registration (see Section 9.4).

CPMP (2001) Points to Consider on Missing Data

The use of various procedures for dealing with missing data, such as LOCF, in conjunction with the choice of analysis sets was covered in this guideline (see Section 7.3). The guideline also contained strong recommendations for avoiding missing data by the thoughtful choice of aspects of trial design. This guideline was revised in 2010 to include, among other things, discussion of the use of new methods for data imputation.

CPMP (2002) Points to Consider on Multiplicity Issues in Clinical Trials

General aspects of multiple testing were considered in this guideline together with discussion on adjustment of significance levels or specific circumstances where adjustment is not needed (see Chapter 10).

CPMP (2003) Points to Consider on Adjustment for Baseline Covariates

It was in this guideline where the use of dynamic allocation was discouraged (see Section 1.4.6). The guideline also covered issues associated with the inclusion of covariates, the handling of centre effects in the analysis, and the investigation of treatment-by-covariate and treatment-by-centre interactions (see Sections 6.7 and 5.4).

CHMP (2005) Guidance on the Choice of Non-inferiority Margin

This much awaited guideline provided some general considerations for the choice of the non-inferiority margin. These considerations were not specific, but nonetheless have given us a way of thinking about the choice (see Section 12.7).

CHMP (2005) Guidance on Data Monitoring Committees/FDA (2006) Establishment and Operation of Clinical Trial Data Monitoring Committees

These documents provided guidance on the set-up, operational and working procedures and the roles and responsibilities of the DMC in a single clinical trial or collection of trials (see Section 14.4).

CHMP (2006) Reflection Paper on Methodological Issues in Confirmatory Clinical Trials with Flexible Design and Analysis Plan

This document has set down some initial thoughts from a regulatory point of view about the issues involved in allowing the design of a clinical trial to be adapted as the trial progresses. Modification of the sample size based on blinded data and stopping for overwhelming efficacy or futility are forms of adaptation that were already well accepted, but this reflection paper considers other possibilities that are more controversial (see Chapter 16).

EMA (2010, 2011a, 2011b, 2012) Benefit–Risk Methodology Project: Work Packages 1–4

These documents have explored various approaches to the quantification of the benefit–risk balance and recommended an approach, multi-criteria decision analysis (see Section 19.4).

In February 2014, a draft CHMP guideline on the investigation of subgroups in confirmatory clinical trials has been issued for public consultation. The need to pre-plan at the protocol stage a strategy for assessing the homogeneity of the treatment effect across subgroups was emphasised in terms of factors that are plausibly predictive of potential heterogeneity based on clinical considerations.

In recent years, we have also seen two additional FDA guidelines on further specific statistical issues:

FDA (2010) Guidance for Industry: Non-Inferiority Clinical Trials (draft)

This guideline contains information on the choice of the non-inferiority margin and also some detailed case studies that can be helpful in thinking through many of the issues associated with the planning of such trials.

FDA (2010) Guidance for Industry: Clinical Trials with Adaptive Design (draft)

There has been a considerable amount of theoretical statistical development in the area of adaptive designs, and this document has incorporated some of those developments, and based its guidance on what can be described as well-understood adaptive designs. The guideline also sets down some less well-understood types of adaptation where the use of such designs remains controversial. The emphasis again is the control of type I error and bias caused by dissemination of unblinded interim results.

FDA (2013) Structured Approach to Benefit-Risk Assessment in Drug Regulatory Decision-Making

The FDA here sets down a plan to develop a tool for a more structured approach to the assessment of benefit-risk.

The regulatory framework is forever changing, and undoubtedly, our statistical methodology will itself change to meet these evolving requirements. Statistics as a subject is also changing, and new innovations are impacting on regulatory thinking.

Other general guidelines such as CHMP (2005) *Guideline on Clinical Trials in Small Populations* contain some statistical considerations. This particular guideline discusses the relaxation of statistical requirements in this setting including the possibility of a less stringent significance level at the trial level, the use of surrogate endpoints, the analysis of data incorporating baseline covariates and the use of meta-analysis as the primary evidence of efficacy.

Both the EMA and the FDA have recognised the need to streamline the drug development process in order to bring new medicines to patients more rapidly (see, e.g. FDA (2004) *Critical Path Initiative*). The FDA raises (FDA (2006) *Critical Path Opportunities List*) a number of statistical issues that need to be resolved in order to help make the clinical trials process more efficient:

- In phase II dose-finding studies, we are beginning to gain experience in the use of modelling to characterise the dose–response curve rather than simply compare a limited number of doses to placebo (CHMP (2013) *Draft Qualification Opinion of MCP-Mod as an Efficient Statistical Methodology for Model-Based Design and Analysis of Phase II Dose Finding Studies under Model Uncertainty*).
- In the design of active control trials, what data should be used to estimate the effect of the active control? Should we look at all previous placebo-controlled trials, how do we deal with inconsistent results, and so on?
- What can be allowed in relation to adapting the trial design based on unblinded data? We need more experience in this area.
- How should we handle missing data? What alternatives exist to LOCF? Again, we have limited experience in using imputation techniques that are now readily available in statistical software, and our views on the appropriateness of those techniques will develop as we gain that experience.
- How to deal with various aspects of multiple endpoints, such as the requirement for success on more than a single endpoint? How to deal with correlated endpoints from the point of view of adjusting the type I error?

Finally, most therapeutic specific guidelines contain recommendations that directly impact on statistical considerations, for example, in terms of the definition of endpoints, the requirement for more than one primary endpoint, the definition of analysis sets and the choice of the non-inferiority margin. In a particular therapeutic setting, it is self-evident that the requisite guidelines should be studied carefully in order to extract relevant information for statistical aspects of design and analysis.

21.3 The statistics process

We have already discussed the role that statistics and statisticians play in the design of clinical trials and programmes of clinical trials. In this section, we will look at the manifestation of that planning in terms of the statistical methods section of the protocol and following on from that what happens from a statistical standpoint once the trial is ongoing through to the final reporting of that trial and the regulatory package as a whole.

21.3.1 The statistical methods section of the protocol

The statistical methods section of the protocol sets down the main aspects of both design and analysis. In particular, this section should contain:

- Justification of the sample size (including the possible re-evaluation of sample size once the trial is ongoing).
- Method of randomisation (although block size will not be specified).
- Clear definition and delineation of the primary and secondary endpoints and how these link with the objectives of the trial.
- Which aspects of the analysis will be viewed as confirmatory and which will be viewed as exploratory.
- How multiplicity will be dealt with within the confirmatory part of the analysis.
- Definition of analysis sets (full analysis set, per-protocol set, safety set).
- How missing data will be handled.
- Detail regarding the methods of analysis for the primary endpoint(s) including specification of covariates to be the basis of any adjusted analyses.
- Overview of statistical methods for the analysis of secondary endpoints.
- Methods for handling the safety and tolerability data; the safety data will be coded using the *Medical Dictionary for Regulatory Activities* (MedDRA; www.meddramsso.com) coding system in order to aid summary and presentation.
- Interim analyses and how the type I error is to be protected within these.
- Software to be used for statistical analysis.

Only methods set down in the protocol can be viewed as confirmatory, and so it is very important to get this section right; mistakes can be costly.

ICH E9 (1998): 'Note for Guidance on Statistical Principles for Clinical Trials'

'Only results from analyses envisaged in the protocol (including amendments) can be considered as confirmatory'.

21.3.2 The statistical analysis plan

The *statistical analysis plan* (SAP) is a more detailed elaboration of the statistical methods of analysis contained in the protocol. The SAP is written as the trial is ongoing but before database lock and the breaking of the treatment codes to unblind those involved in analysing the data. The SAP for studies that are unblinded should be finalised before the statistics team involved in analysing and reporting the data has access to any part of those data to avoid bias potentially introduced by having access to treatment-specific data.

The SAP will also often contain table templates that allow the precise way in which the statistical analysis will be presented to be set down well in advance of running the analyses on the final trial data.

21.3.3 The data validation plan

Once the CRF is finalised, the data management team will be putting together a *validation plan*, which will set down the data checks that will be made in conjunction with the data entry process; for example, are the visit dates in chronological order, are the ages of the patients within the range specified in the inclusion criteria, and so on? It is useful for this plan to be reviewed by a statistician for two reasons and especially in terms of issues that relate to the definition of endpoints. Firstly, it is important that the statistics team is aware of what data checks are being undertaken so that at the data analysis stage they can rule out certain potential data problems and be assured of a certain level of data quality. Secondly, the statistician may be able to suggest other specific checks that will help to increase the quality of those data.

21.3.4 The blind review

There is one final opportunity to revisit the proposed methods of statistical analysis prior to the breaking of the blind or, in an unblinded trial, before the statistics group have seen study data. This so-called blind review usually takes place around the time of database lock, and the following lists some of the aspects of analysis that would generally be considered:

- Precise definition of analysis sets – specifically which patients are to be included and which are to be excluded
- Finalisation of the algorithms for handling of missing data
- Finalisation of algorithms for combining centres should this be required
- Outlier identification and specific decisions taken on how these are to be handled

Under normal circumstances, the blind review should take place over a 24 or 48 hour period to limit delays in beginning the analysis proper. The blind review should be documented, detailing precisely what was done.

Sometimes, the blind review can throw up data issues that require further evaluation by the data management group with data queries being raised, and these perhaps may result in changes to the database. This sequence of events can cause major headaches and delays in the data analysis and reporting, and so it is important in the planning phase to get the data validation plan correct so that issues can be identified and dealt with in an ongoing way.

21.3.5 Statistical analysis

The SAP will have detailed the precise methods of analysis and presentation and should ideally be finalised well before database lock. This enables work to begin in good time on the programming of the analyses. These programs will be tested on *dirty* data from the trial, so that they can be pretty much finalised before the trial ends, enabling, at least in theory, rapid turnaround of the key analyses.

This is not always as simple as it sounds. In particular, working with dirty data can bring its own problems, including illogical data values that the programs cannot handle. Also, when the final data arrives, there may be specific issues and data problems arising that were never picked up at earlier programs. Nonetheless, these aspects of planning and program development and validation are essential if we are going to be in a position to complete the statistical analyses and presentations quickly. Also, working with the database in an ongoing way can avoid any surprises occurring following database lock.

The analyses and tables will be a joint effort involving statisticians and statistical programmers. Quality control (QC) is an essential component of this part of the process and double programming is frequently undertaken, that is, every analysis and all table entries are reproduced independently by a second programmer and cross-checked against the original. Data listings will also be produced and checked, although the level of checking may not be as rigorous as with the tables. Figures and graphs require a different kind of QC, but certainly, the points on these figures and graphs should be verified independently by a second programmer.

21.3.6 Reporting the analysis

ICH E3 (1995) *Note for guidance of the Structure and Content of Clinical Study Reports* sets down the structure, down to the numbering of the sections and precisely what goes in each of those sections, required within the regulatory setting for reporting each study. Medical writers will work with statisticians to put these reports together.

ICH E9 (1998): 'Note for Guidance on Statistical Principles for Clinical Trials'

'...statistical judgement should be brought to bear on the analysis, interpretation and presentation of the results of a clinical trial. To this end the trial statistician should be a member of the team responsible for the clinical study report, and should approve the clinical report'.

There will be a number of areas in the clinical report where the statistician will contribute, but in particular, Section 11, 'Efficacy Evaluation', and Section 12,

'Safety Evaluation', will require statistical oversight. Section 16 of the report contains the appendices, and Subsection 16.1.9 entitled 'Documentation of Statistical Methods' will usually be written by the trial statistician.

Within Section 11, Subsection 11.4.2 entitled 'Statistical/Analytical Issues' contains a series of items covering many of the areas of complexity within most statistical analyses:

- Adjustment for covariates
- Handling of dropouts or missing data
- Interim analyses and data monitoring
- Multi-centre studies
- Multiple comparisons/multiplicity
- Use of an efficacy subset of patients
- Active control studies intended to show equivalence
- Examination of subgroups

Each of these will clearly require input from the statistician.

21.3.7 Pre-planning

A common theme running across almost everything that we do within our statistical analyses is the need for pre-planning.

ICH E9 (1998): 'Note for Guidance on Statistical Principles for Clinical Trials'

'For each clinical trial contributing to a marketing application, all important details of its design and conduct and the principle features of its proposed analysis should be clearly specified in a protocol written before the trial begins. The extent to which the procedures in the protocol are followed and the primary analysis is planned a priori will contribute to the degree of confidence in the final results and conclusions of the trial'.

This pre-planning in terms of both conduct and analysis is predominantly set down in the trial protocol. Pre-planning is one key aspect of the way we design and run our trials that helps to reduce bias. It would be entirely inappropriate to take decisions about methods of analysis based on unblinded looks at the data. Pre-planning also enables us to think through in advance just how we are going to handle the data. This is good discipline and can help us to anticipate problems in advance. A final benefit of pre-planning is a very practical one. Once the trial is complete and the database is locked, there is inevitably a *mad dash* to analyse the data and look at the results. Only with pre-planning and an effective amount of pre-programming and testing of those programs can the statistical analyses be undertaken quickly and without major hitches.

As the trial is ongoing, there is also an opportunity to change some of the planned methods of analysis; for example, information that a particular covariate could be important or that a different kind of effect could be seen in a certain subgroup may have become available based on external data from a similar trial that has been completed and reported. Such changes can be incorporated by modifying the SAP, and if they represent major changes to the analysis, for example, if they were associated with the analysis of the primary endpoint, then a protocol amendment would need to be issued. The reason for this, as mentioned earlier, is that only methods specified in the protocol, including amendments, can be viewed as confirmatory.

In a limited way, there may also be changes in the design as the trial is ongoing, for example, resizing of the trial. Such changes represent major design modifications, and protocol amendments would be needed to ensure that the modifications fall within what could be considered as pre-planning. As pointed out in ICH E9 (1998) in relation to revising the sample size:

ICH E9 (1998): 'Note for Guidance on Statistical Principles for Clinical Trials'

'A revised sample size may then be calculated using suitably modified assumptions, and should be justified and documented in a protocol amendment and in the clinical study report …The potential need for re-estimation of the sample size should be envisaged in the protocol whenever possible'.

The final sentence here again emphasises the need for pre-planning with regard to this process wherever possible.

A change in the statistical methods at the data analysis stage, for example, including unplanned covariates or using a transformation of the primary endpoint when one was not planned, would usually be unacceptable. The danger here is that a method may have been chosen that affects the resulting magnitude of the treatment effect. The choice of statistical method should be pre-specified in the statistical analysis plan and possibly modified at the blind review. Changes to these methods could be acceptable, however, in conjunction with a clearly defined algorithm. For example, the logrank test may be the planned method of analysis for survival data, but if the assumption of proportional hazards is not valid according to some pre-defined assessment of that assumption, then treatment comparisons could be based on the Gehan–Wilcoxon test. Alternatively, it can be stated in the protocol that if on visual inspection of the normal probability plot the data appears to be positively skewed, then the log transformation will be used to recover the normality of the data. These would be examples of clearly defined algorithms leading to a well-defined method of analysis for the calculation of the *p*-value. Of course, *visual inspection* contains an element of subjectivity, but nonetheless, regulators can see a clear way through the decision-making process.

There is one possible area where the rules for pre-planning may be relaxed, and that is in relation to orphan indications/small populations. Regulators recognise that many of these situations are very challenging. For example, even the primary endpoint could be difficult to define in a particular setting, and results for a range of endpoints, without the formal need to control for multiplicity, may be the only way to adequately demonstrate a treatment benefit.

CHMP (2005): 'Guideline on Clinical Trials in Small Populations'

'The choice of the primary endpoint may pose considerable problems. In some cases, the "most appropriate" clinical endpoint may not be known or widely agreed or a validated clinical endpoint may not exist. ... In such circumstances, the usual approach of pre-specifying the primary endpoint may be too conservative and more knowledge may be gained from collecting all sensible/possible endpoints and then presenting all the data in the final study report'.

A further issue concerns new questions that may arise during the analysis of data. These aspects should be clearly distinguished and would constitute only exploratory analyses.

ICH E9 (1998): 'Note for Guidance on Statistical Principles for Clinical Trials'

'Although the primary goal of the analysis of a clinical trial should be to answer the questions posed by its main objectives, new questions based on the observed data may well emerge during the unblinded analysis. Additional and perhaps complex statistical analysis may be the consequence. This additional work should be strictly distinguished in the report from work which was planned in the protocol'.

21.3.8 Sensitivity and robustness

Statisticians and regulators alike, quite rightly, place great store on robustness and sensitivity analyses. All analyses will be based on certain assumptions regarding the data, such as normality and constant variance, or independent censoring in time-to-event data. Analyses could be potentially affected by the presence of single outlying data points or be sensitive to the choice of analysis sets or the handling of missing data. It would be very unsatisfactory if the conclusions drawn from the data were driven by assumptions that were questionable or were unduly influenced by different choices for dealing with specific aspects of the data. Throughout the statistical analysis, the sensitivity of the conclusions to assumptions of the kind discussed should be evaluated. The regulators mention these issues on several occasions and in relation to numerous aspects of analysis and interpretation. Here are just a few:

- Choice of analysis sets
  ICH E9 (1998): 'Note for Guidance on Statistical Principles for Clinical Trials'
  'In general it is advantageous to demonstrate a lack of sensitivity of the principal trial results to alternative choices of the set of subjects analysed'.

- Missing data

  ICH E9 (1998): 'Note for Guidance on Statistical Principles for Clinical Trials'

  'An investigation should be made concerning the sensitivity of the results of analysis to the method of handling missing values, especially if the number of missing values is substantial'.

- Outliers

  The following quote follows on from that on missing data:

  ICH E9 (1998): 'Note for Guidance on Statistical Principles for Clinical Trials'

  'A similar approach should be adopted to exploring the influence of outliers …If no procedures for dealing with outliers was foreseen in the trial protocol, one analysis with the actual values and at least one other analysis eliminating or reducing the outlier effect should be performed and differences between the results discussed'.

In certain cases, more specific guidance is given. The FDA, for example, discusses various sensitivity analyses in relation to the analysis of progression-free survival in FDA (2005) *Clinical Trial Endpoints for the Approval of Cancer Drugs and Biologics*.

A general message coming out of these issues is that where there are doubts regarding how best to handle specific aspects of the data at the analysis stage, consider a range of different approaches, say, two or three, and hopefully demonstrate that the conclusions are unaffected by the approach adopted. If, however, they are affected by this choice, then this lack of robustness could undermine the validity of the conclusions drawn.

21.4 The regulatory submission

The statistics group or groups involved in analysing and reporting each of the trials will have a role in compiling the regulatory submission. Both the integrated summary of safety (ISS) and the integrated summary of efficacy (ISE) will involve the analysis and presentation of compiled results across the whole programme of trials. Formal meta-analysis may be employed or alternatively a pooling of data, and the technical aspects of these methods were discussed in Chapter 18.

Once the regulatory submission has been made, there will inevitably be questions and issues coming back from the regulators. There may be concerns about the way the data has been handled from a statistical point of view. There may be requests for additional specific analyses to resolve uncertainty. There may be more open issues that the regulators are unhappy about that may require a substantial amount of further analysis. At the extreme end, there may be outright rejection and the company may then be back to the drawing board in terms of the product. In all of these cases, there will usually be a need for further statistical considerations.

If certain additional analyses have been specifically requested, then providing these should be fairly straightforward. If the questions, however, are more general, then the company may need to respond by providing a series of reanalyses to address the issues. In this case, the concept of pre-planning is irrelevant; those deciding on what further analyses to present are unblinded to the data. This scenario of itself creates difficulties. There is a temptation to reanalyse in a number of different ways but only present back to the regulators those analyses that support the company's position. The best way to proceed in order to avoid potential criticism is to be open with the regulators and present a wide range of analyses that fit with the questions and issues being raised.

In the USA, the FDA requests, within the submission, an electronic version of the database and this gives them the opportunity to not only reanalyse the data to confirm the results presented within the submission but also to perform their own alternative analyses. This does not happen in Europe. In the USA, therefore, the process following submission is somewhat different, and much of the interchange in terms of requesting and supplying alternative analyses is taken care of by the FDA statisticians.

21.5 Publications and presentations

Outside of the clinical report and regulatory setting, there will clearly be the need to publish the results of trials in the medical literature and to make presentations at conferences.

In recent years, there have been a range of recommendations regarding the structure of publications: how they should be laid out and what they should contain. These have usually been in the form of checklists, and all of this has been encapsulated within the CONSORT statement (Altman *et al.*, 2001; Moher, Schulz and Altman, 2001). The statement has been revised further in 2010 (Schulz *et al.*, 2010). CONSORT is an acronym for *Con*solidated *S*tandards *of R*eporting *T*rials, and increasingly, many medical journals have adopted this guidance in terms of requiring their clinical trial publications to conform to it. There is a web site which provides up-to-date information and helpful resources and examples: www.consort-statement.org.

The guideline breaks down the content of each publication into a series of items, 22 in total, ranging from

1. Title and Abstract,
2. Introduction – Background,
3. Methods – Participants and
4. Methods – Interventions

through to

7. Methods – Sample Size,
13. Results – Participant Flow

and

22. Discussion – Overall Evidence.

The precise content is too detailed to give complete coverage here, but just to give an impression, we will consider two areas: the sample size calculation (item 7) and participant flow (item 13).

The sample size calculation should be detailed in the trial publication, indicating the estimated outcomes in each of the treatment groups (and this will define, in particular, the clinically relevant difference to be detected), the type I error, the type II error or power and, for a continuous primary outcome variable in a parallel-group trial, the within-group standard deviation for that measure. For time-to-event data, details on clinically relevant difference would usually be specified in terms of either the median event times or the proportions event-free at a certain time point.

An important aspect of the reporting of any clinical trial is a clear indication of what happened to all of the patients randomised. CONSORT recommends that each publication should contain a diagram showing the flow of participants through the trial; numbers randomised to each of the treatment groups, receiving intended treatment; protocol deviations by treatment group classified by type of deviation; and patient groups analysed for primary outcomes. See Figure 21.1 for an example of this.

Example 21.1 Natalizumab plus interferon beta-1a for relapsing multiple sclerosis: The SENTINEL study

Figure 21.1 provides the participant flow in relation to this placebo-controlled trial of natalizumab (Rudick *et al.*, 2006).

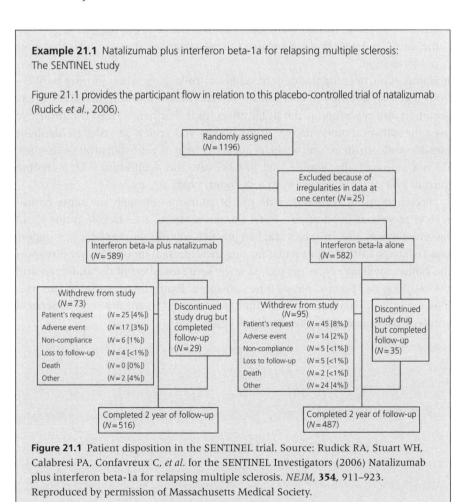

Figure 21.1 Patient disposition in the SENTINEL trial. Source: Rudick RA, Stuart WH, Calabresi PA, Confavreux C, *et al.* for the SENTINEL Investigators (2006) Natalizumab plus interferon beta-1a for relapsing multiple sclerosis. *NEJM*, **354**, 911–923. Reproduced by permission of Massachusetts Medical Society.

The quality of publications is certainly increasing, and in part this is due to guidance of the type already described in this section. It is unfortunately the case, however, that many mistakes in design, analysis, reporting and interpretation are still made, even in leading journals, despite apparently rigorous refereeing procedures. Particular areas of statistics that seem to cause consistent difficulties include:

- Assuming that a large clinical trial necessarily removes bias – large studies have greater precision but precision and bias are different things.
- The correct design, analysis and interpretation of non-inferiority trials – remember conventional p-values have no role.
- Conforming to the principle of intention-to-treat (ITT) to avoid bias – ITT means all randomised subjects or something very close to that.
- Incorrect analysis of time-to-event data in terms of the definition for the origin of the measurement – the point of randomisation is the *only* origin that can be used in a randomised trial that preserves the randomisation.
- Adjusting the analysis for baseline factors – with change from baseline as the outcome variable, include baseline as a covariate to avoid regression towards the mean, and note that it is incorrect to use covariates that are measured after randomisation.

It is important to enlist the help of statistical colleagues when putting publications together, not only in terms of the actual analysis but in terms of the interpretation and reporting in the publication itself. Further, do cast a critical eye over the statistical methodology in the papers you review in order to highlight possible problem areas, and again, request the help of your statistical colleagues. Do not automatically assume that just because the publication is in a leading journal everything is correct from a statistical point of view.

Presentations at conferences do not of course go through the same critical review process as publications. Even though abstracts are often submitted and reviewed in advance, mistakes and bad practice will still slip through. It is important to have statistical input when putting these presentations together. Errors in the statistics will invariably get picked up by some members of the audience, and the resulting bad press could well be damaging. From the opposite perspective, look critically at what is being presented in terms of the statistics and challenge if you feel that inappropriate methods are being used.

References

Altman DG (1991) *Practical Statistics for Medical Research* London: Chapman & Hall.

Altman DG (1998) 'Confidence intervals for the number needed to treat' *British Medical Journal,* **317**, 1309–1312.

Altman DG and Bland JM (1994) 'Diagnostic tests 2: predictive values' *British Medical Journal,* **309**, 102.

Altman DG, Schulz KF, Moher D, *et al.* (2001) 'The revised CONSORT statement for reporting randomized trials: explanation and elaboration' *Annals of Internal Medicine,* **134**, 663–694.

Amit O, Heidberger RM and Lane PW (2008) 'Graphical approaches to the analysis of safety data from clinical trials' *Pharmaceutical Statistics,* **7**, 20–35.

Arani RB, Soong S-J, Weiss HL, *et al.* (2001) 'Phase specific analysis of herpes zoster associated pain data: a new statistical approach' *Statistics in Medicine,* **20**, 2429–2439.

Austin PC and Mamdani MM (2006) 'A comparison of propensity score methods: a case-study estimating the effectiveness of post-AMI statin use' *Statistics in Medicine,* **25**, 2084–2106.

Bauer P and Köhne K (1994) 'Evaluation of experiments with adaptive interim analyses' *Biometrics,* **50**, 1029–1041.

Bellingan G, Maksimow M, Howell DC, *et al.* (2013) 'The effect of intravenous interferon-beta-1a (FP-1201) on lung CD73 expression and on acute respiratory distress syndrome mortality: an open-label study' *The Lancet Respiratory Medicine,* **2**, 98–107.

Bland M (2004) 'Cluster randomised trials in the medical literature: two bibliometric surveys' *BMC Medical Research Methodology,* **4**, 21.

Bradburn MJ, Deeks JJ, Berlin JA and Localio AR (2007) 'Much ado about nothing: a comparison of the performance of meta-analytical methods with rare events' *Statistics in Medicine,* **26**, 53–77.

Breslow NE and Day NE (1994) *Statistical Methods in Cancer Research, Volume II: The Design and Analysis of Cohort Studies,* IARC Scientific Publications, No. 82. New York: Oxford University Press.

Brodie MJ, Richens A and Yuen AW (1995) 'Double-blind comparison of lamotrigine and carbamazepine in newly diagnosed epilepsy. UK Lamotrigine/Carbamazepine Monotherapy Trial Group' *The Lancet,* **345**, 476–479.

Brodie MJ and Whitehead J (2006) 'Active control comparisons: the ideal trial design' *Epilepsy Research,* **68**, 70–73.

Campbell MJ, Donner A and Klar N (2007) 'Developments in cluster randomised trials and Statistics in Medicine' *Statistics in Medicine,* **26**, 2–19.

Cancer Therapy Evaluation Program (2006) *Common Terminology Criteria for Adverse Events* Version 3.0, DCTD, NCI, NIH, DHHS, 31 March 2003. http://ctep.cancer.gov, accessed on 5 June 2014.

Carpenter J and Kenward MG (2007) *Missing Data in Clinical Trials – a Practical Guide.* UK National Health Service, National Co-ordinating Centre for Research on Methodology.

Statistical Thinking for Non-Statisticians in Drug Regulation, Second Edition. Richard Kay.
© 2015 John Wiley & Sons, Ltd. Published 2015 by John Wiley & Sons, Ltd.

Chen JJ, Hsueh H-M and Liu J-P (2003) 'Simultaneous non-inferiority test of sensitivity and specificity for two diagnostic procedures in the presence of a gold standard' *Biometrical Journal*, **45**, 47–60.

Cochran WG (1954) 'The combination of estimates from different experiments' *Biometrics*, **10**, 101–129.

Cohen J (1960) 'A coefficient of agreement for nominal scales' *Educational and Psychological Measurement*, **20**, 37–46.

Coronary Drug Project Research Group (1980) 'Influence and adherence to treatment and response of cholesterol on mortality in the coronary drug project' *New England Journal of Medicine*, **303**, 1038–1041.

Cox DR (1972) 'Regression models and life tables (with discussion)' *Journal of the Royal Statistical Society, B*, **74**, 187–220.

Crawford ED, Eisenberger MA, McLoed DG, *et al.* (1989) 'A controlled trial of leuprolide with and without flutamide in prostatic cancer' *New England Journal of Medicine*, **321**, 419–424.

Cumming G (2009) 'Inference by eye: reading the overlap of independent confidence intervals' *Statistics in Medicine*, **28**, 205–220.

D'Agostino RB (1998) 'Propensity score methods for bias reduction in the comparison of a treatment to a non-randomised control group' *Statistics in Medicine*, **17**, 2265–2281.

de la Taille A, Irani J, Graefen M, *et al.* (2011) 'Clinical evaluation of the PCA3 assay in guiding initial biopsy decisions' *Journal of Urology*, **185**, 2119–2125.

Deeks JJ, Dinnes J, D'Amico R, *et al.* (2003) 'Evaluating non-randomised intervention studies' *Health Technology Assessment*, **7**, iii–x, 1–173.

DeLong ER, DeLong DM and Clarke-Pearson DL (1988) 'Comparing the areas under two or more correlated receiver operating characteristic curves: A nonparametric approach' *Biometrics*, **44**, 837–845.

Doll R and Bradford Hill A (1950) 'Smoking and carcinoma of the lung' *British Medical Journal*, **2**, 739–748.

DuMouchel W (1999) 'Bayesian data mining in large frequency tables, with an application to the FDA Spontaneous Reporting System' *The American Statistician*, **53**, 177–190.

Dunnett CW (1955) 'A multiple comparison procedure for comparing several treatments with a control' *Journal of the American Statistical Association*, **50**, 1096–1121.

Ebbutt AF and Frith L (1998) 'Practical issues in equivalence trials' *Statistics in Medicine*, **17**, 1691–1701.

Eggar M and Smith D (1998) 'Meta-analysis bias in location and selection of studies' *British Medical Journal*, **316**, 61–66.

Eggar M, Smith GD, Schneider M and Minder C (1997) 'Bias in meta-analysis detected by a simple, graphical test' *British Medical Journal*, **315**, 629–634.

Ellenberg SS, Fleming TR and DeMets DL (2003) *Data Monitoring Committees in Clinical Trials: A Practical Perspective* Hoboken: John Wiley & Sons, Inc.

Emerson SS, Levin GP and Emerson SC (2011) 'Comments on adaptive increase in sample size when interim results are promising: a practical guide with examples' *Statistics in Medicine*, **30**, 3285–3301.

Eriksson BI, Dahl OE, Rosencher N, *et al.* (2007) 'Dabigatran etexilate versus enoxaparin for prevention of venous thromboembolism after total hip replacement: a randomized, double-blind, non-inferiority trial' *The Lancet*, **370**, 949–956

Evans SJ, Waller PC and Davis S (2001) 'Use of proportional reporting ratios (PRRs) for signal generation from spontaneous adverse drug reaction reports' *Pharmacoepidemiol Drug Safety*, **10**, 483–486.

Fleiss JL (1993) 'The statistical basis of meta-analysis' *Statistical Methods in Medical Research*, **2**, 121–145.

Fleming TR and DeMets DL (1996) 'Surrogate end points in clinical trials: are we being misled?' *Annals of Internal Medicine*, **125**, 605–613.

Ford I, Norrie J and Ahmedi S (1995) 'Model inconsistency, illustrated by the Cox proportional hazards model' *Statistics in Medicine*, **14**, 735–746.

Gardner MJ and Altman DG (1989) 'Estimation rather than hypothesis testing: confidence intervals rather than p-values' In: *Statistics with Confidence* (eds. MJ Gardner and DG Altman) London: British Medical Journal, 6–19.

Gehan EA (1969) 'Estimating survival functions from the life table' *Journal of Chronic Diseases*, **21**, 629–644.

Geyer CE, Forster J, Lindquist D, *et al.* (2006) 'Lapatinib plus capecitabine for HER-2-positive advanced breast cancer' *New England Journal of Medicine*, **355**, 2733–2743.

Gillings D and Koch G (1991) 'The application of the principle of intention-to-treat analysis of clinical trials' *Drug Information Journal*, **25**, 411–424.

Glasziou P, Simes RJ and Gelber RD (1990) 'Quality adjusted survival analysis' *Statistics in Medicine*, **9**, 1259–1276.

Greenwood M (1926) 'The errors of sampling of the survivorship tables' *Reports on Public Health and Statistical Subjects*, No. 33, Appendix 1. London: HMSO.

Grieve AP (2003) 'The number needed to treat: a useful clinical measure or a case of the Emperor's new clothes?' *Pharmaceutical Statistics*, **2**, 87–102.

Grimes DA and Schulz KF (2008) 'Making sense of odds and odds ratios' American Journal of Obstetrics and Gynecology, **111**, 423–426.

Haybittle JL (1971) 'Repeated assessment of results in clinical trials of cancer treatment' *British Journal of Radiology*, **44**, 793–797.

Helsinki Declaration (2004) *Ethical Principles for Medical Research Involving Human Subjects* WMA General Assembly, Tokyo.

Higgins JPT, Altman DG, Gotzsche PC, *et al.* (2011) 'The Cochrane Collaboration's tool for assessing risk of bias in randomised trials' *British Medical Journal*, **343**, d5928.

Higgins JPT, Thompson SG, Deeks JJ and Altman DG (2003) 'Measuring inconsistency in meta-analyses' *British Medical Journal*, **327**, 557–560.

Hochberg Y and Tamhane AC (1987) *Multiple Comparison Procedures* New York: John Wiley & Sons, Inc.

The ICON and AGO Collaborators (2003) 'Paclitaxel plus platinum-based chemotherapy versus conventional platinum-based chemotherapy in women with relapsed ovarian cancer: the ICON4/AGO-OVAR-2.2 trial' *The Lancet*, **361**, 2099–2106.

Jensen MP, Karoly P, O'Riordan EF, *et al.* (1989) 'The subjective experience of pain. An assessment of the utility of 10 indices' *The Clinical Journal of Pain*, **5**, 153–159.

Jones B, Jarvis P, Lewis JA and Ebbutt AF (1996) 'Trials to assess equivalence: the importance of rigorous methods' *British Medical Journal*, **313**, 36–39.

Jovanovic BD and Levy PS (1997) 'A look at the rule of three' *The American Statistician*, **51**, 137–139.

Julious SA (2004) 'Using confidence intervals around individual means to assess statistical significance between two means' *Pharmaceutical Statistician*, **3**, 217–222.

Julious SA and Mullee MA (1994) 'Confounding and Simpson's paradox' *British Medical Journal*, **309**, 1480–1481.

Kaplan EL and Meier P (1958) 'Non-parametric estimation from incomplete observations' *Journal of the American Statistical Association*, **53**, 457–481.

Kaul S and Diamond GA (2006) 'Good enough: a primer on the analysis and interpretation of non-inferiority trials' *Annals of Internal Medicine*, **145**, 62–69.

Kay R (1995) 'Some fundamental statistical concepts in clinical trials and their application in herpes zoster' *Antiviral Chemistry and Chemotherapy*, **6**, 28–33.

Kay R (2004) 'An explanation of the hazard ratio' *Pharmaceutical Statistics*, **3**, 295–297.

Kay R (2006) Letter to the Editor on 'Phase specific analysis of herpes zoster associated pain data: a new statistical approach' *Statistics in Medicine*, **25**, 359–360.

Landis JR, Heyman ER and Koch GG (1978) 'Average partial association in three-way contingency tables: a review and discussion of alternative tests' *International Statistical Review*, **46**, 237–254.

Landis JR and Koch GG (1977) 'The measurement of observer agreement for categorical data' *Biometrics*, **33**, 159–174.

Lee LL, McNeer JF, Stramer CF, *et al.* (1980) 'Clinical judgment and statistics. Lessons from a simulated randomized trial in coronary artery disease' *Circulation*, **61**, 508–515.

Lehmacher W and Wassmer G (1999) 'Adaptive sample size calculations in group sequential trials' *Biometrics*, **55**, 1286–1290.

Lewis JA (2002) 'The European regulatory experience' *Statistics in Medicine*, **21**, 2931–2938.

Lewis JA (2004) 'In defence of the dichotomy' *Pharmaceutical Statistics*, **3**, 77–79.

Li Z, Chines AA and Meredith MP (2004) 'Statistical validation of surrogate endpoints: is bone density a valid surrogate for fracture?' *Journal of Musculoskeletal Neuron Interaction*, **4**, 64–74.

Liberati A, Altman DG, Tetzlaff J, *et al.* (2009) 'The PRISMA statement for reporting systematic reviews and meta-analyses of studies that evaluate healthcare interventions: explanation and elaboration' *British Medical Journal*, **339**, b2700.

Maca J, Bhattacharya S, Dragalin V, *et al.* (2006) 'Adaptive seamless phase II/III designs – background, operational aspects, and examples' *Drug Information Journal*, **40**, 463–473.

Machin D, Campbell MJ, Fayers PM and Pinol APY (1997) *Statistical Tables for the Design of Clinical Trials* (2nd edn) Oxford: Blackwell Scientific Publications.

Mantel N and Haenszel W (1959) 'Statistical aspects of the analysis of data from retrospective studies of disease' *Journal of the National Cancer Institute*, **22**, 719–748.

Marshall RJ and Chisholm EM (1985) 'Hypothesis testing in the polychotomous logistic model with an application to detecting gastrointestinal cancer' *Statistics in Medicine*, **5**, 337–344.

Matthews JNS, Altman DG, Campbell MJ and Royston P (1990) 'Analysis of serial measurements in medical research' *British Medical Journal*, **300**, 230–235.

Mehta CR and Pocock SJ (2011) 'Adaptive increase in sample size when interim results are promising: a practical guide with examples' *Statistics in Medicine*, **30**, 3267–3284.

Meier P (1978) 'The biggest public health experiment ever: the 1954 field trial of the Salk poliomyelitis vaccine' In: *Statistics: A Guide to the Unknown* (eds. J Tanur, F Mostellor, WH Kruskal, *et al.*) San Francisco: Holden Day.

Miller DH, Khan OA, Sheremata WA, *et al.* (2003) 'A controlled trial of natalizumab for relapsing multiple sclerosis' *New England Journal of Medicine*, **348**, 15–23.

Moher D, Schulz KF and Altman DG (2001) 'The CONSORT statement: revised recommendations for improving the quality of reports of parallel-group randomized trials' *Annals of Internal Medicine*, **134**, 657–694.

Mulrow CD (1994) 'Rationale for systematic reviews' *British Medical Journal*, **309**, 597–599.

Nakamura H, Arakawa K, Itakura H, *et al.* (2006) 'Primary prevention of cardiovascular disease with pravastatin in Japan (MEGA study): a prospective randomised controlled trial' *The Lancet*, **368**, 1155–1163.

O'Brien PC and Fleming TR (1979) 'A multiple testing procedure for clinical trials' *Biometrics*, **35**, 549–556.

O'Brien RG and Castelloe J (2010) 'Sample-size analysis for traditional hypothesis testing: concepts and issues' In: *Pharmaceutical Statistics Using SAS: A Practical Guide* (eds. A Dmitrienko, C Chuang-Stein and R D'Agostino) Cary: SAS Institute Inc.

Okwera A, Whalen C, Byekwaso F, *et al.* (1994) 'Randomised trial of thiacetazone and rifampicin-containing regimens for pulmonary tuberculosis in HIV-infected Ugandans. The Makerere University-Case Western University Research Collaboration' *The Lancet*, **344**, 1323–1328.

Packer M, Coats AJS, Fowler MB, *et al.* (2001) 'Effect of carvedilol on survival in severe chronic heart failure' *New England Journal of Medicine*, **344**, 1651–1658.

Peto R and Peto J (1972) 'Asymptotically efficient rank invariant procedures' *Journal of the Royal Statistical Society, A*, **135**, 185–207.

Peto R, Pike MC, Armitage P, *et al.* (1976) 'Design and analysis of randomised clinical trials requiring prolonged observation of each patient. I. Introduction and design' *British Journal of Cancer*, **34**, 585–612.

Piccart-Gebhart MJ, Procter M, Leyland-Jones B, *et al.* (2005) 'Trastuzumab after adjuvant chemotherapy in HER2-positive breast cancer' *New England Journal of Medicine*, **353**, 1659–1672.

Pocock SJ (1977) 'Group sequential methods in the design and analysis of clinical trials' *Biometrika*, **64**, 191–199.

Pocock SJ (1983) *Clinical Trials: A Practical Approach* New York: John Wiley & Sons, Ltd.

Pocock SJ (2004) 'A major trial needs three statisticians: why, how and who?' *Statistics in Medicine*, **23**, 1535–1539.

Pocock SJ, Clayton TC and Altman DG (2002) 'Survival plots of time-to-event outcomes in clinical trials: good practice and pitfalls' *The Lancet*, **359**, 1686–1689.

Powderly WG, Saag MS, Cloud GA, *et al.* (1992) 'A controlled trial of fluconazole or amphotericin B to prevent relapse of cryptococcal meningitis in patients with the acquired immunodeficiency syndrome' *New England Journal of Medicine*, **326**, 793–798.

Prochaska JJ and Hilton JF (2012) 'Risk of cardiovascular serious events associated with varenicline use for tobacco cessation: systematic review and meta-analysis' *British Medical Journal*, **344**, e2856.

Proschan MA, Lan KKG and Wittes JT (2006) *Statistical Monitoring of Clinical Trials: A Unified Approach* New York: Springer.

Richardson PG, Ho VT, Giralt S, *et al.* (2012) 'Safety and efficacy of defibrotide for the treatment of severe hepatic veno-occlusive disease' *Therapeutic Advances in Hematology*, **3**, 253–265.

Roes KCB (2004) 'Dynamic allocation as a balancing act' *Pharmaceutical Statistics*, **3**, 187–191.

Rosenbaum PR and Rubin DB (1983) 'The central role of the propensity score in observational studies for causal effects' *Biometrika*, **70**, 41–55.

Rosenthal R (1979) 'The "file drawer problem" and tolerance for null result' *Psychology Bulletin*, **48**, 638–641.

Royston P, Altman DG and Sauerbrei W (2006) 'Dichotomizing continuous predictors in multiple regression: a bad idea' *Statistics in Medicine*, **25**, 127–141.

Rubin LJ, Badesch DB, Barst RJ, *et al.* (2002) 'Bosentan therapy for pulmonary arterial hyper-tension' *New England Journal of Medicine*, **346**, 869–903.

Rudick RA Stuart WH, Calabresi PA, *et al.* (2006) 'Natalizumab plus interferon beta-1a for relapsing multiple sclerosis' *New England Journal of Medicine*, **354**, 911–923.

Sargent DJ, Goldberg RM, Jacobson SD, *et al.* (2001) 'A pooled analysis of adjuvant chemotherapy for resected colon cancer in elderly patients' *New England Journal of Medicine*, **345**, 1091–1097.

Schuirmann DJ (1987) 'A comparison of two one-sided tests procedure and the power approach for assessing the equivalence of average bioavailability' *Journal of Pharmacokinetics and Biopharmaceutics*, **15**, 657–680.

Schulz KF, Altman DG, Moher D and CONSORT Group (2010) 'CONSORT 2010 statement: updated guidelines for reporting parallel group randomized trials' *British Medical Journal*, **340**, 698–702.

Senn S (2002) *Cross-Over Trials in Clinical Research* (2nd edn) Chichester: John Wiley & Sons, Ltd.

Senn S (2003) 'Disappointing dichotomies' *Pharmaceutical Statistics*, **2**, 239–240.

Senn S (2007) *Statistical Issues in Drug Development* (2nd edn) Chichester: John Wiley & Sons, Ltd.

Sherman DG, Albers GW, Bladin C, *et al.* (2007) 'The efficacy and safety of enoxaparin versus unfractionated heparin for the prevention of venous thromboembolism after acute ischemic stroke (PREVAIL study): an open-label randomised comparison' *The Lancet*, **369**, 1347–1355.

Smith JG and Christophers AJ (1992) 'Phenoxy herbicides and chlorophenols: a case control study on soft tissue sarcoma and malignant lymphoma' *British Journal of Cancer*, **65**, 442–448.

Solomon S, McMurray JJV, Pfeffer MA, *et al.* (2005) 'Cardiovascular risk associated with celecoxib in a clinical trial for colorectal adenoma prevention' *New England Journal of Medicine*, **352**, 1071–1080.

Spiegelhalter DJ, Abrams KR and Myles JP (2004) *Bayesian Approaches to Clinical Trials and Health-Care Evaluation* Chichester: John Wiley & Sons, Ltd.

Sterne JAC, White IR, Carlin JB, *et al.* (2009) 'Multiple imputation for missing data in epidemiological and clinical research: potential and pitfalls' *British Medical Journal*, **339**, 157–160.

Stokes ME, Davis CS and Koch GG (2000) *Categorical Data Analysis Using the SAS System* (2nd edn) Cary: SAS Institute Inc.

Storosum JG, van Zwieten BJ, Vermeulen HDB, *et al.* (2001) 'Relapse and recurrence in major depression: a critical review of placebo-controlled efficacy studies with special emphasis on methodological issues' *European Psychiatry*, **16**, 327–335.

Stutchfield P, Whitaker R and Russell I (2005) 'Antenatal betamethasone and incidence of neonatal respiratory distress after elective caesarean section: pragmatic randomised trial' *British Medical Journal*, **331**, 662–667.

Szegedi A, Kohnen R, Dienel A and Kieser M (2005) 'Acute treatment of moderate to severe depression with hypericum extract WS 5570 (St John's wort): randomised controlled double blind non-inferiority trial versus paroxetine' *British Medical Journal*, **330**, 503–508.

Tang BMP, Eslick GD, Nowson C, *et al.* (2007) 'Use of calcium or calcium in combination with vitamin D supplementation to prevent fractures and bone loss in people aged 50 years and older: a meta-analysis' *The Lancet*, **370**, 657–666.

van Belle G, Fisher LD, Heagerty PJ and Lumley T (2004) *Biostatistics: A Methodology for the Health Sciences* (2nd edn) Hoboken: John Wiley & Sons, Inc.

van Elteren PH (1960) 'On the combination of independent two-sample tests of Wilcoxon' *Bulletin of the International Statistical Institute*, **37**, 351–361.

van Leth F, Phanuphak P, Ruxrungtham K, *et al.* (2004) 'Comparison of first-line antiretroviral therapy with regimens including nevirapine, efavirenz, or both drugs, plus stavudine and lamivudine: a randomised open-label trial, the 2NN study' *The Lancet*, **363**, 1253–1263.

Viswanathan M, Ansari MT, Berkman ND, *et al.* (2013) 'Assessing the risk of bias in individual studies in systematic reviews of health care interventions' In: *Methods Guide of Effectiveness Reviews*, AHRQ Publication No 10(13)-EHC063-EF. Rockville: Agency for Healthcare Research and Quality.

von Elm E, Altman DG, Egger M, *et al.* (2007) 'The Strengthening the Reporting of Observational Studies in Epidemiology (STROBE) statement: guidelines for reporting observational studies' *British Medical Journal*, **335**, 806–808.

Wallentin L, Becker RC, Budaj A, *et al.* (2009) 'Ticagrelor versus clopidogrel in patients with acute coronary syndromes' *New England Journal of Medicine*, **361**, 1045–1057.

Wang J, Zhao Z, Barber B, *et al.* (2011) 'A Q-TWiST analysis comparing panitumumab plus best supportive care (BSC) with BSC alone in patients with wild-type KRAS metastatic colorectal cancer' *British Journal of Cancer*, **104**, 1848–1853.

Wang S-J, Hung HMJ and O'Neill R (2011) 'Adaptive design clinical trials and trial logistics models in CNS drug development' *European Neuropsychopharmacology*, **21**, 159–166.

Westlake WJ (1981) 'Bioequivalence testing – a need to rethink (Reader Reaction Response)' *Biometrics*, **37**, 589–594.

Wijeysundera DN, Austin PC, Hux JE, *et al.* (2008) 'Bayesian statistical inference enhances the interpretation of contemporary randomized controlled trials' *Journal of Clinical Epidemiology*, **62**, 13–21.

The Xamoterol in Severe Heart Failure Study Group (1990) 'Xamoterol in severe heart failure' *The Lancet*, **336**, 1–6.

The Young Infants Clinical Signs Study Group (2008) 'Clinical signs that predict severe illness in children under age 2 months: a multicenter study' *The Lancet*, **371**, 135–142.

Zhou XH, Obuchowski NA and McClish DK (2002) *Statistical Methods in Diagnostic Medicine* Hoboken: John Wiley & Sons, Inc.

Regulatory Guidelines

ICH Guidelines

ICH E1 (1995) 'Population Exposure: The Extent of Population Exposure to Assess Clinical Safety'

ICH E2E (2005) 'Note for Guidance on Planning Pharmacovigilance Activities'

ICH E3 (1995) 'Note for Guidance on Structure and Content of Clinical Study Reports'

ICH E9 (1998) 'Note for Guidance on Statistical Principles for Clinical Trials'

ICH E10 (2001) 'Note for Guidance on Choice of Control Group in Clinical Trials'

ICH E14 (2005) 'Note for Guidance on the Clinical Evaluation of QT/QTc Interval and Prolongation and Proarrhythmic Potential for Non-Antiarrhythmic Drugs'

FDA Guidelines

FDA (1992) 'Points to Consider on Clinical Development and Labeling of Anti-Infective Drug Products'

FDA (1998) 'Developing Antimicrobial Drugs – General Considerations for Clinical Trials'

FDA (2001) 'Statistical Approaches to Establishing Bioequivalence'

FDA (2004) 'Critical Path Initiative'

FDA (2005) 'Clinical Trial Endpoints for the Approval of Cancer Drugs and Biologics'

FDA (2006) 'Critical Path Opportunities List'

FDA (2006) 'Establishment and Operation of Clinical Trial Data Monitoring Committees'

FDA (2006) 'Guidance for the Use of Bayesian Statistics in Medical Device Clinical Trials'

FDA (2007) 'Guidance for Industry Drug-Induced Liver Injury: Premarketing Clinical Evaluation'

FDA (2010) 'Adaptive Design Clinical Trials for Drugs and Biologics'

FDA (2010) 'Non-Inferiority Clinical Trials'

FDA (2013) 'Structured Approach to Benefit-Risk Assessment in Drug Regulatory Decision-Making. Draft PDUFA V Implementation Plan – February 2013, Fiscal Years 2013–2017'

European Guidelines

CPMP (1999) 'Note for Guidance on Clinical Evaluation of New Vaccines'

CPMP (2000) 'Points to Consider on Switching Between Superiority and Non-Inferiority'

CPMP (2001) 'Note for Guidance on Clinical Investigation of Medicinal Products for the Treatment of Acute Stroke'

CPMP (2001) 'Note for Guidance on the Investigation of Bioavailability and Bioequivalence'

CPMP (2001) 'Points to Consider on Applications with 1. Meta Analyses; 2. One Pivotal Study'

CPMP (2001) 'Points to Consider on Missing Data'

CPMP (2002) 'Points to Consider on Multiplicity Issues in Clinical Trials'

CPMP (2003) 'Note for Guidance on the Clinical Investigation of Medicinal Products in the Treatment of Asthma'

CPMP (2003) 'Note for Guidance on Evaluation of Medicinal Products Indicated for Treatments of Bacterial Infections'

CPMP (2003) 'Points to Consider on Adjustment for Baseline Covariates'

CPMP (2003) 'Points to Consider on the Clinical Development of Fibrinolytic Medicinal Products in the Treatment of Patients with ST Segment Elevation Acute Myocardial Infarction (STEMI)'

CHMP (2005) 'Guidance on the Choice of Non-Inferiority Margin'

CHMP (2005) 'Guideline on Data Monitoring Committees'

CHMP (2006) 'Guideline on Clinical Trials in Small Populations'

CHMP (2006) 'Guideline on Similar Biological Medicinal Products Containing Biotechnology-Derived Proteins as Active Substance: Non-Clinical and Clinical Issues'

CHMP (2007) 'Reflection Paper on Methodological Issues in Confirmatory Clinical Trials with Flexible Design and Analysis Plan'

CHMP (2008) 'Guideline on Medicinal Products for the Treatment of Alzheimer's Disease and Other Dementias'

CHMP (2008) 'Reflection Paper on Benefit-Risk Assessment Methods in the Context of the Evaluation of Marketing Authorisation Application of Medicinal Products for Human Use'

CHMP (2009) 'Guideline on Clinical Evaluation of Diagnostic Agents'

CHMP (2010) 'Points to Consider on Missing Data in Confirmatory Clinical Trials'

CHMP (2012) 'Guideline on the Evaluation of Medicinal Products Indicated for Treatment of Bacterial Infections'

CHMP (2012) 'Addendum to the Note for Guidance on Evaluation of Medicinal Products Indicated for Treatment of Bacterial Infections to Address Indication-Specific Clinical Data (Draft)'

CHMP (2013) 'Draft Qualification Opinion of MCP-Mod as an Efficient Statistical Methodology for Model-Base Design and Analysis of Phase II Dose Finding Studies Under Model Uncertainty'

EMA (2008) 'Guideline on the use of Statistical Signal Detection Methods in the EudraVigilance Data Analysis System'

EMA (2010) 'Benefit-Risk Methodology Project: Work Package 2'

EMA (2011a) 'Benefit-Risk Methodology Project: Work Package 1'

EMA (2011b) 'Benefit-Risk Methodology Project: Work Package 3'

EMA (2012) 'Benefit-Risk Methodology Project: Work Package 4'

Index

Note: Page numbers in *italics* refer to Figures; those in **bold** to Tables.

Statistical Thinking for Non-Statisticians in Drug Regulation, Second Edition. Richard Kay.
© 2015 John Wiley & Sons, Ltd. Published 2015 by John Wiley & Sons, Ltd.